"This lovely book was the final project of WATSU's creator, the genius poet Harold Dull. His inspired reinvention of Zen Shiatsu in the weightless embrace of warm water yielded a discipline that is profoundly connected to the breath, intimate but non-threatening, potentially an ecstatic meditative experience for both giver and receiver. As a practicing physician I find it self-evident that the deep relaxation and inner stillness achieved in a WATSU session can help relieve psychological distress and muscle tension. Less obvious is WATSU's role in treating other medical conditions, and that is the main subject of this well-documented, comprehensive treatise. It begins with an origin story involving hippies in a wine barrel and goes on to provide advice for the practitioner that ranges from the most philosophical to the most down-to-earth. Applications as varied as speech therapy and midwifery, as well as aquatic techniques that evolved out of WATSU, are described in the book's final third. The many case studies are illuminating and often very moving, and a welcome emphasis on ethics and emotional connection permeates the text."

—Susan Levenstein, MD, internist, WATSU® practitioner and author of Dottoressa: An American Doctor in Rome *and the* Stethoscope on Rome *blog*

of related interest

Shiatsu Theory and Practice
Carola Beresford-Cooke
ISBN 978 1 83997 530 1
eISBN 978 0 85701 260 9
Premium eISBN 978 1 78775 845 2

Working with Death and Loss in Shiatsu Practice
A Guide to Holistic Bodywork in Palliative Care
Tamsin Grainger
Foreword by Richard Reoch
ISBN 978 1 78775 269 6
eISBN 978 1 78775 270 2

Intention and Non-Doing in Therapeutic Bodywork
Andrew James Pike
Foreword by Ged Sumner
ISBN 978 1 78775 898 8
eISBN 978 1 78775 899 5

Zero Balancing
Touching the Energy of the Bone
John Hamwee
Foreword by Fritz Smith, MD FCC Ac
Illustrated by Gina Michaels
ISBN 978 1 84819 234 8
eISBN 978 0 85701 182 4

Water Yoga
A Teacher's Guide to Improving Movement and Wellbeing
Christa Fairbrother
Foreword by Ruth Sova
ISBN 978 1 83997 285 0
eISBN 978 1 83997 286 7

The Heart
of WATSU®

Therapeutic Applications in Clinical Practice

Edited by **Harold Dull**
and **Ingrid Keating**

Foreword by **Wataru Ohashi**

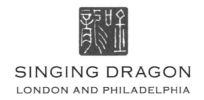

SINGING DRAGON
LONDON AND PHILADELPHIA

First published in Great Britain in 2023 by Singing Dragon, an imprint of Jessica Kingsley Publishers
An imprint of Hodder & Stoughton Ltd
An Hachette Company
1

Foreword © Wataru Ohashi 2023

Chapter 1 © Harold Dull and Ingrid Keating 2023
Chapter 2 © Peggy Schoedinger 2023
Chapter 3 © Ingrid Keating and Dr. Jennifer Olejownik 2023
Chapter 4 © Karen David and Mary Seamster 2023
Chapter 5 © Dr. Cedar Barstow 2023
Chapter 6 © Sheila Pyatt and Dr. David M. Steinhorn 2023
Chapter 7 © Calias Dull, Susan Nachimson and Dr. Rita Alegria 2023
Chapter 8 © Tomasz Zagorski 2023
Chapter 9 © Dr. Ertan Tufekcioglu and Dr. Iftikhar Nadeem 2023
Chapter 10 © Jurgita Svediene 2023
Chapter 11 © Arjana C. Brunschwiler 2023
Chapter 12 © Alexander George 2023
Chapter 13 © Cameron West 2023
Chapter 14 © Karen David and Mary Seamster 2023
Chapter 15 © Elisa Muñoz Blanco 2023
Chapter 16 © Tomasz Zagorski 2023
Chapter 17 © Dr. Jennifer Olejownik 2023

Front cover image source: Jonah Sutherland.

The information contained in this book is not intended to replace the services of trained medical professionals or to be a substitute for medical advice. The complementary therapy described in this book may not be suitable for everyone to follow. You are advised to consult a doctor before embarking on any complementary therapy program and on any matters relating to your health, and in particular on any matters that may require diagnosis or medical attention.

A CIP catalogue record for this title is available from the British Library and the Library of Congress

ISBN 978 1 78775 510 9
eISBN 978 1 78775 511 6

Printed and bound by CPI Group (UK) Ltd, Croydon, CR0 4YY

Jessica Kingsley Publishers' policy is to use papers that are natural, renewable and recyclable products and made from wood grown in sustainable forests. The logging and manufacturing processes are expected to conform to the environmental regulations of the country of origin.

Jessica Kingsley Publishers
Carmelite House
50 Victoria Embankment
London EC4Y 0DZ

www.singingdragon.com

Contents

Foreword

WATARU OHASHI

It was 12:00pm on Monday March 6, 1978 when I met Harold Dull. I was visiting my friend Ryuho Yamada, a Japanese Zen monk who lived in the Russian Hill section of San Francisco. Ryuho said, "This is Dull. He took Masunaga's workshop which I arranged in Sausalito on the houseboat that had been the home of Zen philosopher Allan Watts. Dull is my student; he is interested in Japanese culture, such as Zen and Shiatsu." My first impression of Harold was that of a quiet man but very articulate in language and speech. Later I learned that Harold was also a poet and had published several volumes of poetry.

Starting in 1974, for a period of ten years, I was traveling to California to teach, mainly in Los Angeles and San Francisco where I taught in Japan Town. During this period, I saw Harold a few times. On one of my trips he invited me to come to "soak" in the Harbin Hot Springs. He said, "Let's have a happy time in the water!" He arranged a "hippy" bus, painted with psychedelic pictures on the outside, with lots of bean bags inside. I remember this trip was a three- or four-hour drive in a dilapidated Volkswagen bus. Harbin Hot Springs is many miles north of San Francisco, Sonoma County—yes, wine country. When we were soaking in the hot spring (which from a Japanese point of view was *cold* water), someone found a big, empty wine barrel in the storage house. We put hot water in the barrel, and we hippies (three or four of us) stripped off our clothes and jumped into the barrel. Then we started stretching, rubbing and giving Shiatsu by "accident" because the wine barrel was so deep you had to grab another person in order not to sink down and drown. One person exclaimed, "Hey, this is so groovy," another, "Right-on brother!" Another guy shouted, "This is cool." One girl with long hair said, "This is the Shiatsu in the water—this is *water Shiatsu*," and then someone shouted, "This is *WATSU*."

Those events were more than 40 years ago and perhaps the beginning of Harold Dull's interest in combining Shiatsu and water therapy. I understand that a few years later while teaching at the Harbin School of Shiatsu and

Massage, he began experimenting with giving Shiatsu and other therapies in the waters of the hot springs. I did not communicate with Harold during the many years after we met, but I followed the development and increasing popularity of WATSU. When I was teaching in Italy several years ago, one of my instructors led a session in a convenient swimming pool during a training meeting. I was impressed and delighted.

In February 2022, I received a draft of this *Heart of WATSU®* book from Ingrid Keating, with many excellent clinical studies of aquatic therapy, which absorbed me for one week. This book is well documented, well written, authentic and clinically relevant. I am very impressed with the quality of this book and I feel honored that I witnessed the beginning of WATSU at Harbin Hot Springs in California during the heady and fabulous days of the 1970s. WATSU had its beginnings in a wine barrel with hippies massaging one another while enjoying the benefits of warm water. Like good wine that becomes matured and more valuable, WATSU matured into a valuable therapy through the expertise of the "wine" maker and his staff. They have given society a therapy that has benefited thousands of people worldwide. That is a commendable accomplishment for Harold Dull, his family and all the therapists who have participated in these studies.

Wataru Ohashi

https://ohashi-method.biz
https://ohashi.com
https://ohashiatsu.org

Acknowledgements

We wish to thank all the contributors to this book. Their plethora of experience with clients and hours of work spent on each chapter made this project possible. Thank you to our families for their constant support and patience during the process. During times of Covid-19 we are more aware than ever of the need for human touch and the profound importance of bodywork. Thank you to the Worldwide Aquatic Bodywork family whose hours of practice and dedication make the continued sharing and accessibility of WATSU possible around the world. We lastly want to give thanks and gratitude to our photographer Jonah Sutherland for embodying the heart and essence of WATSU through this book's cover.

About the Contributors

Harold Dull, MFA, BA, was the creator and pioneer of the Aquatic Bodywork therapy WATSU that was born and first taught in the warm waters of Harbin Hot Springs in Middletown, California. Dull's work was inspired by his Zen Shiatsu training in Japan with his teacher, Shizuto Masunaga, as well as the teachings of Wataru Ohashi and Reuho Yamada. He was the founder of the Worldwide Aquatic Bodywork Association (WABA) as well as a poet of the San Francisco Renaissance. Having a deep understanding of energy and the body he authored several self-published poems and titles on WATSU. Prior to his passing, for over 30 years he taught countless WATSU classes in many countries and languages around the world. He co-authored this final swan song manuscript with Ingrid Keating until his death in July of 2019.

This book is a testament to his heart-centered legacy in the water that continues to echo through the work of many contributing clinicians and therapists across the globe. His student predecessors carry forth his water work with new insight continuing to meld the *heart* of Dull's teachings with the present-day and ever-evolving *science* and therapeutic applications within clinical practice. His intention for his final manifest was to illuminate WATSU's reach to adult and pediatric special needs populations, physical rehabilitation, somatics, trauma, palliative care, hospice, pre/postnatal, speech language pathology, life coaching, sports medicine, the evolution of additional Aquatic Bodywork forms and beyond.

Ingrid Keating, LAc, OTR/L, MSOM, FABAA, Doctoral Candidate, is the founder of LOTUS Integrative Therapy LLC and KEATING Equine Acupuncture. She is a NCCAOM board-certified and licensed acupuncturist, Chinese herbalist, occupational therapist, WATSU practitioner and instructor as well as a Fellow of the American Board of Animal Acupuncture with a focus on treating high performance horses. Ingrid has over 20 years of experience working with adults and pediatrics within the WATSU and aquatic therapy fields treating special needs populations in the early intervention, school and hospital settings. Her Chicago-based WATSU program was featured in a variety of publications including *Chicago Tribune, Time Out Chicago, Alternative Medicine and Well Magazine.*

Ingrid integrates her clinical experience in rehabilitative medicine and Chinese medicine within her private practice in Cincinnati, Ohio with humans and horses. She is currently pursuing a Doctorate in Acupuncture and Chinese Medicine (DACM) at Pacific College of Health and Science in San Diego, California, with a focus on Integrative Medicine and continuing her studies in Functional Medicine/Nutrition. Her intellectual curiosity extends to further explore psychedelic medicine and the possible future frameworks for multimodal, interdisciplinary care and how somatic modalities like WATSU, yoga and acupuncture can clinically improve and benefit the therapeutic process of psychedelic integration. Her love of water began at a young age and she later became a US synchronized swimmer and collegiate competitive swimmer. She finds joy in combining heart, science and compassion into practice with her patients.

Dr. Rita Alegria, PhD, SLP, has been practicing speech therapy in Porto, Portugal in private practice. Rita was a high-level competitive swimmer from ages 8 through 22. She represented Portugal many times in international competitions including at the Youth Olympic Games in Fukuoka 1992 at the peak of her swimming career. With a strong background in swimming, she knows how bodies work in water and uses these strategies with clients with severe limitations of voicing, respiration, volume control, oral-sensory hypersensitivity and movement with phonation with children and adults with speech and language disorders. Rita is a professor at the Universidad Fernando Pessoa, Porto, where she practices and teaches graduate students how to use an aquatic setting to treat a variety of speech and language disorders.

Dr. Cedar Barstow, MEd, CHT, DPI, is the founder and director of the Right Use of Power Institute (www.rightuseofpower.org), which provides training, consultation and resources to help organizations cultivate the skills, sensitivities and concepts that will help people develop their personal power and say "yes" to positive use of their role power. Central themes are power with heart and power consciousness. She is the author of *Right Use of Power: The Heart of Ethics—A Resource for the Help Professional* and co-author of *Living in the Power Zone: How Right Use of Power Can Transform Your Relationships*. Cedar lives with her husband in Boulder, Colorado.

Professor Elisa Muñoz Blanco, PT, MSc, is a Professor of Physiotherapy and Master's Professor of Pediatrics at the Universidad San Pablo-CEU (CEU

Universities), as well as an Expert Professor in Aquatic Therapy at Rey Juan Carlos University.

Elisa is an expert in craniomandibular disorders and orofacial pain, manual lymphatic drainage, osteopathy, Craniosacral Therapy, Biodynamic Craniosacral Therapy, Myofascial Induction Therapy™ and traditional Thai massage. She is a Watsupath™ Training Institute Founder and Director as well as Craniosacral Therapy in Water™ concept's creator and instructor. She is also a Certified WATSU 1 & 2 Instructor and Clinical WATSU 3-Free Flow Instructor-in-Training by Worldwide Aquatic Bodywork Association, a certified Ai Chi® Instructor by Aquadynamics Institute, Japan, a Vipassana meditator, Ashtanga Vinyasa Yoga practitioner and instructor, freediver and curious constant seeker.

Arjana C. Brunschwiler, Co-Creator of WaterDance, is a Swiss who has spent the past 35 years involved in teaching thousands of students all over the world in an integrative and holistic way warm-water therapy and a land-based approach to inner wholeness. Her studies include extensive training in body, energy and soul work and in humanistic and transpersonal therapy and group work. After more than 3 decades of teaching and coaching students and clients she still feels deeply connected and carried by the richness, strength and at the same time the gentleness of water—the fundamental and feminine element.

Karen David, RCST®, received her BS and MS at the University of Washington in Seattle with a specialty in Clinical Immunology research in the early 1980s. She raised 4 sons and co-owned a soap and herbal products business, returning to school in 2013, graduating with an MS in Integrative Medical Research at the National University of Natural Medicine in Portland, Oregon. Concurrently, she obtained training and registered as a Biodynamic Craniosacral Therapist at the Colorado School of Energy Studies and practiced until 2020. She is currently retired and living in the Oregon coast and Portland area.

Calias Dull, MS, CCC-SLP, WATSU® Instructor, graduated from the University of Arizona summa cum laude, earning a Master's of Science in Speech-Language Pathology. She completed a Bachelor's degree at the University of California, Berkeley, in Sociology. Calias specializes in pediatric speech therapy and has worked at a private practice in Oakland, California for the last 3 years. Areas of interest include evidence-based assessment and treatment for clients diagnosed with autism spectrum disorder, early intervention, articulation, motor speech, and pragmatic language. Calias provides individualized therapy based on the unique needs of her clients and involves caregivers to deliver culturally sensitive and compassionate care. In addition to direct therapy, Calias has experience mentoring graduate students in the field of speech-language pathology. The daughter of Harold Dull, creator of WATSU, she has been an essential part of the aquatic community since her up-bringing at Harbin Hot Springs in Northern California. Personally trained by her father, Calias has 15 years of experience as a certified WATSU practitioner and is currently certified as a WATSU Instructor. She traveled to numerous countries in Europe and Central America teaching and sharing the many benefits of WATSU with her father prior to his death in 2019.

Alexander George, Creator of Healing Dance, came to the holistic arts in the final third of a 25-year career as a ballet and modern dancer, teacher and choreographer. In 1980 he began the study of holistic massage at the International School of Professional Bodywork in San Diego, completing the 1000 Hour Massage Therapist Training in 1983 and Associate of Science degree in 2004. Alexander qualified as a Trager Practitioner in 1986, subsequently studying with Milton Trager himself. In 1990 he became a WATSU Practitioner at Harbin Hot Springs in northern California under the tutelage of Harold Dull, the originator of WATSU.

In 1993 he studied WaterDance from one of its co-founders, Arjana Brunschwiler. Alexander went on to develop the technique of Healing Dance. He is a certified instructor of the Worldwide Aquatic Bodywork Association, and for nine years taught at the School of Shiatsu and Massage at Harbin Hot Springs. Alexander has led over 300 week-long 50-hour intensives in anatomy, massage, Barefoot Shiatsu, WATSU, Healing Dance and WaterDance. Alexander presently leads trainings in Germany, Italy, France, Portugal and the US. He has written over 90 articles on teaching and aquatic bodywork, a selection of which are available for free download at the official web site for Healing Dance, www. healingdance.org. Alexander lives in Germany with his wife, Kathrin.

Susan Nachimson, MA, CCC, SLP, NDT/C, WATSU® Practitioner, has been practicing speech-language pathology for more than 46 years. She uses water for the treatment of clients with severe limitations of voicing, respiration and volume control, oral-motor hypersensitivity, developmental apraxia of speech (DAS), focusing and attending, and many other clinical issues for infants, children and adults with and without neuromotor limitations. Certified in NDT (NeuroDevelopmental Treatment/Bobath), Hendricks Institute Radiance Breathwork and Prenatal Process, she is also a WATSU practitioner and member of the Worldwide Aquatic Bodywork Association (WABA). Susan works in water heated at or near body temperature (93–96°F) so that clients feel neither chilled nor over-heated enabling them to attain the goals being set. Susan has a private practice in Garberville, California, where she serves a varied population ranging in ages from infant through geriatric.

Dr. Iftikhar Nadeem, PhD, MCC, is an executive leadership coach and director of organizational excellence at a large and prestigious organization in the Middle East. He has more than 30 years of experience marked with excellence in leadership advisory, executive leadership coaching, training & development, enterprise digital transformations, strategy and performance management consulting across various industries including government, higher education, petrochemicals, FMCG and information technology sectors mainly in Saudi Arabia and other Gulf countries. He holds a PhD in leadership coaching from Canterbury Christ Church University in the United Kingdom. He is an ICF Master Certified Coach (MCC), and a certified professional practitioner for various assessments including Hogan, MBTI (Myers-Briggs Type Indicator), Emotional Intelligence (EQi), Global Leadership by Marshall Goldsmith, Kirkpatrick and ELi (Energy Leadership Index). He is also a certified trainer for the Corporate Athlete program.

Wataru Ohashi is a pioneer in holistic healthcare. Ohashi first developed his Ohashiatsu®/Ohashi Method® in 1977. He is the founder and director of the international Ohashi Institute, a cultural and educational non-profit organization. As a teacher and practitioner of Oriental medicine and philosophy, Ohashi has trained thousands of graduates, certified instructors and consultants worldwide. He has lectured widely and authored several books, available in many languages, including *Do-It-Yourself Shiatsu and Reading the Body: Ohashi's Book of Oriental Diagnosis*. His clients have included many notables, such as Liza Minelli, Halston and Henry Kissinger. His website is www.ohashi.com.

Dr. Jennifer Olejownik, PhD, MS, BA, holds a doctorate in Cultural/Somatic Studies from the Ohio State University where she currently teaches courses in Integrative Medicine. She has experience in all phases of qualitative and quantitative research design, sampling and implementation. As a mathematical statistician Jennifer has worked on various projects for local, state and federal agencies from Alaska to Ohio. Prior to receiving her doctorate, Jennifer designed and implemented evaluations for a variety of disciplines and has held research positions for the Academic Collaborative for Integrative Health, US Bureau of the Census, the Ohio Department of Education, and the Ohio State University.

Sheila Pyatt, RN, BSN, grew up in Newton, Massachusetts, a suburb of Boston. Early on, her older sister was diagnosed with cerebral palsy and mental delays. Her parents' faith, skill, courage and humor helped Sheila and her family to care for Mary Ellen, lovingly and effectively. After graduating from Loyola University School of Nursing in 1967, Sheila accepted her first nursing job at Cook County Hospital in Chicago. She was assigned to the Burn Unit, the only unit of its kind in Chicago. Many patients were children and often died from their injuries. After moving to the San Francisco Bay Area, Sheila enjoyed a varied career in occupational, community and mental health settings for over thirty years. Her last nursing position was at the George Mark Children's House, located in San Leandro, California. This first free-standing pediatric palliative care facility in the United States would provide comfort, support, pain and symptom management and quality of life to children with life-limiting and life-threatening illnesses. With the support of management and nursing staff, Sheila developed a palliative aquatic program for children who were medically fragile or dying. This experience was the highlight of her nursing career.

Peggy Schoedinger, Physiotherapist, Senior WATSU® Instructor and Coach Advisor, has taught over 800 aquatic therapy courses for therapists and practitioners at facilities throughout North America, South America, Asia, Africa, Australia and Europe since 1990. She teaches a full range of over 40 topics and techniques including WATSU, The Bad Ragaz Ring Method, The Halliwick Concept in Rehab, Trunk Stabilization, Aquatic Sensory Integration and Aquatic Manual Therapy Joint & Soft Tissue Mobilization Techniques for patients with neurological, orthopedic and rheumatic impairments.

Peggy is the only physiotherapist in the world who is a certified WATSU instructor for levels 1, 2 and 3. She originated the WATSU 3 adaptive and clinical WATSU programs. She specializes in teaching therapists and practitioners how to use and adapt WATSU for clients with special needs. Peggy's frequent international trips allow her to stay abreast with the latest techniques and information from around the globe. She strives to blend the best of East and West into her classes, creating a supportive and joyful environment where each student can explore his or her unique WATSU gifts.

Mary Seamster, LMT, RCST®, Integrative Aquatic Therapist, AMNION®, WATSU® Instructor, currently serves as the Executive Director of White Stone Medical Inc. in La Center, Washington and is the developer of AMNION®. Mary Seamster's first love was art. She spent her early childhood in Florence, Italy surrounded by Michelangelo's sculptures. That early influence of shaping bodies into forms of bronze and wood became a natural progression into shaping live bodies in an aqueous medium. Mary is a life-long learner who has explored a variety of modalities—body-centered psychotherapies, pre and perinatal psychology both on land and in water, cranial sacral, and family constellations to name a few. Daily, she is inspired and honored alongside her clients and students who work toward being embodied and filled with profound joy.

Dr. David M. Steinhorn, MD, FAAP, is an academic pediatrician who practices intensive care and hospice medicine for children. He led the Judith Nan Joy Integrative Medicine Research Initiative at Lurie Children's Hospital in Chicago from 2002 to 2010 and founded palliative care programs at major children's hospitals. Dr. Steinhorn has additional training in energy medicine, yoga, meditation and shamanism and has brought shamanic healing approaches to his critical care practice in children's hospitals across the country. His passion is to find ways of alleviating suffering wherever it may occur and to help patients, families and healthcare providers discover meaning in all of life's experiences. He can be reached at dsteinhorn@gmail.com or www.healingjourneys.life

Jurgita Svediene, Physiotherapist, Midwife, Biochemist, has 30 years of teaching experience in childbirth education, midwifery, pre/perinatal aquatic concepts and infant swimming methods. She holds a Master's degree in Biochemistry and is a midwife, physiotherapist and massage therapist as well as the Founder and Director of Family Center GIMTIS and the Lithuanian Association WATSU° LT. She is the creator of AQVUS (underwater) and MOWE (the movement wonders) concepts. She is a certified WATSU 3 and an underwater instructor with 20 years of experience. She inspires her students to discover precision and freedom in their aquatic sessions. She has served as the Chief of the European Ethical Committee of WABA since 2017. She is a yoga instructor and Birth into Being Facilitator-in-Training. Her education combines her studies of art therapy and pre/perinatal psychology.

Dr. Ertan Tufekcioglu, PhD, PCC, is a faculty member at King Fahd University of Petroleum and Minerals. Since he graduated from the Health Science Institute at Marmara University, Ertan has had 10 years of experience in fitness and is a certified Wellness Champion by ARAMCO. He is an ICF professional certified health and wellness coach. For more than 15 years, he has developed the aquatic bodywork community as the first WATSU® instructor in Turkey. In his PhD, Ertan proved WATSU's efficacy to improve autonomic cardiac modulation followed by many published articles that contributed to the scientific validity of WATSU. He is also a certified trainer for the Corporate Athlete Energy Management program. Ertan can also be credited with his initiative to develop WATSU for Coaching.

Cameron West, LMT, WATSU® Senior Instructor, Creator of Aquatic Integration, is the founder of Aquatic Integration and owner of the AquaZen Center. She has been a practitioner and an internationally known teacher of WATSU for over 17 years and has been instrumental in promoting WATSU and Aquatic Integration into the clinical therapeutic arena. From 1984–1998

Cameron served as the Aquatics Director at Easter Seals Rehabilitation Center in Ventura, California. She also served on the faculty of Oxnard and Ventura Colleges as an Adapted Physical Education teacher from 1987–2001. Her work has been featured in *Massage Today and The Aquatic Therapist* on Aquatic Integration and Substance Abuse. Cameron currently travels all over the world teaching and she maintains a private practice and directs the aquatic programs at the Aquatic Integration Institute in Atascadero, California.

Tomasz Zagorski, WATSU® Senior Instructor and Coach Advisor, has been working in the field of WATSU since 2000 and as a WATSU Practitioner since 2007 and an instructor since 2009. Tomasz mentored many instructors, and brought WATSU to Russia, Singapore, Ukraine and Hong Kong, as well as supported communities in China, Turkey, Slovenia, Slovakia and Iceland. He was the President of WATSU Polska Association from 2008–2020, co-founder of new WABA in 2015, and its vice-president from 2016–2020. He was the creator of the European WATSU Center named after Harold Dull in Dobrociesz, Poland in 2020 and organizer of the International WATSU Conferences in Poland in 2010 and 2015, as well as the first online Instructor Conference in 2020 and annual WABA Community Communication Forum (CCF) in 2021. Tomasz has a background in physical education and athletic coaching and has successfully worked in the sports therapy field. Tomasz is the creator of WATSU for Athletes and Myofascial Release in Water (MRW®) as well as a co-creator of DUO WATSU with Jurgita Svediene and Natalia Ozga.

Chapter 1

The Heart of WATSU®

Therapeutic Applications in Clinical Practice

HAROLD DULL AND INGRID KEATING

On the sources of WATSU

Sitting in the house over a stream in which he slept, listening to the sound of running water, Harold looked back on the sources of WATSU, where his *life aquatic* began as two dragons intertwined, *water* and *poet*. As a child, Harold was surrounded by the water out on the tide flats of Whidbey Island, running up another flock of gulls, following their flight up into the bright sky. He would stoop over to scoop up another handful of sand to build another castle, knowing full well that, like all those before, it would soon disappear under the rising tide. Water takes so many shapes. Water has no shape.

Streams, creeks, lakes and oceans. We can always find ways to *water*.

The origins

After his days as a Renaissance poet in San Francisco publishing a variety of poems, Harold grew a love and passion for hot springs and the poems that could be written in water. In 1980, at Harbin Hot Springs in Northern California, he floated someone in a warm pool and applied the stretches and principles of the land-based Zen Shiatsu he had learned years earlier with its creator, Shizuto Masunaga, in Japan. Harold had no idea that what was coming into being that night would help millions of people of all ages in spas, clinics and backyard pools around the world, and would become a new way to bring people together to come to know and celebrate their connection.

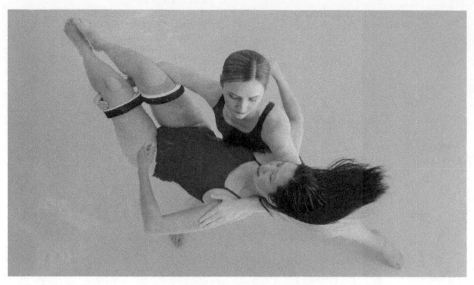

Figure 1.1: The origins

The stretch

In Zen Shiatsu, Masunaga taught that stretches are an older way to access and balance the flow of energy through our bodies than Shiatsu's traditional work with acupuncture points. Stretching increases flexibility, and warm water, which many associate with the body's deepest states of waking relaxation, is the ideal medium for it. The support of water takes weight off the vertebrae and allows the spine to be moved in ways impossible on land. Gentle, gradual twists and pulls relieve the pressure a rigid spine places on nerves and helps undo any dysfunction this pressure can cause to the organs served by those nerves. In WATSU, the receiver experiences greater flexibility and freedom, while a range of emotions can come forward and be released into the process of continuous flow. For both giver and receiver, this work in the water helps us face life out of the water with greater equanimity and flexibility.

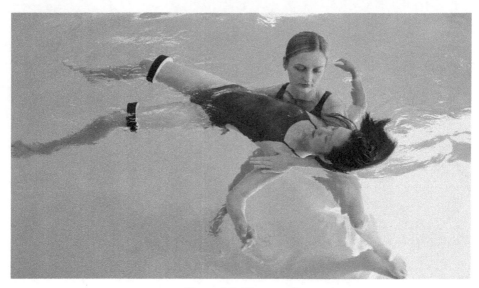

Figure 1.2: The stretch

The breath

In the beginning, WATSU was all about stretching, using our physical close-ness to brace powerful stretches and be moved around the pool by the energy those stretches released. Stretches, and the closeness that facilitates them, will always be important in WATSU, but in its first years of development, another element moved to the forefront—the unique connection to the breath that our closeness in water also facilitates. In water, where the buoyancy lifts our body every time we breathe, our whole body breathes. We begin a WATSU session doing nothing, settling into the water, holding a client with one arm under their occiput, the other arm under their sacrum. When we feel them getting lighter on that arm as they breathe, the therapist's breath is drawn up. Then, we drop back into the emptiness at the bottom of the breath and do nothing. Being drawn up out of that emptiness again and again, up through our core in this *Water Breath Dance*, engages our whole body and establishes a connection that continues through our moves and stretches born in that rhythm. Con-necting through your whole body's response to someone's breathing creates a longer lasting connection than synchronizing your breath by watching or listening, which begins with separation and returns to separation when you stop listening or looking. This connection establishes the rhythm of the moves to follow. Once moves start we do not stop to see if they are still breathing to the same rhythm. Even if they are not, a connection has been established that continues. The *Water Breath Dance* establishes this rhythm of our breathing that we continue to move to.

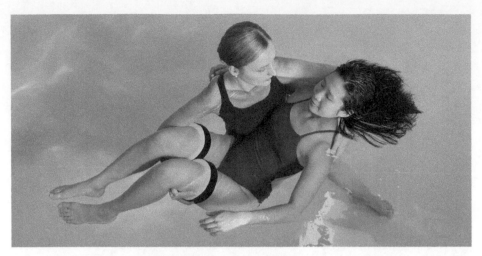

Figure 1.3: The breath

Closeness and holding

The closeness and holding, developed out of necessity when WATSU first came into being because no flotation devices had yet been developed to keep clients fully above water, is still an essential part of the work. Even with the advent of various float devices we use with WATSU today, it's the closeness between giver and receiver that distinguishes WATSU from subsequent forms of aquatic bodywork where practitioners float clients at a distance. Being held accesses an innate level of healing. When infants fall, a mother's response is to pick them up and hold them. Containment creates safety. It allows us to go deeper within and access every level of our being. It is a cornerstone of WATSU.

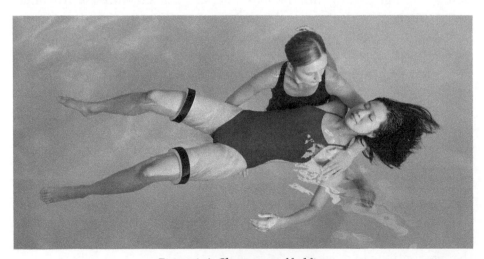

Figure 1.4: Closeness and holding

Lengthening and support

Another essential element of WATSU is the gentle spinal lengthening that, with practice, becomes automatically ingrained in the way we move someone through the water. It protects the neck and lower back from hyper extending. The more relaxed someone becomes lying on their back in warm water, the more their head should be supported as carefully as that of a newborn.

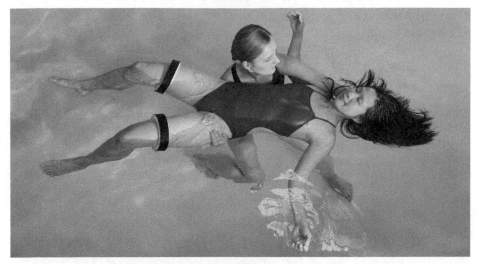

Figure 1.5: Lengthening and support

Another wave, another path

Over many years of being in the water and teaching countless WATSU classes in many languages and countries around the world, we have witnessed the waves of the WATSU create a state of wholeness and a freedom for the body within this safe containment and the deepest pathways to the heart. However, another, extraordinary wave within this one has continued to simultaneously rise, evolve, adapt and flow forward, which represents this book's primary focus. This wave connects the heart to a therapeutic path for those with special needs and medical challenges. This clinical path illuminates a variety of anecdotal, clinical and practical tools for the clinicians who treat those individuals. Its universal translation maintains the heart-centered essence of WATSU's way of being with the one in our arms while integrating a clinically informed framework and lens. This manuscript's purpose and scope is to explore those clinical paths that lead us to shores and oceans of deeper understanding of WATSU's therapeutic applications within the fields of rehabilitative medicine, somatics, trauma, palliative care, Life coaching, midwifery, sports medicine, Chinese Medicine, integrative medicine and more... We will also deepen the *ethics* of how we interact with our clients through this intimate water therapy. Each chapter enlightens practitioners on ways in which WATSU is being used clinically across the globe by expert clinicians, therapists and instructors in a variety of professional settings. Within this exploration to many pools and streams WATSU's unique movements, breathwork, intention, heart and embodiment are steeped in a unifying theme of *adaptation* across a plethora of therapeutic spectrums. These revelations about WATSU will educate the aspiring or seasoned WATSU practitioner as each page, chapter and wave flows to the next.

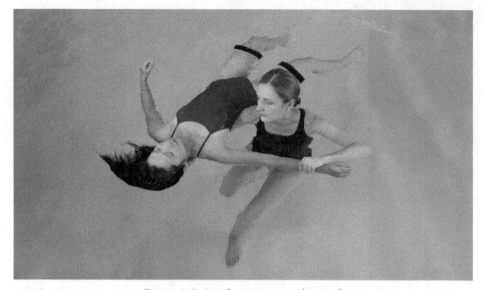

Figure 1.6: Another wave, another path

New aquatic forms

Within the chapters toward the later section of the book we will discover the evolution of aquatic bodywork forms that follow WATSU's birth. These aquatic bodywork modalities enhance WATSU's therapeutic repertoire with great verse and therapeutic depth, like a piece of fine art that continues to inspire. With training and hands-on experience, their teachings can be seamlessly integrated with WATSU, and within existing allied health professions.

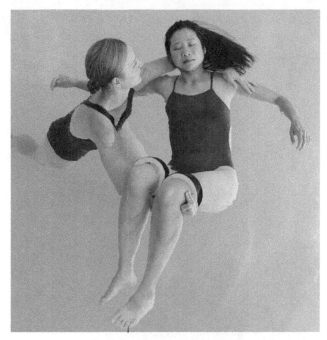

Figure 1.7: New aquatic forms

Proper training is required

This book will not train a therapist or allied health practitioner who has not undertaken a course to learn WATSU or other aquatic bodywork forms that are discussed in this text, from credentialed Worldwide Aquatic Bodywork Association (WABA) training institutes. It will, however, serve as an additional practice companion guide to highlight how WATSU is being utilized for unique clinical populations and within therapeutic settings. Proper training and certification will be essential to obtain and maintain the ethical scope of practice to properly treat medical populations and individuals with special needs or any population that WATSU or its related aquatic bodywork modalities serves. As we continue to advance further into clinical waters, do not forget the *heart* of which our *water family* speaks. The *heart* is the essence of being with and witnessing the one in our arms, holding space for the rise and fall of the breath and ultimately *freeing the body in water*. With additional WATSU coursework, training and proper readiness, a therapist or allied health professional can dive into the waters of clinical practice with *heart* and a unique perspective that is not only outcome driven but *humanistic* in nature, through which our humanity calls us to the *water*. The WATSU practitioner has a unique responsibility and opportunity to expand, innovate and access their current clinical scope of practice while blending the tools of WATSU into daily practice. Their continual role as a water guide is ultimately to provide assurance and safety within the process of a moving meditation and a somatic unfolding. The work of WATSU is indeed an integrative art.

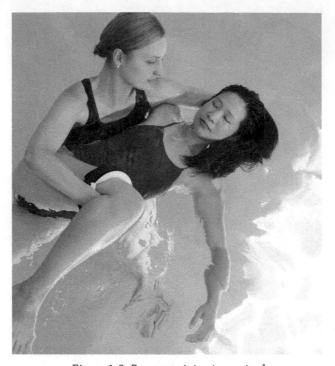

Figure 1.8: Proper training is required

Free flow

Once the clinician has mastered basic WATSU and the courses that follow, they can further expand into the aquatic depths of what is called *free flow*. WATSU free flow is a medium for the therapist or clinician to uniquely follow a client's movement within a safe environment and away from the WATSU sequence to engage further in the somatic unwinding of the breath, tissues, spinal mobility and fascia, and evoke energy or meridian flow. Free flow enhances both the client and practitioner's inclination to go deeper into the internal meditative landscape and deepen the theta brainwave state. We may even find that a client's close or distant memories of joy, pain, grief, anger, sadness or fear may emerge from the depths and be present during or after a session. As these past experiences or traumas float to the surface, WATSU practitioners must remember to somatically listen to the body, track, hold space, maintain healthy boundaries, witness and acknowledge what has been experienced with a non-judgmental and compassionate heart. We must do no harm or re-traumatize, and must uphold our scope and oath to always refer to appropriate professionals as needed. Working in tandem with other clinicians to provide an integrative approach is one of the key components to provide effective treatment for any client or population that we start to work with.

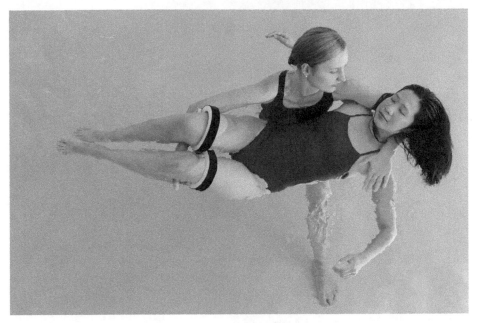

Figure 1.9: Free flow

Somatic benefits

Another contributing benefit of WATSU lies in its somatic and *interoceptive* nature by improving vagal tone, decreasing states of hypervigilance within the central nervous system, and its positive psychological and physiological effects within the areas of post-traumatic stress disorder (PTSD), neuromuscular disorders, pain syndromes, trauma and modulating heart rate variability. Physiologically, we note during WATSU decreases in heart rate and blood pressure, and increased depth of inhalation and exhalation. This improved respiratory response increases our body's ability to communicate with the diaphragm and improves vagal nerve conduction and tonality. The vagus nerve is the longest cranial nerve in the body and regulates our central nervous system responses. Globally, the vagus nerve innervates into the neck, chest and stomach. Vagal conduction is paramount in affecting our stress response, digestion and sleep patterns in heightened or calm transmissions to the brain and the gut, in which the gut is referred to as our "second brain." Other related sub-aquatic forms can also accentuate a client's vagal tone potential through breath-holding and full-body immersion. Somatic research continues to validate WATSU's thera-peutic effects, and more research is needed to forge the clinical path of WATSU to new horizons.

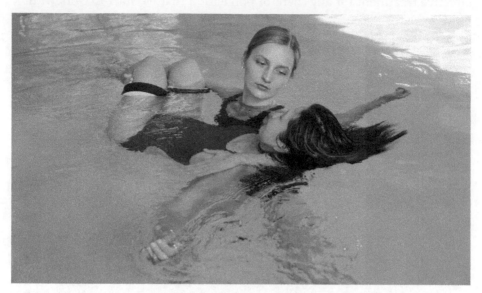

Figure 1.10: Somatic benefits

Heart intelligence

WATSU's utilization of dynamic holding at the heart level is the mainstay of the therapy and the coherence with its Zen-like nature of "being" with the breath and the one in our arms through dynamic holding, following movement and the *heart wrap*. This heart coherence expands at the heart level physiologically as researched by the HeartMath Institute. Its research found that heart-brain connection and the heart's ability to ascend messages to the brain far outweigh the brain's autonomic descending messages to the heart. This heart coherence can be seen in positive emotional states when the heart waves or heart rate variability are more balanced and synchronized; in more stressed states, the heart rate variability and heart waves are more sporadic or chaotic.

Heart intelligence continues to permeate into the scientific research and data that we are finding today within clinical practice. We also understand that compassion-based medicine and whole-person health continues to emerge within interdisciplinary and integrative care models. WATSU is a powerful testament to a whole-person and compassion-driven care movement. As practitioners of WATSU, we listen deeply to the narrative storyline of our client's life experiences as well as having an understanding of how their medical conditions affect the quality of their daily lives and their activities of daily living.

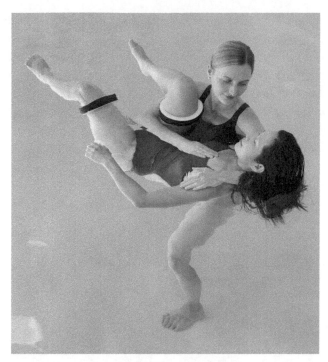

Figure 1.11: Heart intelligence

No separation exists

The National Center for Complementary and Integrative Health (NCCIH) through the National Institute of Health (NIH) would classify WATSU as a mind-body practice, having a combination of both *physical* and *psychological* benefits within the framework of complementary and integrative health since it works in tandem and can be combined with conventional medicine practices. WATSU embraces a larger continuum of care and is not antagonistic to other complementary therapies or allopathic approaches that can ultimately, in combination, improve quality of life through integrative and multi-modal healthcare models. As you begin to learn more about WATSU and its related aquatic forms, you will begin to see that there is also no division between the *coherent heart* and the *interoceptive science*. No separation exists within embodiment. They coalesce as one in the water. The *heart* coherence of holding someone in our arms next to our own beating heart and the quantitative and qualitative effects that manifest within the interoceptive and physiological *body* and psychological *mind* are inseparable. These factors influence each other simultaneously. If we are to learn this dynamic art form of healing we must liken this integration to a colorful, interconnected and moving woven tapestry, always floating at the surface of the water's viscera. As WATSU practitioners we must be in continual communion with our craft, touching each thread and embracing its teachings that heighten and enlighten our ability to understand our client's needs at the most profound levels. Some chapters within this collective manifest and their contributing experts will exude and emulate heavier tones of WATSU's *science*, while others will illuminate the rays of WATSU's *heart*. Moreover, each chapter will always shine the *heart* and *science* forth as one—a union that emerges in the ocean of being, an inseparable truth. A wholeness that transforms our ability to heal the wounds of separation.

Our closing chapter will summarize and fine-tune how we might move forward and embody our next steps into WATSU practice within the current zeitgeist and paradigm of our integrative healthcare system, mapping a path to *whole-person health* and *well-being*.

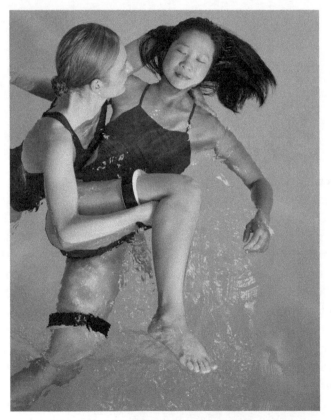

Figure 1.12: No separation exists

Adaptation

Ultimately, WATSU is about adaptation. Sharing WATSU with someone means respecting their limits and adapting to whatever is called for. WATSU allows for the form to evolve and adapt each session, as creativity and authentic movement come into play. WATSU's unique power to reduce stress has made it a treatment of choice in spas and clinics around the world. Many people come out of a session saying it is the most relaxed they have ever been in their lives. WATSU can provide relief from almost any condition related to stress, physical or mental. The anecdotal and research-based evidence surrounding the efficacy of WATSU continues to grow. A practitioner's intention should be to always adapt WATSU to their client's unique health needs, not to adapt their client to WATSU.

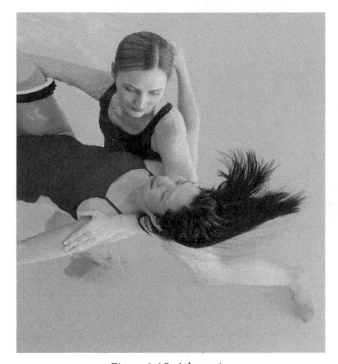

Figure 1.13: Adaptation

The ancestors of our legacy

WATSU was born and cradled in the warm Harbin Hot Springs of Northern California. However, without Zen Shiatsu as its Japanese root, there would be no WATSU. Therefore, we are forever grateful for Harold's masters and teachers Shizuto Masunaga, Wataru Ohashi and Reuho Yamada, who through Zen Shiatsu have shaped this water work with their humble teachings. Our deepest hope is that they may embody the gratitude we hold in our hearts that is expressed through the words and ideas gathered here that collectively pay homage to their teachings.

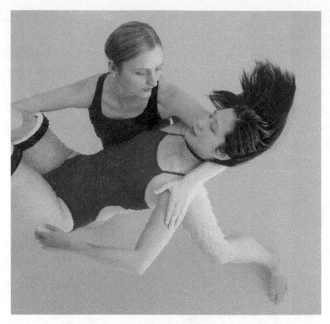

Figure 1.14: The ancestors of our legacy

The water family

We are also grateful for the *water family* as a whole, which includes: WATSU instructors, students, members of the Worldwide Aquatic Bodywork Association, the WABA Board, as well as the therapists and clinicians who have contributed their talents and expertise to this book. We pay tribute to the many practitioners around our blue earth who have created a context of validity and unconditional adaptation while maintaining WATSU's union with the heart. May the words of the storytellers that follow provide a *heart wrap* to all those who engage in the work of WATSU. May this book inform and guide the aspiring WATSU practitioners and clinicians on how the light in the water can be held and passed on to others, from ancestors to predecessors alike. This is the phenomenon of WATSU, its birthright and legacy.

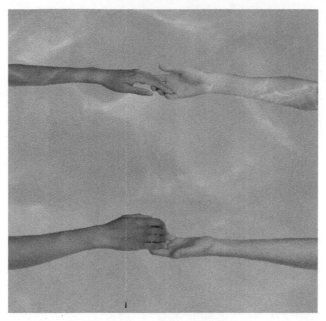

Figure 1.15: The water family

The path of the heart

When WATSU was first created, there was never a goal in mind nor an outcome other than to hold, stretch and be with someone in the water. Floating the receiver at the heart level engages a profound heart coherence. The heart-centered and compassion-based nature of WATSU, coupled with the anecdotal experiences and research that follows, carries us forward. However, the *heart* will always be the centerpiece of WATSU, our greatest treasure. The therapeutic applications branch out, as do the other *new aquatic forms* that sprung forth after its conception, each emanating their own unique stemming pattern from our most superior emperor organ, the *heart*. What evolves next and informs our work is our presence and intuition and our clinical understanding. These pillars raise the energetic field of WATSU to a unique form of therapy that accesses the deepest parts of our being as givers and receivers.

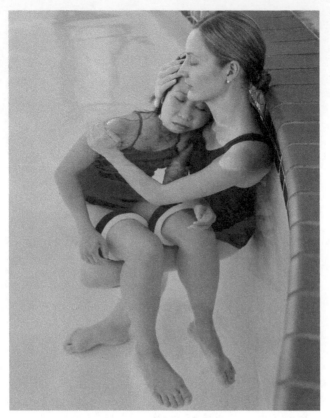

Figure 1.16: The path of the heart

The future

The beauty of WATSU is that it continues to evolve. From water to land, for our communities and a variety of medical populations, WATSU adapts and grows in its ability to connect. The boundlessness felt in warm water is the sheath of *prana*, the warmth within, becoming one with the warmth of the water. During WATSU, when our mind's chatter becomes most stilled, the more spontaneous and intuitive our moves become, the more they are coming out of our body's innate wisdom, and the deeper we move into rapture. It is said that once an opening is made to the rapture, once we know how to access it, we will be able to see it underlying even the greatest of our sorrows. We can imagine no better future goal for WATSU than to help people realize a level of consciousness from which they can face anything, a level as boundless as *water*.

Further reading

Dull, H. (2008). *Watsu: Freeing the Body in the Water.* Middletown, CA: Watsu Publishing.

Chapter 2

WATSU® Meeting the Therapeutic Challenges of Diverse Special Populations

Adult and Pediatric

PEGGY SCHOEDINGER

SECTION 1

Introduction

The intention of this chapter is to inspire WATSU practitioners to broaden the scope of their work to include more clients with special needs and challenges. This chapter is also in response to the countless questions from therapists regarding how to safely use and adapt WATSU for the non-able-bodied clients seen daily in rehabilitation centers, clinics and many WATSU pools around the world.

Think of snowflakes falling softly from the sky. Each one is exquisitely intricate. Every floating white crystal is beautifully unique, having been shaped by its own series of special conditions: changes in air currents, temperature and humidity. Some have floated softly to the ground, others have been blasted by high winds, and some have been slammed into each other.

So it is, also, with each person we hold in our arms. People arrive with their own special set of life experiences, challenges, successes, traumas, joys and sorrows. We will never know all that has shaped an individual, but we can appreciate and celebrate the uniqueness of each person while holding a space of deep compassion for their hardships and challenges.

Information covering a wide range of conditions is included in this chapter so practitioners can feel more comfortable expanding their practice to include clients with various challenges, especially chronic conditions. For practitioners who have professional training in rehabilitation, this chapter is to support and expand the therapeutic benefits of WATSU for their most challenging patients.

The information in this chapter is based on research on a wide range of topics, including the physiological effects of immersion in water and emerging WATSU research. There is also research on other therapeutic techniques that supports the benefits of WATSU's rhythmical, repeated movements, especially spinal rotation, for the body. Research adds to our knowledge base and informs what we do, yet each client remains a unique individual and each session will develop according to the needs and responses of the client throughout the session.

Most of the information in this chapter is based on 40 years of rehabilitation experience, including 30 years and thousands of hours of using WATSU in clinical practice with adults and children with a vast range of orthopedic, neurological and psychological challenges. These clients have been exceptional teachers.

The majority of this chapter will be devoted to suggestions and precautions for using WATSU to address the needs of many health conditions people face. Most of this information will focus on physical needs. The psychological benefits of WATSU are vast for our clients; however, other chapters in this book will address in depth the psychological challenges our clients face.

For the sake of consistency, the words practitioner and client will be used instead of therapist and patient, except in some case reports.

Please note, the information in this chapter is not intended to replace professional medical advice.

Benefits of WATSU for the body
Summary of physiological benefits

WATSU's flowing, rhythmical, repeated movements in warm water promote a deep state of relaxation with extensive changes throughout the body. These changes are readily apparent in the musculoskeletal system and the autonomic nervous system. The net results for the body include an increase in soft tissue and joint mobility, and a decrease in muscle tone, which results in decreases in muscle tension, muscle spasms and neurological hypertonicity. WATSU's movements, combined with the deep presence and the unconditional acceptance of the practitioner, profoundly touch the hearts of those who receive this exquisite bodywork. Many who receive WATSU find it to be transformative on multiple levels.

Physiological effects

The physiological benefits of WATSU are the combined result of:

- The effects of hydrostatic pressure due to immersion in water.
- The gentle warmth of the water.
- The gentle turbulence and flow of water on the skin.
- The slow, rhythmical repetition of many WATSU movements.
- Changes in sensory input, including visual, auditory, tactile, gravitational and vestibular.
- Stretching and soft tissue techniques that are frequently incorporated into sessions.
- Changes within the autonomic nervous system that generally include a quieting of the sympathetic nervous system and enhancement of the parasympathetic nervous system.
- The calming presence, attentive awareness and care of the practitioner.

Physiological benefits include:

- Decreased heart rate.
- Decreased blood pressure.
- Decreased rate of respiration.
- Increased depth of respiration.
- Increased peripheral vasodilation.
- Increased urine production secondary to a decrease in the antidiuretic hormone (ADH).
- Decreased edema due to improved movement of lymph, secondary to the compressive force of hydrostatic pressure.
- Improved smooth muscle activity, including muscles of digestion.
- Decreased activation of striated muscles (less tension in skeletal muscles) resulting in decreased muscle tension and muscle spasm.
- Improved soft tissue mobility.
- Improved range of motion in many joints.
- Decreased reticular activating system activity (often resulting in improved sleep).
- Improved circulation because the heart functions more efficiently when the body is immersed, and hydrostatic pressure increases venous blood return to the heart.
- Decreased joint compression, including decreased spinal compression.
- Decreased pain that is frequently reported by clients.
- Deep relaxation.
- Decreased hypertonicity, especially spasticity, for clients who have neurological conditions with associated hypertonicity. This decrease is the result of rhythmical movements in warm water, coupled with

repeated trunk rotation, trunk elongation, and specific techniques to decrease spasticity that can be incorporated into WATSU sessions.

Each WATSU movement affects the entire musculoskeletal system

One of the benefits of WATSU is that movements are not isolated, as they often are when body parts are moved on land. Because clients are resting in water, every movement tends to affect the entire body.

Example: Near leg rotation—moving toward the head

Some variations, especially rotational movements, will occur with different individuals and with changes in the angle of the client's body in the water.

- Near leg hip is flexed and adducted with a small amount of rotation.
- In the near leg, turbulent drag causes flexion of knee, plantar flexion of ankle and subtle flexion of toes.
- In the far leg, turbulent drag causes gentle extension of hip, flexion of knee, plantar flexion of ankle and subtle flexion of toes.
- Trunk, especially in the lumbar region, is somewhat flexed and the pelvis is rotated toward the far side.
- Near arm remains behind practitioner in shoulder abduction with a small amount of rotation and elbow flexion. Wrist and finger movements depend on the client.
- In the far arm, turbulent drag usually causes shoulder extension with some rotation, and movements for the elbow, wrist and fingers depending on how the body is angled in the water.
- Neck is in a slightly flexed position on the practitioner's arm, and it frequently rotates toward the far side.

CASE REPORTS

Names of all clients have been changed to protect their privacy.

The physical benefits of WATSU have historically been viewed as being related only to passive movements during sessions. However, this view is changing as benefits emerge that are clearly the result of other factors. Some physical improvements strongly suggest that motor learning during sessions is a key factor, especially for some clients with neurological conditions. Neuroplasticity likely also plays a role for some clients. The following case report is an important example of a physical benefit resulting from more than just the passive movements of WATSU.

Case report: Adult with spinal muscular atrophy (SMA)
Benefit: Independent sit to stand following one WATSU session

Judy was an adult female, age 42, with Type 3 SMA who had been unable to rise from her wheelchair independently for more than a year. Judy had extensive weakness throughout her body, especially in her trunk, and required significant assistance to rise from her wheelchair for transfers to her bed or toilet.

Prior to the session, when asked what she would like from the session, Judy said she wanted to "celebrate and feel joyful." She added that she wished she could dance because in her dreams she was often dancing.

Judy was exceptionally weak throughout her body, so the practitioner assumed the session would be slow and gentle. However, Judy began expressing movements as soon as she was brought to supine in the water.

Due to Judy's weakness, especially in her trunk, all she could do was subtly initiate movements. The practitioner followed and gave fuller expression to her movements, while still being mindful of areas of her body that required protection. For example, in daily life outside the pool, the weakness in Judy's trunk resulted in her sitting all day with hyperextension in her lower lumbar spine. Therefore, when Judy went into spinal extension during the session, the practitioner gave gentle extension through most of the spine, but not the lower lumbar spine. Traction and lengthening were simultaneously given to the lower lumbar spine to gently open and protect it from hyperextension.

It was a remarkable session with a great deal of movement, all of which arose from Judy. The practitioner listened, supported, and safely gave more expression to the movements Judy was too weak to do independently.

The majority of Judy's movements during the session were around her central core, including flexion, extension and rotation.

During movements, the practitioner gave subtle tactile facilitation to help enhance activity and motor learning in trunk stabilization muscles that were weak and functioning inefficiently.

Following this one WATSU session, Judy stated that she felt more "alive" in her core than she had in years. She was able to rise from her wheelchair independently without physical assistance. She maintained this ability for nearly two months after the session until she developed kidney stones and had to be hospitalized.

This is one of many examples of clients with improved motor function following WATSU.

Case report: Child with cerebral palsy
Benefit: Increased mobility for dressing

Tyler was an intelligent and verbal seven-year-old boy with cerebral palsy. He had spastic quadriplegia with severe spasticity.

Tyler was seen twice a week for therapy sessions in the pool. WATSU was a portion of every session and was referred to as his "soft time" in the pool.

Each session also included assisted weight bearing on each extremity and initiation of active movements.

During the second month of this program, Tyler mentioned to his therapist that he enjoyed his "soft time" very much. The therapist replied that she enjoyed it, too.

Then Tyler added an unexpected comment. He said, "I like our 'soft time' because it also helps my mommy." His therapist was intrigued and asked him to explain his comment.

Tyler said, "I've always been very stiff and it's hard for mommy to dress me. But now I imagine it's my 'soft time' in the pool and that makes me less stiff so it's easier for mommy to dress me."

The therapist was absolutely stunned by how this child had extended the benefits of WATSU into his daily life to help decrease his spasticity. His mother confirmed everything he had said.

The therapist thanked Tyler and asked if she could share his wisdom with others. The child was delighted.

Over the years, the therapist has encouraged countless clients to use the memories of their felt sensations during WATSU to calm and relax in other situations in life that may be stressful, difficult or painful.

Case report: Adult with cerebral palsy, and a rape victim
Benefit: One session calmed fear, gained shoulder mobility

Lucy was a 57-year-old female with cerebral palsy. She had spastic quadri-plegia with severe spasticity and mental retardation. Lucy frequently vocalized, but only sounds without recognizable words. She was unable to follow any simple verbal, tactile or visual cues. Lucy was abandoned in infancy and had lived all of her 57 years in institutions.

A few months prior to this session, Lucy was raped at night by multiple staff members at the facility where she resided. She was then transferred to a very caring group home with ten residents.

Due to her trauma at the previous facility, Lucy screamed most of each night and frequently during the day. Simultaneously, she would have extremely strong full-body extensor spasticity, including a posterior head thrust.

These strong extensor patterns threw her out of her wheelchair. To keep her safe, the staff had to tie a rolled sheet around her waist to secure her in her wheelchair.

Additionally, her strong spasticity made cleaning and caring for Lucy exceptionally difficult, especially cleaning her perineum and axillae. At the time, she had developed a fungal infection in her axillae, and caregivers were having great difficulty moving her arms enough to adequately care for her.

The staff members at the group home were quite distressed and searching for ways to help Lucy. They were desperate to help calm her fears and gain enough shoulder mobility to care for her axillae.

Socially, Lucy was interactive with grunts and sounds. She fluctuated between appearing to want to interact with others and crying, screaming and appearing terrified.

Two WATSU practitioners had been giving Lucy a WATSU session once a week, but they were uncertain how to help her and felt that they were both needed to work with Lucy safely in the water. They had not seen any improvements.

The only water available was a large but very shallow indoor hot tub. This required practitioners to work in a deeply flexed squat position.

The focus of the session was to help calm Lucy and help her to feel safe and cared for. Additionally, staff members requested a focus on improving the range of motion in her upper extremities, especially her shoulders.

Cooing and rocking with close physical contact were used to help calm Lucy. There were times when Lucy mirrored the cooing back and forth with the practitioner. The techniques used in the session were a blend of WATSU and neuro-developmental treatment (NDT).

The session began with a focus on holding positions of strong trunk rotation while Lucy was swayed and rocked rhythmically. (Strong spasticity prevented the use of typical WATSU rotation moves.)

Lucy's very strong posterior head thrust was managed with combined posterior-inferior pressure on the sternum. (Refer to the section in this chapter titled "Clients with spasticity" for more details.)

Trunk rotation was continued with Lucy in a "tucked or closed saddle" position to stabilize her pelvis. Lucy's legs were tightly flexed and firmly held between the practitioner's legs.

The practitioner then worked with each upper extremity from proximal to distal to increase the range of motion.

When each hand eventually opened, the hand was placed and held on the therapist's thigh while Lucy's body was shifted to create weight bearing on her hand and upper extremity. (Lucy was still held in the "tucked or closed saddle" position.)

All movements required power and strength calmly applied without tension in the practitioner's body and hands.

Any talking increased Lucy's muscle tone, so the practitioner requested everyone to smile warmly but not talk. This was very beneficial for Lucy.

At the end of the session, Lucy sat calmly in her wheelchair smiling. She was equally calm five hours later when the practitioner completed her other sessions at the facility.

Lucy's practitioners ordered a better wheelchair for her and increased her WATSU sessions to three times per week.

Following this one session, Lucy stopped all screaming and crying, even at night. Her spasticity remained diminished, and her shoulder and hip mobility remained in functional ranges for hygiene.

Within a few weeks, Lucy was positioned in healthy alignment in her new wheelchair and was much calmer. She was then able to begin saying a few discernible words.

Case report: Child suffered second- and third-degree burns on 95 percent of her body
Benefit: Gained 70° of shoulder range of motion in one session

Anna was a three-year-old girl who was burned at 18 months of age. In addition to horrific burns, Anna suffered hypoxic brain damage secondary to multiple cardiac arrests in the first few hours after the accident.

Anna's grafted skin was well healed, though her range of motion was limited by tightness and scar tissue in multiple areas, especially her shoulders. Her current therapists reported that both shoulders were limited to 80° of flexion and 65° of abduction.

Anna was receiving physiotherapy, occupational therapy and speech therapy with some aquatic therapy. She was described as tactilely defensive because she strongly resisted all efforts by people to touch or move her arms.

Secondary to the hypoxic brain damage, Anna had hypertonicity in her extremities and trunk. Anna's current therapists reported that when they worked with her in a standing position, she would strongly resist or push into a full and rigid extension pattern.

When carrying Anna into the pool this therapist noticed that Anna "brightened" and became more alert, with slight bouncing movements. The therapist then explored more movements with Anna and discovered she loved the sensory input of bouncing, turning in circles, and being swished strongly from side to side. Although these are not typical WATSU movements, they were Anna's preferred movements, so the therapist used these movements to motivate, engage and sometimes distract Anna when needed.

Songs and playfully modified WATSU movements were used to engage Anna.

Shoulder flexion and abduction stretches were gradually added into the session. Modified WATSU movements were blended with the stretches.

The focus was on inviting Anna's entire body to rotate and elongate from her toes all the way to her fingertips. Using this strategy, plus lots of playfulness, rocking and handling with soft relaxed hands, the therapist was able to fully stretch and elongate Anna's entire body, including full hip extension, trunk rotation and shoulder flexion to more than 150° for both shoulders and nearly full abduction.

High-kneeling and standing activities were also woven through the session. Playfulness kept Anna engaged and encouraged her to stand in the pool in knee-deep water on her knees and then her feet. Firm tapping on her bilateral paraspinal muscles facilitated extension into a healthy upright position versus an extension pattern. Firm tactile facilitation of Anna's gluteal muscles engaged her with laughter and resulted in improved stability in a fully upright and healthy standing position.

Case report: Bedridden elderly man with severe chronic obstructive pulmonary disease (COPD) and multiple comorbidities
Benefit: Client was able to go to party at friend's home

John was an 88-year-old bedridden male. He required multiple personal caregivers around the clock.

John had multiple medical challenges, and was totally dependent on caregivers for all transfers and all activities of daily living, including feeding. He had severe COPD requiring constant oxygen at 2–3 liters per minute, and severe osteoporosis secondary to long-term prednisone use for COPD. He also had bilateral spontaneous hip fractures secondary to osteoporosis and suffered from pain in both hips, his knees and back. He had metastatic cancer with a T_{2-4} spinal tumor, with limited active movement in his legs following tumor and radiation treatment. A mild stroke had left him with residual mild hemiparesis and mild left-side neglect. He also had congestive heart failure and was prone to frequent episodes of pneumonia. John could not sit upright and had been bedridden for two years, with only brief periods of time out of bed in a reclined wheelchair.

These health challenges had left John with depression and he had not been out of his home or seen any friends for nearly two years. He stated, "I don't want people to see me like this."

The therapist discussed quality of life with John, and together they set goals that were meaningful for him. The therapist also met with the caregivers to encourage them to support John's efforts to be more active and do more for himself.

John was seen twice a week for aquatic therapy sessions that included WATSU and practicing functional daily life skills. Oxygen was used at all times during sessions, and John was carefully monitored.

The WATSU portions of John's aquatic sessions were particularly beneficial for improving mobility, decreasing pain and for emotional support. John needed to work on functional skills in the pool; however, he fatigued quickly. Therefore, WATSU was alternated with functional skills training during each session. John enjoyed the WATSU portions of his sessions and said they gave him "relief from pain and great joy."

John was surprised and excited by his early progress, and he became more and more pleased and motivated as he made surprisingly rapid progress toward his goals.

Six-week summary:

- John was much more alert and jovial. His pain was dramatically decreased.
- John was participating in all of his activities of daily living and was independent in feeding himself.
- John was out of bed and in his wheelchair for most of each day (reclined 60% of time, upright 40% of time) and dressed in clothes, not pajamas.
- Friends had been visiting John at his home.
- John had been to a small party at a friend's home. Caregivers were needed for outings, but he was thrilled and proud of his progress.

Benefits of a brief WATSU session used at beginning of active treatment sessions

WATSU is primarily used as either the sole modality during sessions or woven together with other bodywork modalities. However, there are practitioners who work in clinical settings where treatment sessions are significantly limited in number and in the amount of time allotted for each session. The following case report is a valuable example of how beneficial a brief segment of WATSU can be.

Case report: Angry, resistant man, with lumbar pain radiating down his leg, was convinced session would be a waste of time
Benefit: Pain dramatically reduced; able to return to usual activities

Bob was a 52-year-old male, chief executive of a large corporation and an avid kayaker. He had a history of multiple brief episodes over several years of lumbar pain that had been treated with pain medication and muscle relaxants.

His current pain, at time of the session, had lasted nearly three months and he had pain radiating down one leg, which was new and disturbing for him.

Prior to his session in the pool, Bob had seen his primary physician, chiropractor, orthopedic surgeon, neurologist, acupuncturist, physical therapist and massage therapist—each person for only one session.

Bob arrived for his session at the therapy pool, which at that moment was filled with elderly clients. He looked at the people in the pool and rolled his eyes. His therapist approached him to introduce herself, but Bob interrupted her with an angry tirade stating that this session was a waste of his time, and he would *not* do any "stupid exercises" during this session or at home.

His therapist realized his anger was not based on her actions. She listened thoughtfully and wondered about the source of Bob's anger. Her assessment in those moments was that this man was perhaps afraid. He was accustomed to being in charge, in control and successful, but he was now unsuccessful in eliminating his pain, which was getting worse.

The therapist chose to convey strong confidence and to match Bob's body language as much as possible. She said she was glad he had given her this information. She could see he was a man of action, so they would get in the pool immediately and start getting rid of his pain. The therapist was not certain she would be successful, but she felt Bob needed her to be confident and decisive.

The therapist was curious about Bob's strong comments regarding exercise. She thought he might be afraid that exercise would increase his pain or, more likely, Bob might not like exercising. However, she felt he would be uncomfortable admitting either of these. Therefore, she chose to ask him if he didn't like to exercise, or he didn't have time to exercise. She assumed he would state he didn't have time to exercise, which is what he said. She then asked him if he would do an exercise if it took zero time out of his day. He again rolled his eyes but agreed that he would do a "zero time" exercise. This was the response the therapist was hoping for. (The therapist had a wide range of simple exercises that could be incorporated into current activities and required no extra time.)

The therapist chose to start the session with WATSU to calm Bob's autonomic nervous system, decrease his muscle spasms, reduce his back pain, and decrease and centralize the pain radiating down his leg. She briefly described WATSU by choosing words and explanations she felt would give Bob confidence in WATSU.

The therapist moved slowly and calmly and followed Bob's body. She added some gentle stretches to his movements, plus elongation (very gentle traction) for his spine, especially his lumbar spine. The WATSU portion of the session was only 15 minutes, yet the effects on Bob were dramatic. He stared at the therapist in bewilderment and then walked across the pool. When he returned, he said, "The pain in my leg has disappeared, and my back pain has decreased from 8 out of 10 down to 3—but you didn't do anything!" The therapist smiled. Bob kept walking and saying—in a stunned voice—how good he felt.

The remainder of the session was used to do gentle trunk stabilization exercises that did not stress his back. Bob was instructed in one simple exercise he could easily incorporate into his day without requiring extra time.

Bob was seen six times. The first four sessions included WATSU, but when his pain decreased and remained in the 1–2 out of 10 range between sessions, the WATSU portion of his sessions was shortened and then eliminated. Appropriate "no time" exercises were gradually added to his regime. He was able to return to his usual activities.

Bob eventually confided that stress was a major pain trigger for him. The therapist and Bob discussed strategies for this. Bob was taught some simple breathing exercises and visualizations, which he liked. He also chose to continue his "no time" exercises "because they feel good."

Additionally, at the end of his rehab program, Bob chose to schedule a full WATSU session one to two times each month as needed.

Overview of sessions for clients with special needs

This overview contains pertinent information for most clients. For questions regarding specific diagnoses, please refer to the sections of the chapter titled "Additional suggestions and precautions."

Beginning

Our first session with a client begins the moment we meet and make eye contact. From that moment, every little thing we do either creates trust or breaks trust. Let us choose to build trust with every word and tone of voice, every eye gaze, every touch—everything.

For the client's safety, an intake form and an assessment will need to be completed. Clients respond well when we listen to their information and their experiences with sensitivity and respect.

Some clients have conditions that make it difficult for them to speak and convey essential information to us. Acknowledge and speak with the client first. If the client is in a wheelchair, sit or squat down to speak at or below the client's eye level. Take the time to connect with the client, even if they are unable to speak. Look into the client's eyes and smile and hold the client's hand after asking for permission. Then request permission to speak with the client's caregiver. If the client is unable to acknowledge your request, then explain that you now need to speak with the caregiver to gather more information.

Allow extra time, especially in the pool before the session, for deep listening and "being" with unconditional acceptance. People often feel safer and more relaxed in a warm pool, and in this place of comfort they often share more about their lives and challenges.

Clients, especially those with special needs, are accustomed to just relaying the "facts" to others. We need to give our client the time and peaceful space to share more than this. This often means quietly waiting during times of silence without a need to fill the silence. Many clients will then choose to share more about their physical and emotional pain and challenges.

Create a safe emotional space of deep presence and empathetic listening before, during and after each session, without needing to advise or comfort. Often what humans need the most is someone who can just "be" with us with quiet acceptance.

Give the client clear information about the session and the ending of the session. Anticipate questions that might arise for the client during the session. Sharing this information prior to starting the session will create trust, facilitate greater relaxation, and increase the client's sense of safety.

Sessions

Life has brought challenges for each one of us. The truth is that each one of us has some special needs.

There are suggestions for clients but no recipes.

Read research because it provides additional validity to our work. Learn from the experiences and knowledge of other practitioners—their successes and their challenges. These inform and expand our skills and understanding.

Remember that each client is a unique individual who will respond according to a multitude of factors. Every session with each client will develop according to the needs of the client throughout the session. Listen for and follow movements arising from the client. When the client's body speaks, listen.

Follow the client's movements, including subtle movements. Watch for patterns of movement that may emerge. When there is movement, ask yourself, "Is this the client's movement or mine?" "Is this the client's rhythm or mine?" Strive to follow the client's movements and rhythms.

Be especially attentive to rotational patterns. These patterns may be local-ized, but often they flow through the entire length of the body.

Sometimes we give the body an invitation for movement. We listen care-fully, yet we are unattached to whether or not the client's body chooses to follow our invitation. The body will respond to everything we do. What is it saying? How is it responding?

Use the information in this chapter, together with your life and WATSU experiences, the research you read and the information in this book, to inform what you do, but not to dictate your sessions. For our clients with special needs, there are often strategies that have been successful for multiple people with similar needs. These strategies are usually quite beneficial, yet every person is unique.

Be keenly focused on how the client responds to everything you do. How does the client's body respond to everything in the environment and to each subtle movement? Does the response of the client's body suggest that what you are doing is beneficial for the client? If yes, continue what you're doing or build on and expand it.

If the client's body responds in a way that suggests something you did affected the client in a counter-productive way, ask yourself, "Why?" Then test your informed reasoning. Perhaps try doing the same thing but with less ten-sion in your own body and more sensitive awareness of the client. Or perhaps try a movement that's nearly the opposite of what was previously tried but didn't yield positive results. Look at the client with fresh eyes and an open mind to discover a better path.

Expect that everything you do makes a difference—because it does. Let us all be keenly observant.

Suggestions for incorporating WATSU into therapy sessions
Clients with neurological challenges
WATSU is best utilized at the beginning of the session. WATSU will decrease abnormal muscle tone, improve soft tissue mobility, decrease pain and improve respiration. The client will then have greater success at the end of the session practicing functional activities.

For some clients, it may be more beneficial to alternate short periods of WATSU with short periods of active functional movements.

Caregivers also need support. For clients with special needs who require extensive daily care, consider giving one or more free sessions to the primary caregiver, especially if it's a family member.

Clients with orthopedic or medical challenges

WATSU is usually best at the beginning of a session. Benefits include relaxation with decreased sympathetic nervous system activity, decreased muscle spasm, pain reduction, and improved soft tissue and joint mobility.

Some practitioners use WATSU at the end of the session as a "reward" for the client's effort of moving, exercising and addressing functional skills. This is a reward the practitioner gives the client.

Alternatively, if WATSU is used at the beginning of the session to improve symptoms and is followed by active movements by the client, then the "reward" is the client's own successful improvements in their functional skills, strength, mobility and activity tolerance. These improvements are the "rewards" the client earned for themselves, and this puts the emphasis on the client's personal achievements.

Incorporating additional therapeutic techniques

WATSU yields a multitude of benefits for minds, hearts and bodies.

Each practitioner also brings to WATSU a multitude of life experiences, knowledge and skills. All of these will flavor the WATSU sessions of each practitioner in unique ways.

Practitioners are encouraged to incorporate their experience, knowledge and skills into sessions by asking themselves, "What skills, knowledge, techniques and life experiences can I incorporate into this session with this individual?" Elements of other related skills and techniques can be used during sessions to enhance WATSU's benefits. For example:

- Shiatsu
- Massage
- Healing Dance
- AMNION
- Aquatic Integration.

Ai Chi is a related technique that can be used before the start of a session and can also be taught to clients to do independently for relaxation in a pool.

It can also be beneficial to incorporate elements of traditionally land-based therapeutic techniques into WATSU sessions. Here are some examples, though the list of possibilities is nearly endless:

- Sensory integration
- Craniosacral
- Myofascial release

- Neuro-developmental treatment (NDT)
- Rood and Brunnstrom.

In rehabilitation, WATSU is often a portion of the treatment session followed by additional aquatic techniques. Examples of some of the therapeutic aquatic techniques that can be used in the pool following WATSU include:

- Ai Chi
- Halliwick Concept
- Bad Ragaz Ring Method
- AquaStretch
- Burdenko Method
- Functional activities
- Therapeutic exercise.

Techniques that are typically land-based can often be adapted and used in the pool following the WATSU portion of the session. Examples include:

- Neuro-developmental treatment (NDT) (during and after WATSU)
- Rood and Brunnstrom (during and after WATSU)
- Manual lymph drainage
- Proprioceptive neuromuscular facilitation (PNF)
- LSVT Big & Loud
- Mindfulness
- Yoga.

In most therapeutic settings, the focus is on improving function and quality of life—physically, emotionally, every way.

Safety considerations
General safety considerations

- Safety is number one. Keep your client and yourself safe at all times.
- Know your own strengths and limitations in terms of your physical body, your knowledge base, your educational training and your professional scope of practice.
- Refer to "Precautions for aquatic bodywork" later in this chapter.
- If you have any questions about a specific diagnosis or impairment, seek additional medical advice before proceeding. Reschedule the session if you have any uncertainty or concerns.

- Have a plan for getting each individual safely in and out of the pool. Remember that getting someone out of the pool is always more challenging than getting in.
- If you will need physical assistance with a client, arrange for extra help.
- Learn first aid and stay current with CPR certification.
- Have emergency plans and practice them. Plan for cuts, falls, low blood sugar, fainting, vomiting, heart attacks, seizures, and so on.
- Document your emergency plan. Have a sign with the emergency phone number and pool address in your pool area. Remember that a healthy person, including a healthy practitioner, can have a medical emergency. One WATSU instructor fainted while teaching a class, due to acute appendicitis!
- Have some way to contact emergency personnel *while you are in the pool*. A cell phone in a well-sealed clear plastic bag on the side of the pool is one option. If someone is having a medical emergency in the pool, it may be extremely difficult or unsafe to get this person out of the pool until you have additional assistance.
- Locked doors can be a problem. Be certain emergency personnel will have access to your pool from the street.
- A clearly visible clock in the pool area with a second hand will make it possible for you to record pulse rate and rate of respiration. This is important information to give to emergency personnel on the phone or in person.
- If an incident occurs, document exactly what happened, including:
  - Detailed description of what happened.
  - Detailed description of the client's symptoms.
  - Detailed description of specific care given to the client.
  - If family members were contacted, who and when.
  - If physician was contacted, who, when, and what were the physician's recommendations.
  - If emergency personnel were summoned, what time, and what action was taken.
  - If client went home without assistance, at what time, and was this via their own car or other transport.
  - Date and time the client was phoned to verify well-being.
  - Follow-up plan.
- Have emergency equipment available, including:
  - Rescue equipment.
  - First aid kit, including bandages.
  - Latex or other protective gloves.

- Glucose tablets (can be purchased at a pharmacy) or juice for low blood sugar (juice cannot be used if the client is unconscious or unable to safely swallow).
- Ice or emergency cold packs.
- CPR mask with a one-way valve.
- Clock with a second hand for measuring heart rate and respiration.
- Blanket to keep the client warm and dry.
- Cell phone accessible when in the pool with clients—place in a sealed plastic bag.
- Consider purchasing a blood pressure monitor.

Safety considerations before sessions
WATSU client screening questionnaire

- Before the first session, ask the client to fill out an intake screening questionnaire that covers pertinent medical information and emergency information. (Refer to an example of a questionnaire below.)
- Adapt and create your own questionnaire that will be appropriate for your work and your clients. Be certain to ask about acute and chronic medical conditions. Clients often forget to mention chronic medical conditions, such as epilepsy and diabetes. This information can be critically important for safety.
- Follow up with detailed questions about any problem or impairments the client indicates on the questionnaire. Refer to the later section titled "Precautions for aquatic bodywork."
- Know and stay within the *scope of practice* for your specific profession. We are all passionate about this work and sharing it with others. At the same time, we need to keep people safe and protect ourselves by staying within the scope of our own profession.

SAMPLE INTAKE QUESTIONNAIRE

Create your own questionnaire appropriate for your work and your clients.

Name: . . . . Age: . . . .

Address: . . . .

Phone number: . . . . Occupation: . . . .

Emergency contact name, phone number: . . . .

Physician's name: . . . . Phone number: . . . .

Medical history: For your safety, general information about your medical history is needed. Please check any condition listed below that applies to you (past or present):

☐ Any currently infectious condition

☐ Compromised immune system

☐ Current open wounds/rashes/skin conditions

☐ Recent accident or injury

☐ Fractures

☐ Any catheters/ostomies/ports

☐ Sprains/strains

☐ Any respiratory/lung condition

☐ Current fever

☐ High or low blood pressure

☐ Chlorine sensitivity

☐ Joint pain/arthritis/tendonitis/artificial joints

☐ Any heart or circulatory condition

☐ Headaches/migraines

☐ Deep vein thrombosis/blood clots

☐ Epilepsy/seizures

☐ Osteoporosis

☐ Diabetes

☐ Cancer

☐ Any ear problems

☐ Dizziness or motion sickness

☐ Back/neck problems/pain

☐ Heat sensitivity

☐ Difficulty with bowel/bladder control

Are you comfortable in water? . . . . Can you swim? . . . .

Have you had a near drowning experience? . . . . If yes, please briefly

describe. . . . .

. . . .

Are you pregnant? . . . . If so, how many weeks? . . . .

Do you do any type of regular exercise? If so, please describe. . . . .

. . . .

Are you currently being treated for any health condition?. . . . .

. . . .

Have you been given a specific medical diagnosis?. . . . .

When did you receive this diagnosis? . . . .

Current medications?. . . . .

Have you had any surgeries? . . . . If so, what were the surgeries? . . . .

. . . .

Any other medical conditions? . . . .

Is your balance impaired? . . . . Have you had any recent falls? . . . .

Will you need assistance with dressing or getting in/out of the pool? . . . .

Do you use any assistive devices (wheelchair, walker, cane, hearing aids, etc.)?

Please list.. . . . .

Do you have any pain? . . . . If so, where do you have pain? . . . .

. . . .

Do you have any areas of diminished sensation, numbness or tingling? If so,

where? . . . .

Are there any movements, positions or activities that increase your symptoms?

Please describe.. . . . .

Are there any movements or positions that decrease your symptoms? Please

describe. . . . .

Is there any part of your body that is ticklish or sensitive to having pressure applied

or being stretched or massaged? . . . .

Are any of your movements limited because of pain?. . . . .

Have you been told by a medical practitioner not to do certain movements or

activities? Please explain. . . . .

Are your usual daily activities limited in any way due to pain or weakness? Please describe. . . . .

Have you ever received a WATSU session? . . . . Have you ever received a massage? . . . . Have you experienced any significant traumas in the past? If yes, it is your choice whether or not you wish to describe/discuss the incident(s) with your practitioner. . . . .

. . . .

Is there anything else you would like to share about yourself or your specific needs? . . . .

- This is *your* WATSU session. I will do everything possible to make it an enjoyable and relaxing experience. Please wiggle or adjust your head and neck so that you are always in the most comfortable position. Tell me if you wish more or less pressure with any massage or stretch. If there is a move that feels not quite right for you for any reason, gently tap the water so that I will know to move to a different position/movement.

- There will be periods of stillness and movement. If you would like more stillness at any time, let me know.

- WATSU sometimes awakens emotions and memories (positive and sometimes negative). You can choose to simply allow these to arise, observe them and allow them to flow. I will be with you to calmly support you. At the end of your session, you may wish to talk about your experience, or you may wish to be quiet. I will respect your wishes.

- If your medical condition changes in any way, please be sure to inform your practitioner prior to your next session.

I (your name) . . . . have read this form and discussed all of my relevant health information with my WATSU practitioner. My WATSU practitioner has described this modality to me and answered my questions regarding WATSU. I assume full responsibility for my health and understand that there may be a risk of injury despite all of the safety precautions taken by the WATSU practitioner.

Signature . . . . Date . . . .

THANK YOU FOR TAKING THE TIME TO COMPLETE THIS QUESTIONNAIRE!

Safety considerations before sessions (continued)

- Anticipate problems or barriers your client may encounter. Proactively mitigate potential problems, including:
  - Wet, slippery pool deck—the most common cause of falls and injuries.
  - Wet, slippery or cluttered floors and small rugs in hallways and changing areas.
  - Doors that are too heavy to open.
  - Steps and door thresholds that may be difficult or cause tripping.
  - Inadequate lighting.
  - Need for a place to sit while changing clothes.
  - Need for safety bars and possibly a bench in the shower.
  - Need for assistance with changing clothes and/or toileting.
  - Accommodations needed for pain, vision, hearing or mobility challenges.
  - Encourage your client to be comfortable throughout the session. "Move or wiggle your head or move my arm so that your head and neck always feel supported 'just right,' like your pillow when you go to sleep."
- You will want to know during a session if your client feels any motion sickness or discomfort at any time. Here are some examples of positive ways to convey this to the client:
  - "During your session there will be times of movement and times of stillness. If you wish to have more stillness, please say, 'Stillness.'"
  - "If there is a move or position that feels not quite right for you for any reason, just tap the surface of the water gently a few times, and I'll know to move on to something else." This statement is a particularly useful one. The client is not required to speak or to specifically state if the movement is physically uncomfortable or feels emotionally uncomfortable. Most clients will clarify later, but it is their choice.
- Let the client know that if they want to stop the session at any time for any reason, they can just say, "Stop."
- Begin each session in an appropriate position for that individual's condition. Begin by standing next to the client's healthier (less injured, less painful, less stiff, etc.) side. Clients perceive it to be safer and less invasive when we begin the session close to their healthier side.

Safety considerations after sessions

- Ask all clients to drink water and walk/move around in the pool before exiting. Make sure the client is fully alert and safe before leaving the pool.
- Most clients are in an extremely relaxed condition after a WATSU session. Guard clients closely when they are exiting the pool and while walking on the deck, to be certain they are moving safely. The number one risk in all pool areas is falls, even for healthy, typically abled individuals.
- Be sure to have a towel(s) within easy reach so that your client can wrap up as soon as they leave the pool. A heat lamp installed in a safe location can be used to keep clients warm while changing into clothes after the pool. Most clients with special needs require more time for dressing, and it's essential to keep them adequately warm.
- Be certain that all clients with special needs safely reach their caregiver or their transportation home. We are responsible for their well-being until they leave the property.
- Write a brief summary of the session, including before/after comments from the client and/or caregiver. This will be valuable information for you to have when the client returns for a session, and it will be essential for you if there are legal concerns.

Precautions for aquatic bodywork
Precautions versus contraindications

The term *precautions* has been purposely chosen rather than *contraindications*. A contraindication is something that absolutely should not be done. A precaution means that a condition or activity may have associated risks, yet have the potential to be done safely, if one is well-informed and considers all aspects carefully. Depending on our profession, knowledge and skills, some situations may be too risky. Practitioners need to use good clinical reasoning and critical thinking. Additionally, it may be necessary to seek qualified medical advice/support before working with some clients. Some clients may require the support of two or more practitioners in the pool for safety. Some clients may be outside your scope of professional practice.

Think before bringing each person into a pool, and then decide if it will be a safe, moderate risk or high risk for this person, and whether you can safely manage the risks. You must carefully consider all risks and potential benefits of aquatic bodywork for each individual.

As an example, consider open wounds. Aquatic therapy, hydrotherapy and aquatic bodywork books frequently list "open wounds" as a "contraindication" for going into a pool. The reality, however, is that all of us often go into pools with open wounds—open blisters, small cuts, open abrasions, torn hangnails, and so on—without endangering our health.

When our clients have open wounds, we need to consider the size, depth, location, type of wound and our ability to safely protect it if needed. We must also carefully consider the overall health and risks for every individual.

Let's consider two clients:

- A 42-year-old male has been receiving sessions in the pool for his lower back pain. During the weekend, he buys a new pair of shoes. On Monday, he comes to the pool with a small torn/open blister on his heel. This blister is an open wound. Should he stay out of the pool? If this man is in good health with no medical problems (except for his back pain), then clinical reasoning suggests the risks for him coming into the pool with his small open wound are very low. However, if this same man has diabetes, then his risk of infection is much greater. In this case, he should only come into the pool if his open blister can be completely protected. Bio-occlusive dressings often do not form an effective seal around the curved surface of heels. If the seal is not complete, a spray-on dressing could be considered (see note below), though it may not provide an adequate seal. For the best protection, place his lower leg and foot in a cast guard (cast protector), or securely place his foot and ankle in a durable plastic bag securely taped to his leg. Whatever method of protection is used, the goal would be to keep his blister completely dry during his session in the pool.
  Note: Bio-occlusive dressings are gas permeable but not water permeable. There are several products widely available internationally. Two of the most common are Tegaderm™ and Opsite™. Liquid and spray protective dressings are also available, though they can be messy and are often not as effective as dressings when in the pool.
- A 54-year-old female has been receiving sessions in the pool for fibromyalgia. During the weekend, she goes for a walk one evening and is bitten by mosquitoes. She scratches one bite on her hand, and it is slightly open and oozing when she comes for her session. If she is in good health, except for fibromyalgia, then it would be reasonable for her to be in the pool with this tiny open wound. However, if she has had a mastectomy with some lymph nodes removed on that side of her body, even if it was many years before, this is a significant concern. There is too much risk of infection and possibly lymphedema that could last for the rest of her life. The same options to protect

the wound, as described for the previous client, could be used. Additionally, care must be taken to not apply anything to this client's arm that might limit or obstruct lymph drainage from her arm.

General precautions for aquatic bodywork

It is impossible to predict all possible problems or conditions our clients may have. Refer to the four sections later in this chapter titled "Additional suggestions and precautions" about various conditions. Please seek further medical advice as needed. The information in this chapter is not intended to replace professional medical advice.

- Fever over 38° C (100° F). Wait until the client is feeling well and their temperature has returned to normal.
- Cardiac failure, unstable angina, severely compromised cardiovascular system—check with a physician.
- Excessively high blood pressure, depending on the acceptable blood pressure levels established by the client's healthcare provider.
- Excessively low blood pressure can also be a concern because immersion in warm water causes vasodilation, which lowers blood pressure. Light-headedness or fainting can occur when the client exits the pool. (Without the supportive force of hydrostatic pressure on the body, blood pressure drops when exiting the pool.)
- Significantly limited vital capacity (below 1000ml) due to a spinal cord injury, pulmonary disease, and so on. Consider the size of the client. A very petite client will naturally have a lower vital capacity. The inability to tolerate a 10 percent decrease in current vital capacity is a better indicator of safety. ("Vital capacity" is the maximum amount of air a person can breathe in and breathe out in one breath.)
- Absence of cough reflex or difficulty managing oral secretions due to a stroke, brain injury, amyotrophic lateral sclerosis (ALS), cerebral palsy, and so on. Absolutely *must* keep the nose and mouth above water at all times.
- Unpredictable bowel incontinence. Use a swim diaper (available in pediatric and adult sizes). It's best if babies wear plastic pants with elastic at the legs and waist over the swim diaper. Children and adult clients can wear snug pants (bike shorts or leggings) over the swim diaper. This is aesthetically more acceptable for clients, and the snug pants also provide extra security from fecal matter leaking into the pool.
- Significant open wounds and small open wounds on a person very susceptible to infection secondary to diabetes, and so on. It may be

possible to cover a small, clean wound with a bio-occlusive dressing such as Tegaderm or Opsite that is gas permeable but not water permeable. A cast guard (cast protector) or a securely taped plastic bag (with excess air inside expelled) can also be used to cover a limb.

- Contagious water or air-borne infection or disease. Wait until the client has completely recovered.
- Sensitivity to chemicals used in pool (chlorine, bromine, ozone, etc.). Chloramines (chlorine bonded with organic material) are a common source of irritation for skin and respiratory systems.
- Diabetes:
  - Keep glucose tablets or juice available at pool for emergencies due to low blood sugar. Encourage clients to eat a healthy snack or small meal containing protein approximately one hour before the session, and to drink water. Remember that people cannot be given any liquids if they have lost consciousness due to the high risk of aspiration into the lungs.
  - Give extra care to skin to prevent infection, which can lead to the loss of a limb. Suggest that clients wear a thin pair of socks to protect feet from abrasions on the pool floor, steps and pool deck. Thin socks will not create excess drag on the legs during WATSU. Remind clients to thoroughly dry and carefully inspect their feet before donning socks and shoes.
- Perforated eardrums. Keep all water out of ears. May require custom earplugs made by an audiologist.
- Severe kidney disease, especially if the client is unable to adjust to fluid loss. Speak with the client's physician.
- Clients with severely impaired ability to regulate body temperature are at risk for over-heating or chilling or both during a session. Adapt the session to the needs of the client. Severe cases may require an alternative treatment modality.
- If the client is on long-term steroids or has had recent deep x-ray therapy, water tends to make already delicate skin even more fragile. Dry skin thoroughly by gently patting dry. Allow skin to dry completely before donning clothes.
- Tracheostomy. Uncapped and capped tracheostomies are extremely high risk for getting pool water into lungs. Head floats exacerbate the risks because they lower the neck more into the water.
- Deep vein thrombosis. Do not proceed until the problem is resolved or cleared for movement in the pool by a physician. People who have been bedridden, recently completed long international flights or have some specific medical conditions are at increased risk for developing

thrombophlebitis. This can be in a superficial vein or a DVT (deep vein thrombosis). There is a risk of the clot breaking free and becoming a pulmonary embolism, which can be life threatening.

- Varicose veins. Be very gentle when working near these veins.
- Impaired sensation, especially in legs, secondary to stroke, brain injury, spinal cord injury, diabetes, and so on. Care must be taken to avoid the client sustaining an abrasion injury on the feet on the bottom or side of the pool or steps. A thin pair of socks can provide extra protection without causing drag during a WATSU session. Underwater lights generate considerable heat, so be careful that clients with impaired sensation do not lean against them.
- Intravenous lines, hep locks, Hickman lines, and so on may be able to come into the pool if adequately protected to keep water out. You will need to cover with gauze and Tegaderm or Opsite for waterproof protection. Check with the client's healthcare provider.
- Acute ligamentous instability (following trauma). Use extreme caution. Depending on the location of the instability, WATSU may be contraindicated unless the area can be stabilized with a splint. Check with the client's healthcare provider.
- Gastrostomies, colostomies, ileostomies, and so on can usually come into the pool if the skin around the stoma is well healed. Drain the bag first. Check the seal around the stoma before entering the pool.
  - Urinary catheters can usually come into the pool. Drain the bag first. Attach the bag to the client's leg. Don't move the leg to a position that would cause urine to flow from the bag back into the bladder. Check with the client's healthcare provider if the client has a suprapubic catheter.
- Autonomic dysreflexia. Anyone with an upper motor neuron injury has the potential to develop autonomic dysreflexia, but it is most common with spinal cord injuries above T6. If it occurs, it can be extremely serious. Discuss with client and physician. (For additional information, refer to the section in this chapter titled "Spinal cord injuries.")
- Avoid pressure or excessive movement of any area where inflammation is involved, such as a sprain, tendinitis or rheumatoid arthritis flare.
- Osteoporosis. Be gentle with stretches and rotations with anyone who may be at risk for osteoporosis. (For additional information, refer to sections in this chapter titled "Elderly clients" and "Osteoporosis.")
- Range of motion precautions. Check with the client and speak to their physician if necessary. (For additional information, refer to the section in this chapter titled "Specific joint range of motion precautions.")

- Epilepsy/seizures, especially if uncontrolled.
  - Discuss type and frequency of the seizures. Many seizures are petit mal, which are generally not difficult to manage if you know what to expect.
  - Grand mal (tonic-clonic) seizures require considerably more precaution and care. Ask questions regarding how well the seizures are managed with medication. How frequent are seizures, and when did the last seizure occur?
  - Inquire whether there is anything that precipitates a seizure for this client, and if the client has an aura or other indication that a seizure is imminent.
  - If flickering lights are a precipitating factor, lights reflecting off the water may increase the probability of seizures for some of these clients. If so, turn off as many lights as possible, especially overhead lights.
  - Only proceed if you are confident you can safely manage a grand mal seizure if it occurs.
  - The most critical and most challenging focus of care is maintaining the client's airway and keeping it completely free of water.
  - You must also be able to keep the client safe while summoning assistance if needed.
  - After a grand mal seizure, clients are tired and may be somewhat confused, agitated and embarrassed. Check for any injuries and provide calm reassurance and compassion. Allow the client to rest. Make sure the client has safe transportation home provided by someone else.
- Cancer and chemotherapy.
  - It is generally recommended to wait four days to two weeks after a chemotherapy treatment, depending on the type and duration of the chemotherapy and the client's response to chemotherapy.
  - For a period of time after chemotherapy (length of time depends on multiple factors), toxins are released in all bodily fluids/solids. This includes the sweat released into the water during sessions.
  - For a period of time after chemotherapy there are also added risks for the client, which may include extreme fatigue, nausea, increased risk of infection, fungal/yeast infections, and digestive problems, especially diarrhea. Allow time for these issues to mostly resolve prior to a session in the pool.
  - WATSU is often the treatment of choice, especially in late-stage cancer when relaxation, pain reduction, improvement in sleep and emotional support become the primary goals.

    – When it is safe for the client to have WATSU sessions, the physical and emotional benefits are immeasurable. It is profoundly touching and an honor to be a support person for people during their cancer journey.

- For additional precautions for babies and children please refer to the section titled "Additional suggestions and precautions for babies and children."

SECTION 2

Additional suggestions and precautions for special medical considerations

The following information is based on professional education, extensive reading of medical research, and thousands of hours giving sessions to people with special needs.

Pregnancy

- Due to the increased risk of miscarriage during the first trimester, many massage therapists choose to not give massages, or they are selective with the areas being massaged during the first trimester. Many WATSU practitioners also choose to not give WATSU sessions during the first trimester. Although there is no evidence to suggest that WATSU sessions during the first trimester increase the likelihood of miscarriages, many practitioners choose to err on the side of caution.
- Encourage women to eat a small meal or a healthy snack containing protein approximately one hour before their session.
- Encourage women to drink more water. As the baby grows and puts increased pressure on abdominal organs, including the bladder, women sometimes begin to decrease their water consumption, so they won't need to urinate as frequently. This causes dehydration, which can cause multiple problems, including increased constipation and increased muscle cramps, including more Braxton Hicks contractions. Dehydration during pregnancy increases oxytocin levels. Brief rises in oxytocin during pregnancy are not a problem, but a prolonged rise in oxytocin can increase contractions and sometimes start premature labor.
- Hormonal changes cause ligamentous laxity as the pregnancy progresses, especially during the third trimester. Be gentle with

movements that might stretch the sacroiliac and symphysis pubis joints. Avoid any strong lumbar extension. Lumbar flexion is greatly appreciated by healthy pregnant women, especially in their third trimester.

- Gentle, prolonged stretches, especially for muscles that tend to shorten (pectorals, lumbar extensors, upper trapezius, etc.), are appreciated by women. Invite chest/thoracic opening and expansion, and lumbar flexion.
- If a pregnant woman experiences any vaginal bleeding, she needs to speak with her healthcare provider before receiving a session.
- If pre-eclampsia develops, it is advisable to avoid WATSU. If the woman wishes to continue Watsu sessions, it's essential to discuss this with her obstetrician first.
- If a woman has lost her mucus plug or her waters have broken, then she can be in a clean bathtub, but not in a pool due to the significant risk of infection.
- Women and the babies they are carrying, including babies in a breech position, benefit from WATSU sessions.
- The flowing, fluid movements of WATSU and the unloading of joints due to buoyancy are a gift for women during the second and third trimesters.
- Giving a WATSU session to a woman (and her fetus), especially during the final trimester of a pregnancy, is an experience to be cherished.
- Please refer to the chapter titled "A Water Journey Through Pregnancy and Parenthood" by Jurgita Svediene for detailed information.

Vestibular hypersensitivity (dizziness, tendency to develop motion sickness)

- A problem for many people, and common following a traumatic brain injury and various conditions such as Meniere's disease.
- Ask clients about their tendency to develop motion sickness.
- Ask clients to say "stillness" during the session whenever they wish to have stillness.
- Schedule a session for a time when the pool is quiet and calm. Dim the lights, if possible, to decrease sensory input.
- Ginger (pills or fresh ginger tea) prior to the session may help.
- Wristbands with small acupressure knobs help some people. They are available at most pharmacies.
- Watch for possible signs and symptoms of motion sickness,

including pale and clammy skin (or suddenly flushed skin), increased swallowing, sudden change in rate of respiration (usually an increase but may also decrease, especially in children who may start to yawn), and so on.

- Some clients prefer to keep their eyes open.
- Use movements that are slow and more linear.
- Avoid rotational movements that cause the head to turn/roll from side to side. Avoid turning and spiraling movements.
- Movements, including rotation of the body, may be well tolerated if the head and neck are maintained in good alignment and not being rolled from side to side or bounced due to movement or turbulence.
- Change positions extremely slowly, especially during multiplanar movements (standing to starting position in supine, supine to open saddle, etc.).
- Use of appropriate Shiatsu points may help. Speak with a Shiatsu practitioner for suggestions.
- Joint approximation techniques during and following WATSU may help. A physical therapist or occupational therapist can give suggestions.
- For extreme cases in children or adults:
  - Decrease all types of sensory input (dim all lights, no noise, no music, no echo, no light reflecting on pool water, no itchy or uncomfortable clothes, not too hot, not too cold, etc.).
  - Choose a time with no one else in the pool.
  - Practitioner: calm, limited talking, slow talking, no moving hands when talking, stay within same focal distance from client.
  - Start with sitting on step in very shallow water with feet flat on lower step.
  - Just watching the movement of the pool water may be challenging for some people.
  - Moving from standing to a supine position may aggravate symptoms. Initially, may need to start with the client in a more upright position (make sure the head is supported) and do more soft tissue work and less movement. Upright positions to consider include side saddle, open saddle and upright with the client's head, neck and back supported by your chest (client in a sitting position facing away from you).
  - Transition extremely slowly from vertical to horizontal and from horizontal to vertical.
  - Move "slower than grass growing."
  - Be calm and without tension in your own body.

- When supine is tolerated, begin with a very short session.
- Water Breath Dance is usually enough for the first time supine.
- Call the client the next day to ascertain how well they did for the remainder of the day and the following day.
- A brushing and joint approximation program (Wilbarger Protocol) prior to the WATSU session may help. Discuss this with an occupational or physical therapist with specialized sensory integration training.
- For additional suggestions, refer to "Sensitivity to sensory stimuli (sensory defensiveness)" in the babies and children section.

Post mastectomy

- Wait until the client has been cleared for the pool and movement by a physician. Check if there are contraindicated movements or a range of motion limitations for the client.
- Start by standing on the client's non-surgical side.
- Encourage a gentle range of motion of the shoulders.
- Encourage trunk rotation and gentle extension of the thoracic spine.
- Gently invite the lengthening of the pectoral and axillary (armpit) muscles within the ranges recommended by the surgeon.
- Avoid soft tissue mobilization in the area of surgery unless approved by a surgeon.
- If lymph nodes have been removed, protect from anything that might interfere with lymph drainage and therefore cause lymphedema.
  - Avoid any constricting grasp.
  - Avoid under arm pressure in armpit.
  - Avoid over stretching tissues.
  - Protect arm from infection.
- If the client has had reconstructive surgery, follow the surgeon's protocol for movement and gentle stretching.

Respiratory conditions, including COPD (chronic obstructive pulmonary disease)

- If the client's vital capacity is less than 1000ml, be cautious. Check with the client's physician. Immersion in water causes approximately a 10 percent decrease in vital capacity.
- Watch during your session for any sign of shortness of breath, increased heart rate, adverse changes in skin color, or any other sign of distress.

- Ask the client to report any dizziness or light-headedness.
- Be aware of the risk of respiratory infection. Do not work with the client on days when either of you have any signs of illness.
- Be extra careful to ensure that water doesn't go into the mouth or nose of the client.
- Stay with your client after the session until they are out of the pool, and you are completely sure the client is not experiencing any ill effects.
- Choose movements that encourage fuller inhalation, which will bring air down into the lower lobes of the lungs.
- Choose movements that encourage fuller exhalation. Most clients with COPD have difficulty completing a full exhale to release air out of their lungs, so improvements in exhalation are beneficial.
- Encourage movements that gently mobilize the ribs and thoracic spine.
- If the client is using oxygen:
    - Place a portable oxygen tank on side of pool.
    - Use extra-long respiratory tubing during session.
    - Make tubing more visible for you and for everyone else in the pool. One option is to cut slits in small colored foam rubber balls. Then place the balls onto the tubing for flotation and visibility.
- After the session, encourage clients to gently exercise or at least walk in the pool before exiting. Exercise is crucial for people with COPD. Exercise in water is especially beneficial, because the hydrostatic pressure of the water gives gentle resistance to inhalation and assists exhalation. If the client is using oxygen, they need to continue to use oxygen while walking/exercising.

Fibromyalgia

- Fibromyalgia affects 2–6 percent of people throughout the world, across all ages, races and genders. The World Health Organization lists fibromyalgia syndrome (often referred to as FMS, or sometimes FM) as the number one cause of chronic, widespread musculoskeletal pain.
- Ninety-five percent of people with FMS experience:
    - persistent widespread pain
    - non-restorative sleep with decreased delta wave sleep cycles.
- Additional problems frequently include:
    - incapacitating fatigue
    - irritable bowel syndrome
    - irritable bladder syndrome

- low exercise tolerance
- anxiety, depression
- headaches
- challenges with memory and concentration, often referred to as "fibro fog."

- The client's autonomic nervous system is often unbalanced with high activation of the sympathetic nervous system for much of the time. A large percentage of clients with FMS have a history of significant trauma. They may alternate between times of high sympathetic nervous system activation and times of parasympathetic collapse and freeze.
- Clients with FMS often seek WATSU for relief of symptoms.
- During initial intake, ask clients what their goals are. If they say, "Get rid of the pain," ask, "If you hurt less, what would you be doing that you are not doing now?" This helps the practitioner and the client to understand and focus on what is most important for improving the quality of the client's life.
- FMS symptoms can be lessened or managed with:
  - healthy psychosocial and mental health support, usually including a mental health professional
  - mindfulness, meditation, Ai Chi, Tai Chi or related techniques
  - healthy restorative sleep with delta wave cycles
  - good pacing skills for daily activities
  - healthy nutrition tailored to the needs of the client
  - healthy body mechanics and ergonomics
  - consistent exercise started extremely gently and progressed very gradually
  - cardiovascular exercise.
- Pacing is essential throughout daily life. Acknowledge that it can feel frustrating at times, but good pacing skills will ultimately enable clients with FMS to accomplish more in their lives.
- Simple example of pacing skills: When you go grocery shopping, make sure all the products that require refrigeration are packed together. Ask someone to carry groceries to your car and to position them in your car so they can be easily removed, with cold items most accessible. When you arrive home, first remove all the cold items and put them away. Then rest for a few minutes. Later, you can bring the remainder of the groceries inside. Rest again for a few minutes. Then put away the remainder of the groceries.
- The goal with pacing is to have frequent, brief rests to prevent over-doing. Over-doing causes increases in pain and fatigue. Frequent brief

rests are usually more beneficial than occasional long rests. Lying down provides more beneficial rest than sitting.

- People with fibromyalgia may have to reduce their activity level to such a low level that they feel they are doing nothing, and this can have a negative impact on their self-esteem. Encourage them by helping them understand they are making gains when they are being as consistent as they can be, even if their activity level is low. Consistency is more important than quantity.
- Clients benefit from Ai Chi as part of their gentle exercises in water.
- Encourage clients to initiate a daily "movement routine," which may include some walking and some very gentle exercises. Encourage clients to commit to a daily program that is significantly *less* than what they think they can accomplish. Again, consistency is more important than quantity.
- As practitioners, we want our clients with FMS to be able to enjoy life more. Our sessions may contribute to their success, yet ultimately, we want our clients to feel empowered by knowing their progress and success are the result of *their* efforts.
- WATSU can be helpful for decreasing pain and improving the amount and quality of sleep. By helping to decrease FMS's most debilitating symptoms, our clients are then more able to begin making necessary lifestyle changes.
- Clients with FMS generally respond well to WATSU. Be very gentle with all stretching and soft tissue work. Ask the client to tap the surface of the water if any movement, position or pressure feels "not quite right for you."
- Periodically, especially in the first one or two sessions, raise the client's head slightly and ask if there has been any change in *symptoms*. Asking about symptoms gives a broader perspective and feedback than inquiring about pain. It also helps direct the client's perspective to a bigger picture, instead of just pain.
- It is often better for clients to only receive a 20-minute WATSU session the first time. Remember, a little too little is better than a little too much. This is especially true for clients with FMS when they are pacing their life activities, including receiving WATSU sessions.
- Do a little slow relaxed walking in the pool before and after each session. Walking backward in water is usually less effortful and more relaxing than walking forward.
- Everything needs to be gentle. Slow down your WATSU. Then slow it down more. Also, keep your arms and hands relaxed and without

tension. People with fibromyalgia are exquisitely sensitive to touch, pressure and stretching. Have clarity with your touch, yet be cautious, and avoid firm or deep pressure or strong stretches.

- Let clients know that *any* movement in water (including slow walking) causes our muscles to work against the resistance of the water, so we get stronger. Because water is constantly moving, we continually need to make adjustments when we walk, and this improves strength, balance and core stability.
- Even when people with fibromyalgia progress to cardiovascular conditioning, they need to begin at 50 percent of their maximum heart rate (maximum heart rate is 220 minus their age). If they continue to be consistent with their exercise/activity program, they can very gradually begin to increase their heart rate during daily activities and exercise.
- People need to be actively involved in their health program. We want to empower them by knowing their progress and success are the result of their own efforts, not the practitioner's.
- WATSU is helpful for clients with FMS. However, WATSU is only part of a larger program, which may include mindfulness (or other body mind practice), pacing, healthy ergonomics and body mechanics, consistent gentle exercise/movement, healthy restorative sleep, healthy diet, and appropriate psychosocial and mental health support.
- We cannot cure FMS, but we can contribute to improving quality of life.

Chronic fatigue syndrome

- Chronic fatigue syndrome (CFS) is a debilitating disorder characterized by:
  - extreme fatigue that lasts for at least six months
  - fatigue that can't be explained by an underlying medical condition
  - fatigue (sometimes extreme exhaustion) that worsens with physical and mental activity
  - fatigue that does not improve with rest
  - unrefreshing sleep
  - challenges with memory and concentration
  - symptoms that vary widely and unpredictably from day to day, and even hour to hour.
- Additional symptoms may include:
  - unexplained muscle and joint pain

- headaches
- enlarged lymph nodes in neck or armpits
- unexplained muscle or joint pain
- unexplained numbness or tingling
- dizziness (sometimes caused by postural hypotension) that worsens with moving from lying down or sitting to standing.
- There is considerable overlap of symptoms among people with fibromyalgia and people with chronic fatigue syndrome. WATSU practitioners working with clients who have CFS will find the approach used for fibromyalgia similarly beneficial for clients with CFS.
- As with fibromyalgia, our goal is to support quality of life.

Lyme disease

- Lyme disease is the most common disease spread by ticks in the Northern Hemisphere, especially in the United States. It is estimated to affect 300,000 people a year in the USA and 65,000 people a year in Europe. Infections are most common in the spring and early summer when ticks are most active. Lyme disease was diagnosed as a separate condition for the first time in 1975 in Lyme, Connecticut. It is currently found in more than 80 countries worldwide.
- Lyme disease can often be successfully treated if treatment is initiated early enough. Unfortunately, the vast majority of people don't know they've been infected until many months or even longer after being infected. This can result in chronic Lyme disease.
- Chronic Lyme disease may include:
  - fatigue that is not relieved by rest
  - arthritis (Lyme arthritis) with joint pain and swelling, particularly in the knees and other large joints
  - severe headaches and neck stiffness
  - muscle aches
  - sleep impairment with non-refreshing sleep
  - neurological symptoms (fascial palsy, nerve pain, numbness, hot/cold sensations, shooting pains, numbness or tingling, especially in hands and feet)
  - cognitive challenges, especially impaired memory and "brain fog"
  - psychological symptoms, including depression, anxiety, mood swings
  - gastrointestinal symptoms
  - cardiac rhythm irregularities (Lyme carditis)

- episodes of dizziness or shortness of breath
- inflammation of the brain and spinal cord.
- There is considerable overlap of symptoms among people with Lyme disease, fibromyalgia and chronic fatigue syndrome. WATSU practitioners working with clients who have chronic Lyme disease will find the approach used for fibromyalgia will be similarly beneficial for these clients. However, extra care and caution will be needed if the client has Lyme arthritis (refer to the section titled "Rheumatoid arthritis") or other more serious symptoms, including severe headaches, Lyme carditis and inflammation of the brain and/or spinal cord.
- As with fibromyalgia and chronic fatigue syndrome, our goal with Lyme disease is to help improve quality of life.

Chronic regional pain syndrome (previously known as reflex sympathetic dystrophy)

- Complex regional pain syndrome (CRPS) is excessive and prolonged pain and inflammation that follows an injury to an arm or leg. The pain experienced, even with gentle touch, is much greater than normal.
- Multiple additional symptoms include changes in skin color, temperature and texture of skin, plus changes in bone and nail growth and swelling of the arm or leg distal to the site of injury. Skin on the affected limb may change color, becoming blotchy, blue, purple, gray, pale or red.
- CRPS is typically caused by dysfunction of the peripheral C-nerve fibers that carry pain messages to the brain. Their excess firing also triggers inflammation. Skin symptoms fluctuate because the opening and closing of the small blood vessels under the skin are controlled by the C-nerve fibers that are injured in CRPS.
- It's essential to keep the painful limb or body part moving to improve blood flow, lessen circulatory symptoms and maintain flexibility, strength and function.
- WATSU can be beneficial for CRPS. The neutral warmth and hydrostatic pressure of the water are both calming and pain reducing.
- The affected limb is frequently exquisitely painful. Touch below the knee or elbow of the affected limb may not be tolerated. Move the client slowly in the water to limit the amount of turbulent flow on the extremity. Addressing needs, especially muscle tension, in other parts of the body can have a calming and balancing effect on the autonomic nervous system.

- Walking and gentle movements of the extremities in the water at the end of the session are beneficial.

Elderly clients

- Elderly clients, especially those who live in nursing homes, sometimes are only touched and moved for cleaning and feeding. They are deeply affected by WATSU. Most have such a yearning to be held and loved that they become tearful during WATSU sessions, even if they are confused. It is a deep joy to give them sessions.
- Engage their humor and be respectful.
- Balance may be impaired due to weakness, lack of exercise and decreased proprioception that naturally occurs as we age. Allow plenty of time at the end of the session for the client to reorient and walk around before exiting the pool. Provide guarding for safety, and assistance if needed, when getting in and out of the pool and possibly in the locker room.
- Clients are often more sensitive to temperature changes, so protect them from over-heating and from chilling.
- Many have vision challenges. Have a safe container for glasses on the side of the pool, so you can return them to the client as soon as needed after the session.
- Many have hearing challenges. Avoid speaking loudly to clients. This usually creates more echo in the pool area and makes hearing more difficult. It is more effective and respectful to speak more slowly and enunciate words more clearly and separately. Allow more pauses for your words to be processed. If the client uses hearing aids, these must be removed and left in a safe place with the client's belongings. They are expensive and easy to lose, so be certain the client has them before leaving your facility.
- Many elderly clients have comorbidities. For additional health considerations, refer to the section "General precautions for aquatic bodywork" from earlier in the chapter.
  - Renal (kidney) responses occur faster and are more intense in the elderly. The increase in urine output is more likely to lead to dehydration. Additionally, many elderly clients don't drink water regularly during the day, especially those who worry about urinary incontinence. Have water at the poolside and recommend the client drinks a full cup of water before exiting the pool. Explain to clients that immersion in water causes an increase in urine production, so it is important to drink water following a session.

- May have cardiovascular disease. If in doubt, check with the client's healthcare provider.
- May have diabetes. Refer to the section in this chapter titled "Precautions for aquatic bodywork."
- May wear hearing aids, and these must be removed before coming into the pool.
- May be osteoporotic, especially females, but also those who have been inactive for a long period of time. Refer to the section on "Osteoporosis."
- Likely to have osteoarthritis. Refer to the section on "Osteoarthritis."
- May have dementia. Refer to the section on "Alzheimer's disease/dementia."
- Respiratory vital capacity will probably be decreased. Watch for any signs of respiratory distress. If the client has any lung disease such as COPD (chronic obstructive pulmonary disease), refer to the section on "Respiratory conditions."

Inappropriate behavior (physical, verbal, sexual)

- On very rare occasions, clients exhibit inappropriate physical, verbal or sexual behavior by touching or speaking in ways that are unacceptable for the practitioner. This may occur for various reasons, including:
  - a misunderstanding of expectations for the session, especially in a private setting. Many practitioners working alone in private settings include a clarifying statement on their intake form
  - a desire for intimacy with the practitioner
  - neurological conditions. Clients with a variety of neurological challenges, particularly those with traumatic brain injuries, may act impulsively and without a behavioral filter. Redirect these clients with neutrality and clarity, without anger. Redirection may need to be repeated several times with firmness, but without anger. Additionally, choose positions and movements that are less intimate. If necessary, choose a different treatment modality.
- The practitioner needs to be clear about their own boundaries and redirect the client.
- A simple change in positioning during a session is usually adequate.
- If a more direct approach is needed, start by owning your own feelings rather than blaming the client. "I am noticing your hand is…"

"I am not comfortable with..." "It would be better for me if..." "Are you willing to comply with...?" "Do you agree to receive without...?"

- If the client is unable or unwilling to change their behavior, either for neurological or other reasons, or you continue to feel uncomfortable, choose the option below that is best for you:
  - Select a different therapeutic modality with less physical contact.
  - Refer to another practitioner after explaining the situation to the practitioner.
  - End the session. Calmly state that the client's behavior is unacceptable for you and ask the client to leave.
  - These are clear decisions that are respectful of your own boundaries and will yield better outcomes rather than an angry outburst directed at the client.

Psychological support in conjunction with WATSU

- Frequently sessions evoke old sorrows, injuries and psychological wounds, sometimes very strongly with tears, laughter and movement. As practitioners, we are there to hold the space with calm, unconditional acceptance and without intervening, giving advice, "mothering" or rescuing.
- However, working with significant psychological challenges, such as multiple personalities, requires compassion and strong boundaries. Additional professional training is strongly recommended. It is also recommended to work closely with the client's mental health provider. (For detailed information regarding psychological support please refer to the chapters by Karen David and Mary Seamster.)
- Some clients are very apprehensive due to pain, fear of the water, difficulty trusting others, past abuse or other severe trauma. Go slowly. Seek outside professional guidance for clients and for yourself.
- WATSU can be a beneficial adjunct to psychotherapy. It is advantageous to work with the client's mental health provider (with the client's *written and signed permission*). For most clients, it is helpful to schedule WATSU prior to the client's psychotherapy sessions, either the same day or the day before.
- Allow enough time at the end of the session for the client to talk (or not talk), and for you to listen and be fully present. Your supportive, unconditional acceptance will benefit your clients enormously.
- When clients cry during a session, hold the space for the tears to flow. We are there to unconditionally accept, listen and be present. Wanting/ needing to "comfort" or hug the client is unhelpful and generally not

healthy for either the client or the practitioner. Stay well grounded and calmly "hold the space" for the client with acceptance and deep compassion for whatever the client is feeling and experiencing.

- Stay within your scope of practice. Do not offer advice or counseling unless you are a qualified healthcare professional, and the client has specifically come to you for psychotherapy.
- Encourage all clients to tap the water to let you know immediately if any movement or position is uncomfortable or unwelcomed in any way.
- Ask the client to say "stop" if needed at any time for any reason, and the WATSU session will immediately stop. Let clients know it is their session and their choice to stop if they choose to.
- Discover and utilize positions of physical and psychological comfort for your client even if it means being positioned on a head float so there is less physical contact with the practitioner.
- Many of the clients who come to us have suffered severe traumas. Many suffer from PTSD. Here are some additional suggestions:
  - Progress slowly. Get to know the client. Listen with an open and compassionate heart, without judgment, advice or counseling. The first session may not progress to WATSU.
  - Keep sessions simple and safe. The client needs to feel safe.
  - Follow the client's movements, including subtle movements. Watch for patterns of movement that may emerge. When there is movement, ask yourself, "Is this my client's movement or mine?" "Is this the client's rhythm or mine?" Follow the client's movements and rhythms without imposing your own.
  - Guided imagery can be helpful for some clients. Find something that gives your client a sense of peace and safety. This will probably be a place (mountains, seashore, favorite chair, etc.). Involve the client's senses in imagining this place. ("What sounds do you hear?" "What do you smell?" "How does the sunshine feel on your skin?") Use this safe place as a starting point for your WATSU and as a place to return to when needed.
  - It can also be helpful for some clients to begin by identifying a part of their body that feels comfortable and safe. This may be an arm, a leg or just a part of one finger. Ask your client to focus on this safe body part. How does it feel in this portion of themselves that is safe and comfortable? Invite your client to allow this feeling to slowly spread out to include larger portions of their body. Come back to the place of comfort if your client begins to feel

overwhelmed. Do not push to continue. It's always better to do less than to do too much.

– Clients' bodies may twitch and jerk as they discharge energy that may be related to past traumas. Simply allow this to happen. If the movements increase and become very irregular, this may signal that the client is going too far into the past trauma. You may need to return the client to the wall and utilize techniques for safely grounding and returning to the present.

– Safe grounding. It is often helpful to gently turn clients toward the wall. Let the client know what you are doing. Position the client facing the wall with the client's hands on the wall and feet on the pool floor. The practitioner can then place the palm of their hand gently on the client's lower lumbar spine—ask for the client's permission first. The practitioner can then press gently down through the lumbar spine to direct pressure down through the client's sacrum, legs and feet to assist grounding and returning to the present. Continue to monitor the client's color, respiration and other signs of their emotional and physical state. Gently bring the client's awareness to their breathing, and, when appropriate, join with the client's breath and gradually invite deeper, calmer breaths. When inviting a client to orient to the here and now, it may be helpful to ask them to look around and identify things that are green, or some other color. This can help the client differentiate between "then" and "now." Ask permission before any touch.

• Encouraging clients to reach a big "emotional release" can be detrimental. There is a significant risk of further traumatizing the client.

Additional suggestions and precautions for orthopedic conditions

The following information is based on professional education, extensive reading of medical research, and thousands of hours giving sessions to people with special needs.

Arthritis

There are over 100 different types of arthritis. Here are suggestions for three of the more common forms of arthritis. Ankylosing spondylitis is also included because WATSU is exceptionally beneficial for this form of arthritis.

Osteoarthritis

- A localized degenerative condition that is the result of increased wear and tear on particular joints. Though it may produce some inflammatory symptoms, it is not considered an inflammatory disease. It primarily destroys joint cartilage over time.
- Can occur in any joints, though most commonly in weight-bearing joints, especially hips and knees and the small joints of the fingers and thumbs.
- Stretching is essential for maintaining mobility, and mobility is essential for function. Stretch slowly. Allow time for muscles and soft tissue to relax.
- This population generally tends to be older, so be aware of other possible risk factors, including osteoporosis and various cardiac conditions.

Rheumatoid arthritis

- A systemic and complex autoimmune disease that affects the entire body causing fatigue, fever, weight loss, malaise and loss of appetite.
- Affects joints all over the body, including hands, fingers, elbows, knees and hips, and can lead to severe joint damage.
- Other conditions may develop, including respiratory diseases, cardiovascular diseases, lymphoma and lupus.
- People need plenty of restorative sleep, good nutrition, some exercise and appropriate medication.
- Strive to maintain mobility but protect joints which are currently inflamed. If a joint is significantly inflamed, encourage movement at other joints and avoid movement of the inflamed joint. May need to use a splint to support an inflamed joint during WATSU.

Systemic lupus erythematosus—the most common form of lupus

- An autoimmune disease that can cause inflammation and pain in any part of the body.
- Lupus affects joints, but also skin and internal organs, including kidneys and heart. It's essential to know what regions and organs are affected.
- May additionally have blood disorders, including anemia, low levels of white blood cells or low platelets.

- Very sensitive to ultraviolet light and sometimes indoor lighting, too. LED lights are better.
- May have Raynaud's phenomenon and be very sensitive to cold, especially in the hands and feet.
- Clients with lupus respond well to gentle WATSU sessions to maintain mobility and decrease pain.
- Discuss chemicals used in the pool with the client before the session to assess the safety of using this pool for a session.

Ankylosing spondylitis

- An inflammatory disease that is more common in men. Some joints, especially in the spine, may gradually fuse (ankylose). Pain and inflammation may occur in multiple areas of the body.
- A primary risk is fusing of joints, especially in the spine. The tendency for clients is to gradually adopt a flexed posture. This can eventually affect breathing and daily life activities if the joints fuse in this position.
- Treatment is most successful before the disease causes irreversible damage to joints.
- Goals are to relieve pain and stiffness and prevent or delay complications and spinal deformity.
- Focus of care is on pain relief plus improved strength and flexibility. Extension movements are important, especially for the thoracic spine. Hips and shoulders also benefit from stretching.
- Maintaining optimal sleeping and walking positions and doing abdominal and back exercises are essential for maintaining an upright posture.

Osteoporosis

- Use extra care, especially with spinal movements.
- Use slower, more gentle movements.
- Avoid strong movements and stretches at the end of range of motion, especially with spinal rotation.
- Avoid movements that might cause spinal compression.
- Keep movements smooth. Quick movements may cause sudden loading of joints and bones.
- Be aware that other joints, especially hips and wrists, may also be osteoporotic in addition to the spine.
- WATSU is helpful in decreasing the stiffness, muscle spasm and pain that often accompany osteoporosis.

- WATSU is most helpful for maintaining mobility, especially in the spine. This will result in less pain and better function in life, including better depth of respiration.
- Include walking and gentle exercise in the water following the WATSU portion of the session.

Specific joint range of motion precautions

- Total hip replacement—posterior surgical approach: Typical movement restrictions include no internal rotation or adduction past neutral and no flexion past 90° to reduce the risk of dislocation. Movement restrictions are for approximately eight weeks. WATSU is usually contraindicated during this time due to the risk of dislocation. Check with the surgeon.
- Total hip replacement—anterior surgical approach: Usually few movement restrictions. Check with the surgeon.
- Post laminectomy, spinal fusion and other spinal surgeries: Check with the surgeon regarding specific movement restrictions.
- Spinal stenosis: Most clients do better with spinal flexion, worse with extension. Be aware that spinal stenosis is more common in elderly clients who may also have osteoporosis.
- Bulging or herniated spinal disc: Most clients whose symptoms are truly from a disc gain more relief from extension than flexion. For these clients, work more in neutral or mildly extended positions for that area of the spine and avoid flexion.
- Recent bone fracture: Protect fracture site from further injury. Depending on the site and severity of the fracture, WATSU may be contraindicated. A cast guard (cast protector) can often be used to protect a cast on a limb. The casted extremity will sink or float more than the other side depending on the weight of the cast and the amount of air held inside the cast guard.

Amputation

- An amputation will influence a receiver's position in the water. Most receivers will tend to roll away from the side of the amputation. If the client's intact limb is very buoyant, then the client may tend to roll toward the side of the amputation.
- In the legs, especially with an above-knee amputation, it will help to put a float on the intact leg to prevent excessive rolling toward that leg.

- Check the range of motion of the residual limb. Above-knee amputees frequently develop contractures in the hip flexors, so stretch hip flexors during the session.
- Ask the receiver about sensation, numbness, pain and phantom limb pain in the residual limb.
- Remind the receiver to dry the end of the residual limb thoroughly after WATSU. Prolonged exposure to warm water makes skin more fragile and susceptible to breakdown. If possible, leave the prosthesis off for 20 minutes after the session to allow water to completely evaporate from the skin.

Pain

- We don't always know, and clients may not disclose or even know if there is a history of trauma. If the client shows signs of a release, neutrally follow and support the client without the need to "make" something happen. Allow the movements to be the client's movements, not the practitioner's. If needed, return the client to the wall with feet on the floor. Breathe. Guide the client to "ground" and gently return to the present. For additional suggestions, refer to the section on "Psychological support."
- If possible, know the cause of the pain. Be certain you have the necessary knowledge to work with this client without exacerbating their condition. Seek further medical advice if necessary.
- Know if there are any specific precautions. If in doubt, consider not doing WATSU at this time.
- Prior to WATSU, find out which positions/movements relieve symptoms (flexion, extension, rotation) and which positions/movements aggravate symptoms.
- Ask your client questions. People can tell us a great deal about their own bodies if we ask the right questions and listen carefully.
  - Progress slowly. Get to know the client. Listen with an open and compassionate heart, without judgment or counseling. The first session may not progress to WATSU.
  - "Where is your pain?" Ask them to show you on their body. If the client reports pain with movement in a joint, do some testing. Is the pain only during active movements by the client, or do passive movements also cause pain? Ask to hold the client's extremity, and then ask the client to let go (relax) and let you hold the arm/leg. Support the extremity and slowly move the joint that is painful. If there is pain, remember what specific range in movement

elicited pain. During the session, avoid letting water passively move the extremity into the painful range of passive movement.

- "What movements or positions increase your symptoms? What movements or positions decrease your symptoms?" The answers to these questions will guide you in the type of movements you use during the session. Many clients have difficulty answering these questions, so ask them about their symptoms during specific daily activities. The client's answers can guide you toward or away from specific movements.
- Examples:
  » If a client says sitting increases/decreases their symptoms, then bring your awareness to movements which cause spinal loading or flexion.
  » Pain in standing suggests lumbar extension and weight bearing.
  » Pain with walking suggests weight bearing, spinal rotation, lumbar extension, cervical extension.
  » Tying shoes (spinal flexion and hip flexion with rotation).
  » Arching backwards (lumbar extension).
  » Stomach sleeping (lumbar extension, cervical rotation).
  » Sleeping/resting on the back with a pillow under the knees (lumbar flexion).
  » "Is there anything else you can think of that changes your symptoms in any way?" Positions? Activities? Work? Stress?
  » "Is there anything else you would like to share with me about yourself or your needs?"

- Begin the session with movements that decrease symptoms or at least don't increase symptoms.
- During the early portion of the session, focus the movements and bodywork on non-painful areas of the body. As the client's body relaxes, you can then begin to gently address painful areas.
- If pain is related to muscle tension, sensitively applied pressure can be very beneficial.
- As the session develops, you can gently invite other movements. If you sense any reluctance within the body to accept the invitation, return to safer movements.
- Gently follow the client's movements. Keep asking yourself, "Am I following my client's movements and rhythms, or my own?" Follow the client's movement and rhythm.
- Give extra attention to the alignment of the client's body throughout the session, especially the client's head and neck.

- If the client is very slow and guarded when moving their own head and neck before getting into the pool, keep the client's head low and calm in the water with gentle opening/lengthening for the neck provided by the subtle opening of your chest and arms.
- Move slowly! It is better to do too little than too much.
- It can be helpful to check in with the client from time to time, especially early in the session, to assess whether what you are doing is changing the client's symptoms in any way. Inquire about "symptoms" vs. "pain." This will give you more complete feedback, and it will also broaden the focus to multiple changes within the body.
- Appropriate use of flotation devices (noodles, soft head floats) can be useful for some clients. Be certain the client's body, especially the neck, is in good alignment and is well cared for.
- Ask for feedback if any position, movement or hand/finger pressure increases symptoms. Again, using the word "symptoms" will yield more complete information than the word "pain," and will also help to shift the primary focus from pain to the "bigger picture" of overall function.
- Incorporate your other bodywork knowledge and skills into your WATSU session. Nearly all types of therapeutic bodywork can be modified, adapted and utilized during WATSU.

Muscle tension and holding patterns in necks

Tension in the neck is common in the modern world for a variety of reasons—long hours sitting at computers, long hours driving, daily life tension, pain, stress, anxiety, poor postural habits, worries and past traumas, the list is long. For tension in the neck without significant pathology, there are many ways to invite clients to relax. Here are a few suggestions:

- We protect our heads and necks most of all. Give your client's head precise attention, care and respect. Give the head exquisite care from the very start of the session, and the client will trust you and be more likely to relax their neck.
- Keep the head low in the water to allow buoyancy to help support the weight of the head. The lighter the head feels for the client, the safer it will feel, and they will be more likely to relax. Keeping the head low in the water also makes the head lighter on the practitioner's arm, so the practitioner can relax their arm more.
- Allow your own body to relax and let go of holding patterns. The more we relax, the more our clients will relax and let go.

- Use all the therapeutic skills you use on land for alleviating tension in the neck. Almost every skill can be adapted to the water.
- The neck is one of the most common places for bodies to unwind to help release tension and past experiences. When you feel subtle movement in the head and neck (or anywhere in the body), follow these movements and allow them to release.
- Head thrust:
  - Some clients hold their head forward but tipped backward with a tremendous amount of tension. Providing some traction and soft tissue techniques for the neck can help some of these clients. Some necks, however, do not release with traction or soft tissue techniques. For these clients, the technique below can often quickly invite the neck to release safely and comfortably. This gives relief from pain and tension for the client.
  - Continue to support the head on your elbow or your hand if you are positioned at the client's head. Keep the head comfortably low in the water. Continue to provide length for the neck. Place your foot-hand on the client's sternum, avoiding any contact with the throat. Give gentle, sustained, steady pressure posterior on the sternum combined with a gentle inferior pull (press on the sternum and pull gently toward the client's feet). This technique is gentle and often remarkably effective for releasing pain and tension. The receiver's neck and body often spontaneously release and unwind.
  - For more details about this technique, refer to the "Spasticity" section of this chapter.

Additional suggestions and precautions for neurological conditions

The following information is based on professional education, extensive reading of medical research, and thousands of hours giving sessions to people with special needs.

There is a vast array of neurological conditions. Some of the most prevalent include stroke (cerebral vascular accident—CVA), traumatic brain injury, cerebral palsy, spinal cord injury, multiple sclerosis, Parkinson's disease and Alzheimer's disease. Although it is generally safe to bring people with these conditions into the pool, there are sometimes medical reasons why immersion in water would not be safe. Think carefully before bringing a client into the pool and discuss concerns with the client's healthcare provider.

WATSU can be enormously beneficial for most clients with these conditions. It is especially helpful for decreasing various neurological challenges in muscle tone (spasticity, rigidity, athetosis, chorea, etc.) to improve overall mobility and quality of life.

Most clients tolerate WATSU quite well if their overall health is good. The primary risk with WATSU for clients with more severe neurological challenges is aspirating water. If you keep the nose and mouth out of the water, most clients will tolerate being in the water and benefit from receiving WATSU.

Many clients who are more severely affected are cleaned and fed by caregivers, but they rarely have the opportunity to be tenderly held for an extended time. Your genuine caring and unconditional acceptance will profoundly touch their hearts and improve their well-being.

Clients with spasticity

- Spasticity is a common challenge for people with a wide range of conditions, including traumatic brain injuries, strokes (CVA), spinal cord injuries, multiple sclerosis and cerebral palsy. Although there are multiple neurological challenges in muscle tone, spasticity is the most common. For information about rigidity please refer to the section titled "Parkinson's disease."
- Plan ahead for how you are going to get the client safely in and out of the pool. Will the client need assistance showering, dressing, walking or toileting?
- Keep your client warm before and after the session. Be sure to have towels ready to wrap around the client immediately as they exit the pool. If you frequently work with clients with significant spasticity, consider having a heap lamp on a timer above the changing area. Be certain it is out of reach from clients.
- Start with the client leaning against the wall or sitting down if his/her balance or mobility are impaired. Clients who enter the pool via a lift or hoist will likely already be in a sitting position.
- If the client enters via a lift, put any needed flotation straps on the client before he/she enters the pool. You will need both of your arms available to assist the client when he/she enters the water.
- Positioning leg floats above the knees will be beneficial for clients with spasticity. Floats positioned below the knees tend to limit movement at the knees and increase spasticity, especially in the legs.
- Begin the session next to the client's healthier side. Start with your foot-arm under the client's knees instead of under the pelvis.
- The following are suggestions based on sessions with more than one thousand clients with spasticity. Each person is unique. There are no recipes. Use the following information to guide and inform what you

do, but always listen to and observe the subtle changes and responses of the body in your arms.

- Focus first on spinal movements. Emphasize rotation of the trunk. Rotation of the spine helps decrease spasticity and improve mobility. Rotation movements for people with stronger spasticity will need to be stronger and more sustained. Typical WATSU rotational moves tend to cause "log rolling" instead of spinal rotation.
- Spinal rotation combined with elongation for the trunk is also helpful.
- Some extension of the thoracic spine (with lumbar spine maintained in flexion) can be beneficial, especially for breathing and sitting posture.
- Gradually progress to the extremities:
  » Begin with the proximal joints and then progress to the more distal joints.
  » If you are working on the upper extremity, start first with the trunk, then the scapula, then the shoulder, then the elbow, wrist and finally the hand and fingers.
  » Use a similar progression with the legs (hip, knee, ankle, foot, toes).
  » Open each joint in the opposite direction to its holding pattern of spasticity. Example: Arms are often in a position of shoulder internal rotation and adduction, elbow flexion, forearm pronation, wrist flexion and finger flexion. Therefore, externally rotate the shoulder, then add elbow extension, next add supination, then wrist extension and then open the fingers. Avoid pressing directly on the palm of the hand because that may stimulate a palmar grasp reflex.
  » Use firm, steady pressure to slowly open the client's joints. For some clients, you will need to use strength while maintaining your own alignment.
  » Use the strength and power of your body with good alignment and without tension in your body. The less tension there is in the practitioner's body, the less tension and spasticity the client will have in their body.
- As the session progresses and muscle tone begins to soften somewhat, you may be able to use your soft tissue skills for additional improvements in mobility in areas where soft tissue has shortened as a result of the holding patterns of spasticity.
- During the session, include weight bearing through the legs and

also the hands and arms as this helps to decrease spasticity and improve function.

- Consider including time at the end of the session for practicing walking and other functional skills according to the abilities of the client. Water is a safe place to practice the skills that are difficult to do on land.

- Practicing functional skills is more challenging for the practitioner when working with clients with strong spasticity or more cognitive challenges.

  » You may need to use your legs to give stability to your client's legs, and you may need to do so one leg at a time.

  » Weight bearing through the upper extremities can be onto a bench or chair placed in the pool.

  » If the client is unable to follow directions, you may need to position the client for weight bearing. Stabilize the client's shoulder and elbow. Position the client's hand on a bench, chair or (more often) your thigh. Then shift the client's weight over their hand for weight bearing.

- Head thrust:

  » This backward head thrust is the Moro startle reflex seen in typical babies. However, in typical babies this reflex is gradually integrated. It is still seen in adults, especially in extreme startle situations and holding patterns from tension and trauma.

  » The head thrust can be strong and head collars and floats can rarely keep the head above water. The head must rest on the practitioner's arm.

  » A calm, quiet environment will help decrease the frequency and strength of head thrusts, but they will still occur.

  » To release the backward force of the head thrust, continue to support the head on your elbow. Place your foot-hand on the client's sternum, avoiding any contact with the throat. Give sustained, steady pressure posterior on the sternum combined with an inferior pull (press on the sternum and pull gently toward the client's feet). This is very effective. The pressure needs to be steady, but does not need to be strong. Share this technique with caregivers. It will make it easier for them to bathe and dress the client.

  » This technique is based on the use of key points of control in NDT (neuro-developmental treatment) training.

- Strong extensor spasticity:

  - For some clients, the strong spasticity may cause the client's body to push into a full pattern of extension, especially through the entire spine and legs.

– Use the above steps for spasticity in addition to the following suggestions.

– Start in first position with your foot-arm under the client's knees and firmly maintain flexion in the hips, knees and spine. Keeping the chin slightly tucked and neck slightly flexed can also help.

– When working with the trunk and upper extremities, both of your hands will be needed. It will be imperative to stabilize the client's body and also maintain some flexion. One very useful position is similar to an open saddle, with the client in a vertical position but with the legs tightly flexed and held firmly between your legs. This position will allow you to use both of your hands, and the client's pelvis will also be stabilized. (You may need to stabilize the client's pelvis between your knees. And you may need to use your head to support your client's head.) Then use your hands to firmly rotate the trunk to help decrease spasticity. Then progress proximal to distal with each upper extremity to help decrease spasticity and improve mobility.

– Maintain some flexion and avoid allowing bilateral hips and knees to fully extend simultaneously.

– If a joint needs to be stretched into extension, avoid stretching multiple joints or bilateral joints at the same time.

– Example:

  » Hip flexors become shortened if the client is in a wheelchair all day, so these flexors benefit from stretching. Stretch one hip into extension while maintaining the other hip in strong flexion. Keep one hip and knee tightly flexed while pushing the opposite leg into hip extension. This will prevent hyperextension of the lumbar spine. One position to use for this stretch is the cradle position. In this position it is possible to hold one knee tightly to the client's chest while extending the opposite hip. You may need to stand on one leg and use your opposite leg to wrap around the client's free leg and pull it down into hip extension. You can lean against the side of the pool if necessary for balance.

  » When changing sides, maintain the hips and knees in flexion to prevent a strong full body extensor pattern. Do this by flexing the client's hips and knees firmly to their chest. Then hold the client's tightly flexed legs between your legs (similar to a closed saddle position, but with stronger flexion and a firm hold with

your legs). You will then be able to shift the client's head to
your other arm.

Shoulder subluxation following a stroke (CVA) or traumatic brain injury

- For some clients, the humerus tends to sublux and drop down slightly out of the shoulder joint.
- Start by standing on the client's healthier side in first position. Your head-hand can then be used to provide additional support for the far shoulder (the subluxated shoulder) by holding the humerus and gently supporting it in the glenohumeral (shoulder) joint.
- Avoid movements which push the involved arm far out into abduction or cause the humerus to drop down out of the shoulder joint.
- When gravity is pulling the humerus down out of the shoulder joint, apply gentle compression up through the flexed elbow to the shoulder. This will help move the humerus into the glenoid fossa to help approximate and realign the shoulder joint. This will be especially helpful when the client exits the pool. They will be relaxed, and the shoulder will benefit from your extra care and support.

Traumatic brain injury

- Each brain injury is unique. There are often orthopedic as well as neurological problems. Consider all of your client's challenges and needs, including orthopedic, neurological and psychosocial.
- Because WATSU addresses so many needs at once, it is an excellent treatment choice for at least part of a client's treatment program.
- WATSU often has a beneficial calming effect on brain-injured clients that can be especially helpful for people with mild brain injuries.
- For additional information, refer to these other sections in this chapter:
  - Clients with spasticity
  - Sensitivity to sensory stimuli (sensory defensiveness)
  - Specific joint range of motion precautions
  - Vestibular hypersensitivity.

Multiple sclerosis

- Clients with multiple sclerosis may be very sensitive to heat. Heat may exacerbate their symptoms and/or decrease their functional abilities for several hours due to a drastic reduction in muscle tone. Check first to see if your client tolerates warm weather, hot showers, and so on. If heat is a problem, work in a cooler water temperature. Each person is unique. Some may need a much cooler water temperature of approximately 31° C (88° F), while others with MS can tolerate warmer temperatures of 32.8–33.9° C (91–93° F), and a few will tolerate a typical WATSU pool temperature.

- Each person with MS has a unique collection of symptoms depending on what regions of the central nervous system are affected. Among the many possible challenges, vision, hearing, bladder control, pain and cognition may be affected. Fatigue and spasticity are very common.
- WATSU has the potential to help people with MS by decreasing spasticity, increasing range of motion, decreasing pain and improving sleep, in addition to all the other remarkable benefits of WATSU sessions.
- It is helpful to use WATSU at the beginning of each session and then use the remainder of the session to work on functional skills, including transfers, sit to stand, walking, movements for dressing and other activities of daily living, and high-level balance and coordination tasks depending on the abilities of the client.
- Please refer to the above section about "Clients with spasticity."

Spinal cord injuries

- Injuries vary widely depending on the level of the injury and the completeness of the injury at that level.
- WATSU has been very effective in the treatment of both new and old injuries. Note: Spinal fractures must be healed and stable or surgically stabilized before WATSU.
- The higher the client's level of injury, the greater the likelihood of diminished vital capacity, especially if the level of injury is C5 or above, because the diaphragm will be impaired. If vital capacity is less than 1000ml, monitor the client's breathing and color carefully. Immersion in water generally causes approximately a 10 percent decrease in vital capacity. Progress slowly. The client's mouth and nose absolutely must be kept out of the water. It's advisable to check with the client's healthcare provider prior to the first session.
- Stretching needs to be done with gentle and sustained stretches because clients often develop osteoporosis and sometimes heterotrophic ossification (bone deposition around a joint).

- Don't over stretch flexed fingers if they have been allowed to develop flexion contractures so the client can use their fingers to hook objects. Discuss this with the client before the session.
- Empty the urinary catheter bag before entering the pool. Keep the bag strapped to the client's leg. Don't move the client's leg in a way that might cause urine to flow from the bag back into the bladder.
- Special care must be given to the skin. Protect from scrapes on steps, sides and bottom of pool and lifts. Thin cotton socks provide good protection for feet. Leggings can be used for extra protection for legs and for extra warmth, if needed.
- Check for decubitus ulcers (pressure sores) before the session. If the skin over a newly forming decubitus ulcer has broken open, the client is at risk for infection and should not come into the pool until the area is healed.
- After the session, dry skin thoroughly, especially between the toes.
- Watch for signs of autonomic dysreflexia (sudden severe headache, sudden increase in heart rate, sudden increase in blood pressure). Autonomic dysreflexia doesn't happen often, but when it does, it can quickly develop into a medical emergency. It is usually triggered by a noxious stimulus (distended bladder, increase/decrease in body temperature, etc.). Immediately determine the cause and remedy it. If symptoms worsen or don't improve quickly, seek medical help. Autonomic dysreflexia is more common with injuries at T6 and above.
- Listen to your client. Most have an excellent understanding of their body, its needs, and how to move it safely. Listen to what each person wants/needs before, during and after the session.
- During the session, be aware of where the client does/doesn't have sensation. If you have both hands in locations without sensation, the client may not know where you are. Some clients may keep their eyes open or may want to be told where you are. This is especially true early in the first session. As trust develops, there are usually fewer concerns.
- Please refer to the section about "Clients with spasticity."

Parkinson's disease

- Tremors are extremely common in distal segments of limbs, especially in the hands. They occur during movement and at rest. Because of the distinctive movement, these tremors are often referred to as "pill rolling tremors."
- Rigidity also develops in all voluntary muscles, including muscles for

breathing, speech and facial expression. Rigidity feels quite different from spasticity, so different WATSU adaptations are needed.

- Begin the session with slow, calm movements.
- Gradually progress to slow, gentle yet sustained trunk rotation movements using all the different rotational WATSU movements in different positions. This will help improve trunk mobility and respiration, and decrease the rigidity that develops with Parkinson's disease.
- Continue to return to trunk rotation and trunk elongation throughout the session.
- Respiration tends to become shallow, and the trunk begins to round forward, so explore opening the thoracic spine and ribs. Be aware that older clients may have osteoporosis. Avoid strong stretches. Instead, use gentler, sustained stretches.
- People with Parkinson's disease develop shallow respiration which interferes with speech and also makes them prone to respiratory infections. Explore chest/thoracic expansion and deep breathing.
- Pectoral muscles tend to shorten, so gentle, sustained stretches are beneficial.
- Hip and knee flexors also tend to tighten and shorten, so invite lengthening.
- Passive movements are not enough for Parkinson's disease. People with Parkinson's disease greatly benefit from doing big, active movements, and the pool is the perfect (and safe) environment for movement with much less risk of falling. Consider allowing time at the end of the session especially for walking. The tendency will be for clients to struggle somewhat with initiation of any movement, especially walking. They often shuffle when walking. Strongly and enthusiastically encourage them to take big steps and lift their knees high and swing their arms. Strongly encourage large, fast movements with quick changes after two or three repetitions, instead of multiple repetitions. You can also encourage clients to take deeper breaths and speak loudly with lots of facial expressions. Be enthusiastic and fun. Many of these suggestions are based on the principles of the Parkinson's disease treatment program *LSVT Big and Loud*. Discover more information about this program online.
- Be especially careful to protect from falls when dressing, walking across the pool deck and pool entry/exit.

Amyotrophic lateral sclerosis (ALS)

- ALS is a progressive neurological disorder that affects motor neurons, leading to loss of muscle control and function. All muscles needed to move, speak, eat and breathe gradually deteriorate, often to complete paralysis.
- In the earlier stages of ALS, many clients benefit from the calming, soothing, repetitive movements of WATSU and the gentle stretching.
- As weakness and paralysis progress, contractures often develop. Gentle stretching is beneficial.
- When there is bulbar ALS onset, there are increased difficulties with speech and swallowing. The risks of aspiration greatly increase, including aspiration of saliva. The risks associated with WATSU become high. It is then recommended to discontinue WATSU.

Post-polio syndrome

Working with clients with post-polio requires a very delicate balance. They have fewer muscle fibers available in the regions affected by polio. They are often using (and over-using) every fiber they have.

- Avoid any chilling. Have towels immediately available when exiting the pool. Over-heating is also a concern.
- Prevent falls on wet, slippery decks and changing areas.
- Avoid stretching of muscles affected by polio.
- Avoid massage, especially point pressure. Instead, sandwich an area between both of your hands to nurture and invite it to let go of stress.
- Have the client do some walking in the pool (only a little is needed) before exiting.
- Keep the first session short; 15–20 minutes is enough. Call the client the day after and the day after that to assess their response to WATSU.
- Symptoms that suggest too much was done in session include:
  - muscle cramps or spasm
  - muscle twitching
  - muscle pain
  - extreme fatigue.
- Clients need to be exceptionally cautious with exercising. Muscle strength is graded on a 0 to 5 scale. A grade 3 muscle is able, with maximum effort, to move the full range against gravity. Grade 3 muscles must work all day to fight gravity in basic activities of daily living. Attempting to strengthen these muscles may cause overuse

damage, resulting in increased weakness. No strengthening should be done unless a muscle is at least a grade 3+, preferably a grade 4. Many muscles may be grade 3 or less. These muscles need to be used in daily life to prevent atrophy, but only used gently to avoid overuse and further damage to muscle fibers.

Alzheimer's disease and other forms of dementia

- Be kind, empathetic, calm, patient and respectful. Talk less and speak more slowly, allowing increased time for processing information.
- Singing is also a great way to connect with the client. Focus on the client's favorite songs (ask family members) and childhood songs. Clients who are non-verbal will often sing.
- Use appropriate communication skills, including accepting whatever the client tells you. Guide and redirect the client when needed, but do not discount or contradict what they say. Even if something sounds illogical or untrue to you, remember that this is the client's current reality, so acknowledge it. Be patient and respectful.
- WATSU has been beneficial, especially in the later stages of dementia. Clients respond well to the tender, nurturing aspects of WATSU. The gentle, repetitive trunk rotation movements of WATSU are particularly helpful in improving the range of motion and general mobility. Caregivers report that clients are less confused, more verbal, less agitated, and also walk and sleep better after receiving WATSU.
- Choose a quiet time of the day in the pool. This will help the client to be less distracted, overwhelmed or agitated. This will lead to a better, more peaceful outcome for the client with less likelihood of resistance or anxiety.
- Be mindful of other possible medical precautions (respiratory, cardiac, etc.) as well as common problems such as incontinence and increased risk of falls on the deck and in changing rooms.
- Include walking and other simple movements in the pool at the end of the session.
- The water provides a safe environment for clients with dementia to move and exercise without risk of injury due to falls.
- Movement in water provides resistance in all planes of movement, so any movement in the water will improve strength, balance, ambulation and functional skills.
- Keep your words to a minimum. Use visual and tactile cues, singing and plenty of smiles.

Additional suggestions and precautions for babies and children

The following information is based on professional education, extensive reading of medical research, and thousands of hours giving sessions to people with special needs.

General precautions for babies and children

- Review the section in the chapter titled "Precautions for aquatic bodywork."
- Do not allow babies and children to drink the pool water. Among other problems associated with drinking pool water, there is the risk of severe hyponatremia (dangerously low sodium level in the blood), especially with babies and very small children. This can lead to mental confusion, seizures and even death.
- Watch for overstimulation and over-fatigue.
- Young children cannot temperature regulate as well as adults. Watch for any signs of chilling (blue lips, shivering) or over-heating (skin flushing, yawning, sleepiness). Over-heating is more of a concern than chilling, so it is usually better to work with children in water at a slightly cooler temperature than what would be used for an adult with a similar impairment. However, if the air temperature is cool and/or the humidity is low, children will need to be kept warm until they are fully clothed. Immediately wrap the child in a towel when exiting the pool. If needed, add an extra heat source, such as a heat lamp, above the changing table and out of children's reach.
- The high humidity and chloramines in the air may be a problem for some children with asthma.
- For children with compromised immune systems, be especially aware of avoiding waterborne and airborne pathogens.
- Children with athetoid movements or cerebellar ataxia may experience more difficulties, especially when sitting, standing or walking in the pool, because of visual distortions (light refraction) and decreased proprioception (awareness of the position and movement of body parts) secondary to decreased joint compression forces due to buoyancy.
- Check with the child's healthcare provider about perforated eardrums and tubes in ears. Most children with these require adequate earplugs, possibly custom-made earplugs from an audiologist.
- Be sensitive to the fact that pools can be big, scary and overwhelming places for children. Watch for anxiety and overstimulation. You may

need to initially work with the child when the pool is quiet and lights are turned down or off. Additionally, you may need to begin with extra time connecting with the child while sitting on the top step and gradually progressing down the steps. Working in a small area in a corner of the pool may also feel less overwhelming for the child.

- Encourage all children (and adults) to use the restroom before each session. Encourage all children to drink water at the end of the session. If there is any doubt about bowel continence, use a good quality swim diaper. Wearing plastic pants with elastic at waist and thighs (or snug shorts/leggings for older children) over the swim diaper will provide additional containment for feces. Children should not come into the pool if they have had diarrhea that day. If the child has watery stools more than one time in a day, wait at least 48 hours after the last watery stool before coming to the pool. Adhere to your local health codes and pool policies.

Overview: Typically abled and special needs

- Children tend to be less inhibited and much more spontaneous than adults. They are wonderful for teaching us to be playful and 100 percent present. If we can just "be" with them, our sessions become exceptionally joyful. Be free of expectations because a child may sing, talk, be completely relaxed, or suddenly flip over to reach for a ball that has caught their attention—all in the same session.
- Babies and young children are wonderful to work with in the water, and they often respond very differently from adults to WATSU. Babies are totally honest in their responses. If they are in any way uncomfortable, frightened, frustrated or bored, they will let you know immediately. Take time to connect with each child.
- WATSU sessions with babies and young children are very spontaneous and generally playful. Babies/children often don't want to be put directly onto their back when they come into the water. You may have better results if you start by holding the baby/child close to you in a vertical position facing away from you when the child is ready to do so. Then sway from side to side and do additional rhythmical movements similar to WATSU together with the baby/child. Gradually angle your body backward toward supine, which will also progress the baby/child to supine, but with the support of your torso.
- Allow the baby to squiggle and squirm if they want to. Follow the child's movements. Be prepared for sudden quick movements. Infant massage can also be incorporated into your session.

- Try to keep exciting toys and colorful objects out of the child's view to decrease distractions. However, if the child suddenly chooses to do a different activity, it's often better to follow the child's interests. If the child chooses a toy, find ways to include the toy or another toy in your session with the child.
- With many children, WATSU sessions are a joyful dance of WATSU and play. Meet the child wherever the child is and be spontaneous with the dance.
- Calm humming often helps. Be joyful and open to whatever the baby or child presents to you.
- Give the baby/child extra fluids after the session to prevent dehydration.
- Picture Exchange Communication cards (commonly referred to as PEC cards or PECS) are a valuable tool when working with children with various challenges. Anyone can order these cards or you could make your own. These cards have simple drawings (or you can use simple, uncluttered photos) to depict activities, toys, animals, foods, short phrases and anything else that is pertinent to the child's life and interests. The cards are helpful for communicating with the child and decreasing their frustration. Use these cards to give the child choices and to prepare the child for the progression of activities, including preparing the child for leaving the pool at the end of the session. Even children with good speech and language skills can benefit from having activity cards to choose from.
- If you are working with children with special needs, it's especially helpful to coordinate with other professionals (occupational therapist, physiotherapist, speech therapist, psychologist, doctor and others) who are working with the child. Speak with them, and, if possible, do some shared sessions together in the pool. Of course, it's essential to discuss this sharing of information and co-treating with the child's legal guardians first, and receive written permission.
- Singing your instructions to children is also helpful. You can use specific songs for specific activities, but any simple instruction can be sung using a few notes. These don't need to be specific tunes—and they definitely don't need to be tuneful. Children will enjoy and follow your requests more readily. Have fun! Be fun!

Cerebral palsy (CP)

- The challenges children with CP face are widely varied. Some degree of spasticity is one of the most common difficulties faced by kids with CP. Refer to the section in the chapter titled "Clients with spasticity."

- Ask if the child has seizures. If yes, review information regarding seizures in the section titled "Precautions for aquatic bodywork."
- WATSU is beneficial for decreasing tone so the child with spasticity can experience what it's like to "feel soft." Please refer to the case study of a child with cerebral palsy. Use WATSU at the beginning of your treatment session and intermittently during the session as needed. Functional and therapeutic activities can be woven through the session.
- For a "floppy" child with extremely low tone, WATSU will make an already low tone child even more hypotonic. This may decrease the child's functional abilities. Carefully consider your rationale for choosing WATSU. Some possible reasons might include psychological benefits, improvements in respiration and in soft tissue mobility. Consider if the potential benefits outweigh the potential for decreased function, or if you can add other therapeutic techniques to your session to enhance function.
- Most children with athetoid movements respond well to WATSU. Benefits will include relaxation, improved soft tissue mobility and improved normalization of tone. It is helpful to incorporate joint compression into the session to increase proprioceptive input. Also include functional skills, disguised as play, as part of the session.
- Children with ataxia generally respond well with improved relaxation and soft tissue mobility. Be aware that these children may be seizure prone. Also be aware that these children are often sensitive to vestibular stimulation. Refer to the earlier section in this chapter titled "Vestibular hypersensitivity."
- Refer to the case report of child with cerebral palsy earlier in this chapter.

Spina bifida

- Symptoms of spina bifida vary widely. There are three primary classifications:
  - Children with spina bifida occulta generally have no symptoms, and WATSU is safe.
  - If there's a meningocele, there may be some symptoms and the child may have had surgery. Following surgery, it is generally safe to do WATSU. Learn more about the child's specific needs and possible precautions.
- Myelomeningocele (meningomyelocele), also referred to as spina bifida cystica, is the most serious form. Most children have surgery soon after birth. Many also need shunts to manage hydrocephalus. Learn more

about the specific needs of the child and how to avoid pressure on the shunt. Many of these children have neurological challenges similar to a spinal cord injury. Many are incontinent. Babies will need a swim diaper covered by plastic pants with elastic at the legs and waist. Children will need a swim diaper covered by snug shorts or leggings to contain any fecal matter.

- Children with spina bifida generally respond well to the relaxation and gentle stretching benefits of WATSU to maintain mobility and to alleviate pain if needed. However, there are many variations with spina bifida and its associated complications. Each child will need to be carefully evaluated and the benefits as well as precautions for WATSU assessed.
- Incorporation of functional skills will be highly beneficial. Find playful and engaging ways to incorporate these activities.

Muscular dystrophy

- There are different types of muscular dystrophy (MD). Becker and Duchenne are two of the most common. Spinal muscular atrophy (SMA) is a related, though different, process. Carefully consider the potential benefits versus the potential risks for each child. Consider the medical risks, including potential respiratory complications for the child.
- Benefits for the child may include improvements in soft tissue and joint mobility, increased depth of respiration, decreased pain, improved sleeping at night, and psychological benefits.
- WATSU will decrease the child's muscle tone. This may decrease their functional abilities. Therefore, include games that incorporate functional skills.
- Keep sessions short, especially the first few sessions, and assess the effects on the child and their specific needs.

Attention deficit hyperactivity disorder

- Keep the WATSU portion of the treatment session short initially. Gradually lengthen the WATSU session according to the tolerance of the child.
- Choose a quiet and calm time of the day in the pool with the lights dimmed.
- Remember that "attention deficit" does not mean a lack of attention. The challenge for most children is that they attend to everything and have difficulty focusing on one topic, one thought or one activity.

- Not all of these children are hyperactive.
- You will likely need to do other activities in the pool before progressing to WATSU.
- Many of these children respond well to joint compression. Use games that involve jumping up and down in waist-deep water at the beginning of the session.
- Slightly firmer pressure is usually more effective than light touch.
- For some, it will require time before they can progress to WATSU, and for most children, WATSU will need to be at the end of the session.
- Talk with the child and work as a team with the child to discover what is most beneficial.
- You may need to use quicker movements at the beginning of each session to mirror the child's energy level. Then begin to use slower, rhythmical movements to calm the central nervous system and invite the child to slow down and focus.
- Slow, rhythmical humming often helps. (If you sing words, children will often lift their head out of the water to listen to you.)
- A brushing and joint compression program (such as the Wilbarger Protocol) at the beginning of a session may help. Talk with an occupational or physical therapist trained in this technique.
- Be sensitive to the fact that many of these children have difficulty with emotional self-regulation.
- Many of these children also have sensory challenges. Refer to the section titled "Sensitivity to sensory stimuli (sensory defensiveness)."

Autism spectrum disorder

- There is an enormous variation in children with autism. Avoid generalizing.
- The child will likely have some social and communication challenges, which may include the following and more:
  - Difficulty recognizing and expressing emotions in self and others.
  - Overwhelmed in social situations.
  - Difficulty with spoken language, although many do well using a keyboard for communication.
  - Difficulty with emotional self-regulation.
- The child may have repetitive behaviors. Learn what these are.
- The child will almost certainly have some sensory challenges. These typically involve over-sensitivity or under-sensitivity to sounds, lights, touch, tastes, smells, pain and other stimuli. Learn what the

child's specific challenges are, and what strategies are currently being used to help the child.

- Learn as much as possible about the child: likes, dislikes, triggers and the strategies the child's parents/caregivers/teachers use.
- Depending on severity of autism, the child may resist you if you try to make verbal or eye contact too soon.
- Progress slowly. Choose a quiet time of the day in the pool. If possible, choose a time when no one else is in the pool. The child may scream or make other loud noises.
- Observe the child's behavior in the water. Mirror the child's behavior near the child.
- Gradually move closer to the child. If your touch is permitted or is essential for safety, slowly begin to make contact.
- Progress to gently lifting the child while supporting and allowing them to stay in their preferred position, whatever it is.
- Give the child your unconditional acceptance. At the same time, have clear boundaries regarding acceptable and unacceptable behavior. Have consequences for unacceptable behavior, such as hitting you or pulling your hair. Have clarity around your boundaries, not anger.
- Be consistent and stay calm. Discover what activities the child likes. Use these as rewards. "We'll do three…, and then we'll do…"
- Talk less. Use fewer words and be more direct in your speech.
- Children with autism often have difficulty mirroring movements or activities, so you may need to use other strategies.
- Children with autism often have difficulty following directions. Songs with a simple, repeating theme can be paired with activities to help the child. Repeat the same music paired with the same activity each session. PEC cards (or PECS) are a valuable tool for children who struggle with communication. As mentioned above, a keyboard can also be a helpful aid for communication for some children. For information about PEC cards refer to the earlier section titled "Overview: Typically abled and special needs."

Sensitivity to sensory stimuli (sensory defensiveness)

Some children are especially hypersensitive or hyposensitive to light, sound, touch, smells and/or movement. Sensory hyper- or hyposensitivity may fluctuate at times, except for vestibular, which usually remains either hypo or hyper. For more detailed information, speak with an occupational therapist or physical therapist with specialized sensory integration training. The following may aid children who exhibit these challenges.

Light
Hypersensitive:

- Have the child wear dark glasses (if tolerated) to the pool and in the pool if desired, even an indoor pool. A baseball cap can also be helpful, if tolerated.
- Decrease the amount of light, especially reflected light off water, in the pool area.
- Keep your hand gestures to a minimum when talking.

Hyposensitive:

- The child may want to keep their eyes open.
- The child may seek additional visual stimulation, including hand movements in front of their face.

Sound
Hypersensitive:

- Select a quiet time of the day in your pool for the WATSU session.
- Turn off the music in the pool area.
- Keep your voice calm and quiet, but avoid whispering, which is noxious for many children.
- Try ear plugs during WATSU if water in the ears and/or the pool noise is a problem.
- Many children cannot tolerate earplugs. Instead of earplugs, try using a headband that is made for wearing over earplugs in the pool.
- Try putting your mouth under the water and singing to the child. Sometimes this is enough to engage the child and help them to tolerate ears being under water.

Hyposensitive:

- The child may seek additional input from specific sounds.
- The child may create additional input by hitting water, screaming, yelling, striking equipment against side of pool, and so on.

Touch
Hypersensitive:

- Gentle yet firm pressure is generally better tolerated than very light touch.

- The child may be very sensitive to specific textures.
- The child may not tolerate specific clothes, fabrics, pool toys.

Hyposensitive:

- The child may seek additional tactile stimulation, including self-stimulating, repetitive movements.
- The child may seek additional oral stimulation, including biting self, practitioner or pool equipment, especially leg floats, kickboards.

Smell
Hypersensitive:

- Keep the pool area as free as possible of any strong smells.
- No perfume, cologne, scented hair products or strongly scented mouthwash.
- Brush teeth after eating. Avoid coffee, onions and garlic.

Hyposensitive:

- The child may seek additional input with specific materials and equipment.

Movement and vestibular stimulation
Hypersensitive:

- The child may seek the comfort of gentle compression under water.
- Refer to the section in this chapter titled "Vestibular hypersensitivity."

Hyposensitive:

- The child may seek additional input through movement, especially jumping, spinning, and so on.
- The child may seek extra input through active underwater play.

Abused children

- If possible, work in conjunction with the child's mental healthcare professional. You will need written permission from the child's legal guardian.

- Seek out information about the child prior to meeting them.
- Explain *every* step to the child. Allow the child to make choices.
- When the child is ready for you to touch them, slowly begin by using the child's position of choice. Request the child's permission before you touch them, unless touch is needed for safety.
- It may take time before the child is ready to move out of their position of comfort. Remember that just breathing with and slowly rocking a child or an adult can be a profoundly moving experience and lay the groundwork for trust.
- As you progress, you can use the water to gently invite, but not impose, movement.
- If the child ever wants to stop for any reason, they should just say "stop" and you will stop the WATSU immediately.
- WATSU can also be used for bonding with a foster parent or adoptive parent. The parent/guardian can easily be taught a few simple moves including simply holding the child gently in the warm water and rocking.
- For more information and suggestions, refer to the section titled "Psychological support in conjunction with WATSU."

A personal message to the reader

Thank you for exploring this chapter. I hope I've given you support for the ways you've been using WATSU, and also expanded your use of WATSU into new possibilities for your most challenging clients. I encourage you to reach out to more people with special conditions who will benefit from your knowledge and skills in sensitive, adaptable sessions where the needs of each client can be uniquely met. Keep your clients safe, and share your open heart, compassion and deep empathy with each one. They will touch your life in profound ways.

With love and gratitude,
Peggy

Further reading

Childre, D. & Martin, H. (1999). *The Heartmath Solution*. New York, NY: HarperCollins Publishers.

Chon, S.C., Oh, D.W. & Shim, J.H. (2009). WATSU approach for improving spasticity and ambulatory function in hemiparetic patients with stroke. *Physiotherapy Research International*, 14(2): 128–136.

Corcoran, R.P., Cheung, A., Ross, S. & Toner, R. (2014). An evaluation of the Wave Academy approach to reducing post-traumatic stress disorder. *The Center for Research and Reform in Education (CRRE)*, Johns Hopkins University, August 17, 2014.

Dougherty, L., Dunlap, E. & Mehler, S. (2004). The Rehabilitative Benefits of Watsu. In H. Dull, *Watsu: Freeing the Body in Water*. Middletown, CA: Harbin Springs Publishing.

Faull, K. (2005). A pilot study of the comparative effectiveness of two water-based treatments for fibromyalgia syndrome: Watsu and Aix massage. *Journal of Bodywork and Movement Therapies*, 9(3): 202–210.

Jamison, L. (2000). The therapeutic value of aquatic therapy in treating lymphedema. *Rehab Management: The Interdisciplinary Journal of Rehabilitation.* Aug.–Sept.

Levine, P. (1997). *Waking the Tiger: Healing Trauma*. Berkeley, CA: North Atlantic Books.

Maczkowiak, S., Hölter, G. & Otten, H. (2007). WATSU—the effect of differently accentuated movement therapy interventions on clinically depressive patients. *Bewegungstherapie und Gesundheitssport*, 23(2): 58–64.

Marafon, G. (2008). Techniques of body mediation from alternative medicine—WATSU. *Sexologies*, 17(1): 29.

Morris, D.M. (1994). Aquatic rehabilitation for the treatment of neurological disorders. *Journal of Back and Musculoskeletal Rehabilitation*, 4(4): 297–308.

Morris, D.M. (1997). Aquatic Rehabilitation of the Neurologically Impaired Client. In R.G. Ruoti, D.M. Morris & A.J. Cole (eds), *Aquatic Rehabilitation*. Philadelphia and New York, NY: Lippincott.

Morris, D.M. (2011). Aquatic Rehabilitation for the Treatment of Neurologic Disorders. In A.J. Cole & B.E. Becker (eds), *Comprehensive Aquatic Therapy* (third edition). Pullman, DC: Washington State University Publishing.

Nakamoto, B.V., Acosta, A.M.C. & Couto, M.B. *The Effectiveness of Watsu® Therapy for Fall Prevention Among the Elderly: A Case Study*. This is a case study submitted to achieve a Specialist Degree in Theories and Techniques for Integrated Care, at the Federal University of São Paulo-UNIFESP. The study was approved by the Ethics Committee for Human Research, UNIFESP (CAAE: 45425115.2.0000.5505).

Scaer, R. (2001). *The Body Bears the Burden: Trauma, Dissociation, and Disease*. Binghamton, NY: Haworth Medical Press.

Schitter, A.M. & Fleckenstein, J. (2018). Passive hydrotherapy WATSU for rehabilitation of an accident survivor: A prospective case report. *Complementary Medical Research*, 25(4): 263–268.

Schitter, A.M., Fleckenstein, J., Frei, P., Taeymans, J., Kurpiers, N. & Radlinger, L. (2020). Applications, indications, and effects of passive hydrotherapy WATSU (Water Shiatsu)—A systematic review and meta-analysis. *PLoS One*, 15(3): e0229705. doi: 10.1371/journal.pone.0229705.

Schitter, A.M., Nedeljkovic, M., Baur, H., Fleckenstein, J. & Raio, L. (2015). Effects of passive hydrotherapy WATSU (Water Shiatsu) in the third trimester of pregnancy: Results of a controlled pilot study. *Evidence-Based Complementary and Alternative Medicine*, 2015: 437650.

Schoedinger, P. (2008). Adapting Watsu for Clients with Special Needs. In H. Dull, *Watsu: Freeing the Body in Water*. Middletown, CA: Harbin Springs Publishing.

Schoedinger, P. (2011). Watsu in Aquatic Rehabilitation. In A.J. Cole & B.E. Becker (eds), *Comprehensive Aquatic Therapy* (third edition). Pullman, DC: Washington State University Publishing.

Tufekcioglu, E., Erzeybek, M.S., Kaya, F. & Ozan, G. (2018). The effect of 12-week passive aquatic bodywork on sympathovagal balance of obese youth. *Journal of Education and Training Studies*, 6(2): 166–176.

Tufekcioglu, E., Konukman, F., Kaya, F. & Arslan, D. (2021). The effects of aquatic Watsu therapy on gross motor performance and quality of life for children with cerebral palsy. *Montenegrin Journal of Sports and Science Medicine*, 10(2): 25–30. doi: 10.26773/mjssm.210904.

Useros-Olmo, A.I., Martinez-Pernia, D. & Huepe, D. (2018). The effects of a relaxation program featuring aquatic therapy [Watsu] and autogenic training among people with cervical dystonia (a pilot study). *Physiotherapy Theory and Practice*, 36(4): 488–497.

Vogel, W.A. (2005). Self-perceived benefits of receiving sessions for 18 months by residents of a continuing care retirement community. *Journal of the Aquatic Exercise Association*, 19(4). Accessed on 21/11/2022 at https://massagelanzarote.com/resources/watsu%20with%20 elderly.pdf.

Weber-Nowakowska, K., Gebska, M. & Zyzniewska-Banaszak, E. (2013). Watsu: A modern method in physiotherapy, body regeneration, and sports. *Annales Academiae Medicae Stetinensis*, 59(1): 100–102.

Chapter 3

Interoceptive Embodiment

The Ocean Within

INGRID KEATING AND DR. JENNIFER OLEJOWNIK

A call to the blue

As human beings, we have been crafted with the innate intelligence of the entire universe within our bodies. Our somatic relationship with water nestles deep within our humanity and within the watery amniotic sac of our first home. Ancient Chinese Medicine and acupuncture texts proclaim that energetic waterways or meridians begin as *wells*, bubble to *springs*, flow toward *streams*, ripple into *rivers* and courses toward the ultimate home, the majestic *sea*. This *sea of energy or ocean within* encompasses the surface of the white-capped waves to the seabed depths of our body wisdom and primordial and interoceptive sense of self. The microcosm of water permeates our internal organs as 80 percent of our body is made of water and thus is mirrored through the waters that flow within the macrocosm of our blue earth. Our fascination with water is really no mystery, it is cellular and our biology calls us back to our watery formation and birth. When our clients seek out water as a form of therapy to better navigate their earthly everyday lives, they may also be fulfilling a desire to embody an earlier stage of their human development. There is an instinct to balance some aspect of their inherent yin and yang energies and meridians within the aqueous environment where their DNA coded and formed. It is a need to shift the epigenetic predisposition and process past traumas that occlude their ability and birthright to feel their essence as *whole beings*. Water rituals and therapies may help us to remember whence we came and speak softly to our humanhood—a portal back to our first beginnings, our primordial lore and our amniotic story. Within our first cellular breath and sensory awakening we reminisce how our bone, muscle and inverted cortex sprung forth. Consciously and subconsciously, water serves as a healing environment to help us examine, reconcile and process some aspect of our *ocean within* and become more of what we are intended to be: *whole beings*. As practitioners we witness our clients with eyes closed sink down to this childhood past with optic cortexes that paint strokes of shadows and teal hues amidst a crimson chasm, swallowing the nourishment of life. Sinking deeper and deeper toward the bottom of the energetic breath, they float into the void. On their exhales yang forces grasp the home within. The tide rising up again, they inhale yin energy while this cycle of knowing begins and ends again and again. The ability for our clients to recalibrate and integrate these powerful experiences of breath, movement and conscious awareness back to the gravitational pull of their daily lives with a renewed outlook and perspective makes WATSU and its other related aquatic forms a lasting experience, not an isolated one.

In this chapter, we invite you into the deep blue, a coursing and flowing abyss of the unknown at the very bottom of the breath. What we postulate in this chapter is that the healing properties of water and the evolving art form of WATSU and aquatic bodywork in its many forms gives us a knowing, an understanding and an alignment with our own uniquely individual embodiment processes, rituals, birthright and ultimate wholeness. The *ocean within* is so vast and sometimes an unknown discovery of *self*. Our primary intent in this chapter is to display the elevating somatic art of WATSU and aquatic bodywork and provide tools that inform practitioners on key areas of somatic processes, practitioner awareness, client safety and proper therapeutic integration so that clients can continue to process through the many healing stages beyond the aquatic setting. Practitioner introspection, analysis and continued somatic study is warranted to further uncover the many streams toward an embodied somatic practice.

Interoceptive embodiment

As WATSU practitioners, we journey to take a deep dive with our clients, providing safety nets, visible and invisible in the water, holding a container so they can experience and remember the wholeness of their humanhood. From shore to sea and back again we journey towards their "felt" sense and alignment with coming home to the vast ocean of self.

What we encounter in our water explorations with our clients are the stimuli, processes and past experiences that shape the present moment within a session. This unfolding process is in real time and happening right in front of us in the present moment as we hold our clients in warm water. However, how our clients process, regulate, integrate and transform through many archetypes of movement and breath is a culmination of many years of conditioning, traumas, triumphs, and a complex constellation of somatic experiences. In turn, these remarkable observations are revealed through verbal exchanges, non-verbal language, movement, and holding patterns in the body and usually provide some clue to how our clients are currently navigating their internal (*intero-ceptive*) and external (*exteroceptive*) world. Encouraging and guiding them to fine-tune their renewed self-awareness is a primary goal in somatic practice.

Researchers are now finding a major key factor to better understanding how we process and feel the world from the inside out. Our experiences and this deep ocean within may reside in the science of *interoception*, a growing topic of interest as evidenced by the decision by the National Center for Complementary and Integrative Health in 2021 to fund initiatives to study basic mechanisms of interoception (Chen 2021). The National Institutes of Health (NIH) created a strategic plan to further research and better understand how deeper levels of interoceptive awareness can influence our mental, emotional and physical health and well-being (National Institutes of Health n.d.). While this reductionist approach will certainly be useful in providing foundational scaffolding needed to understand how interoception contributes to neurologi-cal, psychiatric and behavioral disorders, it is only a portion of what is required to unpack the ancient wisdom of contemplative embodiment. It is essential to understand the effect interoception has on our overall well-being and what ongoing steps we must take to understand and safeguard our clients' mental health. As water informs our clients' understanding of their interior landscape, we must take our responsibility quite seriously and realize the multidimen-sionality of our clients' narrative and story.

Interoception is a complex innate body wisdom that directly connects us to our emotional experience, self-regulation, decision making and consciousness. It is a palpable sense of the experience of the internal functions of the body and provides an awareness of our visceral processes. Ceunen, Vlaeyen and Van Diest (2016) trace the origins of the term interoception and highlight the distinction between restrictive and inclusive meanings, where restrictive definitions of interoception state that only sensations from viscera are introspective. Inclusive meanings, in contrast, are broad in scope and represent phenomenological expe-riences of the body through the actions of the central nervous system (p.743). In this chapter, we are incorporating an inclusive meaning of interoception and how it contributes to the subjective perceptions of body states.

The shifting sense of self

To give shape to the deep meaning and complexities that occur through the process of WATSU, it is useful to briefly identify some concepts and ideas that describe the ways the body is understood or viewed during a clinical encounter. While it is not within the clinician's scope of practice to interpret or psychologically analyze what comes forth during a session, it is of the utmost importance for clinicians to recognize that a client's sense of self shifts through movement and embodied experience. With this understanding, clinicians over time cultivate an awareness and a skill for knowing how to have a relationship with clients' changing sense of selves and the somatic cues that guide their evolving sessions with clients.

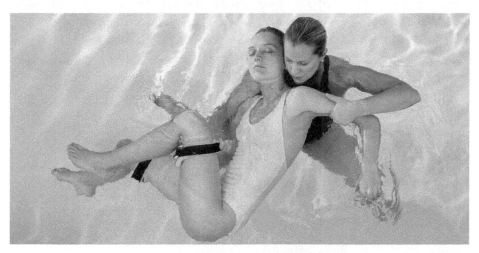

Figure 3.1: Arm leg rock (WATSU)

Although WATSU and its related aquatic modalities offer many *physical* and *psychological* benefits that can be measured, observed or verified by a third party, there exists another stream of data that relates to how a client experiences changes related to their sense of self during a session. This type of data is made possible only through a first-person perspective, a witnessing of the self as experienced through movement and body position. This distinction clearly underscores the somatic aspects of the practice. Somatics generally refers to the body as experienced from within (Hanna 1986). A somatic perspective is not unique to the art of WATSU as many of the contemplative movement forms such as yoga, Tai Chi and breathwork impact the experience of self through the actions of watching, witnessing, noticing, sensing and allowing. Proprioception and interoception are physiologic constructs that impact and inform one's own somatic awareness.

Less understood is a theoretical lens to explain how individuals come to understand a sense of embodiment. Therea Silow (2010) posits that the experience of self is a normative process that follows a developmental trajectory grounded in direct and embodied experience (see Table 3.1). As humans grow and mature, they ascend through several developmental stages spanning different levels of awareness shaped and informed by different stimuli. As individuals grow, develop and change, over time "...with the amplification of the meaning making, language, and abstract faculties, the actual experience of body senses becomes less conscious to the point where it moves into the background of the perceptual field" (Silow 2010, p.87). Today, the increased use of technological devices in all sectors and segments of society further competes with access to a more intimate relationship with embodiment. Disruption from the embodied experience is often attributed to traumatic experiences, and Silow proposes that disconnection is actually another stage in the developmental process, often resulting in a fragmented sense of self. The experience of fragmentation is the impetus or awakening of a desire to return to sensory and somatic experiences. Simply put, reconciling the felt sense of disembodiment is actually another developmental stage toward wholeness.

Table 3.1: Ascending stages of development of self (Stern 1990)

Stage of self	Experience of embodiment
Emergent sense of self (0–2 months)	Self-based on reoccurring organismic experiences (feeling tones, pleasure, discomfort, discrete affects, motor experiences and perceptions across different sensory channels)
Core sense of self (2–6 months)	Experience of self-related to embodied experience stemming from dyadic interaction
Subjective sense of self (7–9 months)	Movement away from direct experience to subjective mental states
Verbal sense of self (24 months)	Use of language increases distance from direct experience

WATSU provides an opportunity for clients to reconnect with their internal experience and to appreciate or perhaps even reclaim a sense of embodiment. There are few places in our culture where we can truly amplify our internal experience while muting any competing external stimuli. Being submerged in water naturally allows a client to disengage from all competing sources of information, turning one's attention and awareness to the sensations, or changing sense of self. Continual movement is the vehicle for this as:

> [It] continues to inspire sensation via activating the kinesthetic, proprioceptive, and interoceptive elements of the somatosenses. Movement in its potentially wide spectrum, from extrinsic, volitional, and high energy movement, to subtle and intrinsic movements, including pulsations and micromovements, is a fundamental element in the pursuit of cultivating body awareness. Particularly non-habitual and nonlinear movements, such as wave motions and micromovements, in concert with a rich array of breaths and subtle sounds, allow us to deeply touch ourselves. (Gintis in Silow 2010, p.89)

WATSU, with its unique, fluid and highly creative movement patterns within the neural warmth of water, represents an opportunity to experience non-habitual forms of movement. Clients experience the ability to engage in deep attention to an embodied sense of self no matter where they fall on the embodiment continuum in their everyday lives. In this view, the experience of WATSU takes us back to a primal stage in utero, connecting us to deeper ways of knowing and experiencing the self, allowing us to notice and observe our somatic patterns through movement of the physical body. The aquatic aspect of the practice amplifies connection to our fluid body where movement "becomes a felt reality" (Conrad in Silow 2010, p.91).

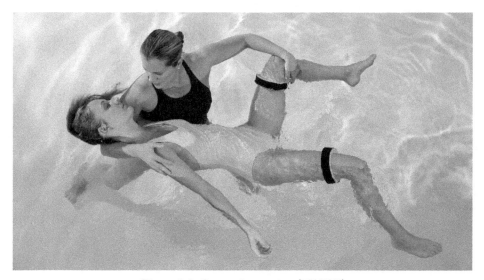

Figure 3.2: Over grip rotation (WATSU)

Interoception and vagal tone

Studies continue to examine the complex relationship between improvements in interoception via vagal tone stimulation through breathing, yoga, meditation and other related practices. Aquatic therapists are not limited to WATSU techniques alone as they have the ability when properly trained to also utilize and integrate other modalities that are spoken about in later chapters. Modalities that emerged and grew after WATSU's birth incorporated sub-aquatic and full-body immersion with the entire head going underwater while a client wears a nose clip. Examples of some of these sub-aquatic therapies that integrate these techniques to elicit the dive reflex include WaterDance, Healing Dance, Aquatic Integration or AMNION. Others may, in addition, tap into the cranial sacral and the fascial systems. These aquatic forms combined with the existing vagal tone effects of WATSU may also create enhanced respiratory changes, altered states of consciousness or non-ordinary states due to activating and accentuating the power of the vagus nerve through the added technique of client breath-holding and bringing the entire body into the three-dimensional underwater environment. Vagal tonality is further explored in Chapter 11. WaterDance images that help to illicit and deepen a vagal tone response are represented in Figures 3.3–3.8.

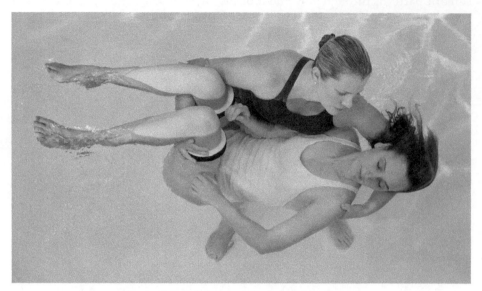

Figure 3.3: Submerging the face (WaterDance)

The science of floatation: An active interoceptive process

Historically, WATSU and even some of its other related modalities are referred to and marketed as "passive" forms of aquatic bodywork. These modalities do indeed have moments of stillness where the therapist is manually moving the client's upper and lower extremities and manually rotates the spine. However, the internal interoceptive and motor learning processes that are happening while being moved are most certainly "active" in nature. Some clients may even feel a need to move or stretch physically, specifically in what we call "free flow" where a practitioner follows the client's movement patterns. Even when we sit quietly in deep meditation we are not experiencing a passive process, even within stillness, we are participating in an active interoceptive experience and path to improved internal awareness.

We can look at interoception without any form of external movement or proprioception applied by a practitioner to see that improvements in interoception can be observed through flotation without exteroceptive interruption.

Justin Feinstein (Feinstein *et al.* 2018) researched:

the elicitation of relaxation and interoceptive awareness in individuals with high anxiety and sensitivity using floatation therapy. Floatation-REST (reduced environmental stimulation therapy), an intervention that attenuates exteroceptive sensory input to the nervous system, had been found to reduce state anxiety across a diverse clinical sample with high levels of anxiety sensitivity (AS). To further examine this anxiolytic effect, Feinstein's study investigated the affective and physiological changes induced by Floatation-REST within sensory deprivation tanks and assessed whether individuals with high AS experienced any alterations in their awareness for interoceptive sensation while immersed in an environment lacking exteroceptive sensation. Using a within-subject crossover design, 31 participants with high AS were randomly assigned to undergo a 90-minute session of Floatation-REST or an exteroceptive comparison condition. Measures of self-reported affect and interoceptive awareness were collected before and after each session, and blood pressure was measured during each session. Relative to the comparison condition, Floatation-REST generated a significant anxiolytic effect characterized by reductions in state anxiety and muscle tension and increases in feelings of relaxation and serenity (p< .001 for all variables). Significant blood pressure reductions were evident throughout the float session and reached the lowest point during the diastole phase (average reduction >12 mm Hg). The float environment also significantly enhanced awareness and attention for cardiorespiratory sensations. Floatation-REST induced a state of relaxation and heightened interoceptive awareness in a clinical sample with high AS.

Within a sensory deprivation tank, floating quietly with no exteroceptive interruption we are actively changing our ability to align ourselves with improved interoceptive awareness and decreasing states of anxiety. This is indeed an active change and another portal that opens toward a new neural pathway to increasing interoceptive awareness.

Practitioner awareness

In WATSU, we utilize the science of floatation, properties of warm water that provide deep proprioceptive input, Shiatsu point work, intentional movement, spinal buoyancy, intuition and close dynamic holding to elicit a deepened body awareness. This powerful combination creates an ideal healing space for a client. However, without proper *practitioner awareness* the space will not manifest healing in the heightened forms that we might anticipate. Practitioners must strive to create a therapeutic environment where their client's exploration and deep dive into the iceberg of self and the subconscious can be journeyed safely and with care, pause and proper modulation. The WATSU practitioner, through the act of witnessing and holding space, enables a client to experience regulation and attunement. "The quality of the relational experience has an effect on the individual's capacity to experience, tolerate, and regulate states of arousal" (Silow 2010, p.86). Preparing them for the session and letting them know what to expect can decrease the amount of fear or anxiety that can sometimes be exhibited in a first session or sessions thereafter. Where we might begin is within ourselves as the practitioner and also our intent. Having proper intention and boundaries before, during and after a session is of extreme importance as we become witnesses to our client and is indeed, our ethical duty.

Practitioner self-care and grounding rituals

As therapists or clinicians working in warm water, one of the key components before stepping into the therapy pool with clients is not only having solid professional boundaries but also maintaining proper practitioner boundaries for self-care, including grounding rituals. The warmth of the water and buoyancy can be dehydrating or even disorienting. Drinking plenty of water during sessions and taking breaks between clients is essential. Working long hours in the water can also physiologically change bone density due to the decreases in gravity for prolonged periods of time. This is why it is necessary for both one's physical and emotional well-being to have specific rituals or exercises that a practitioner engages in outside the pool.

What you recommend to your clients may also mirror the mind-body, self-regulating activities that promote grounding and centeredness within ourselves as practitioners. Weight-bearing and meditation practices such as hiking, walking, yoga, Tai Chi, meditation, prayer, journaling and breathwork are just some of the outlets for a therapist or practitioner to engage in to provide stress reduction and to tap into their own unique interoceptive capabilities. Experiencing the same verbal and non-verbal cues, movement and patterns of holding in the self, may serve as an instructional guide to recognize and notice these changes in others.

In Chapter 5, Dr. Cedar Barstow provides an informative section that covers a practitioner self-care assessment using a rating scale of 1–10. This assessment helps the practitioner to track and assess their self-care needs and how these relate to their therapeutic relationships in the areas of *balance, rest, satisfaction* and *support*. Understanding our own self-care needs as practitioners and clinicians and making our needs a priority has a ripple effect not only for our own individual well-being as the practitioner but also for the well-being and proper alignment of the boundaries we maintain with our clients.

Client and practitioner boundaries within somatic practice

For transformative healing to take place, practitioners must understand and empathize with what their client's experience means to them. Empathy is a productive tool, but practitioners must not take on or pathologize the constructs of someone else's pain as their own. This can be extremely non-productive for both the practitioner and client. Practitioners must have boundaries within the framework of empathic care. Some practitioners may have a ritual that they engage in before and after a session that helps maintain healthy client/practitioner mind-sets and frameworks. Leading with a sense of compassion can help practitioners maintain professional boundaries whilst being keen to their own practitioner self-care needs before and after a session. We continue to speak more about how ethics and these specific boundary constructs impact ethical client/practitioner scenarios in Chapter 5.

Practical somatic tips for beginning a session

- Start at the wall and conduct a very thorough medical intake while on land.
- Track your clients while in a vertical position in the water.
- Explain specifically how the session will begin and end and give permission to state if there is anything that needs to be adjusted during the session.
- Suggest that your client focuses on their breathing and closes their eyes to get more in tune with the internal world of their body.
- Apply proper leg floats as needed.
- Gently transition your client to a horizontal position on the water's surface, so as not to elicit a startle reflex.
- Observe some of the first micro-neurodevelopmental movement patterns that are reminiscent of the first motor patterns from conception. Movements can be seen in the neck and the mouth and reach deep into the coccyx bone and undulate up the spinal column.
- During a session, never make assumptions about what was felt, expressed or experienced.
- While witnessing, do not project your own experiences onto your client.
- Maintain healthy boundaries.
- Somatic listening does not only include the sense organ of the ears but the use of your kinesthetic and visual awareness.
- Engage your sensory awareness as a practitioner by utilizing a soft gaze that not only sees and feels directly in front of you but encapsulates and surrounds you and your client.

Client safety

While doing somatic-based or interoceptive practices, there are many emotions that can rise to the surface like *grief*, *sadness*, *joy* and *pain*. One of the most common emotions is *fear*. Referring back to our Chinese Medicine texts, we understand that the water element is associated with the organs of the Kidney and the Urinary Bladder meridians and the emotion of fear. Being in water and being floated on your back requires a great deal of trust in your practitioner and even a form of self-trust within the client's mind. The water can be a healing place but also a vulnerable one as well. We also must assess and determine if there are any past near-death drowning episodes as a child or adult because these experiences can also cause fear and sometimes those experiences that have been numbed can come back up in a session. Water represents the unknown and what may or may not happen within the moment due to its flowing and ever-changing nature. The other obvious safety precautions that would preclude a client from receiving treatment are covered in Chapter 2, as well as a variety of special needs and neurodiverse populations that a practitioner may encounter in somatic aquatic practice.

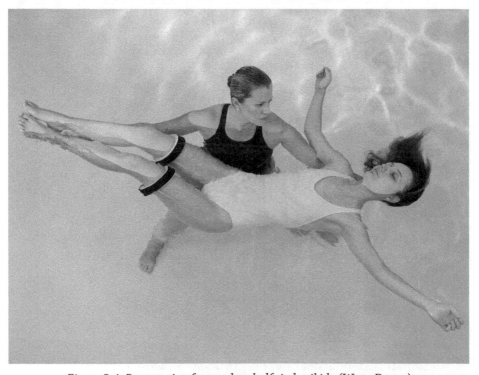

Figure 3.4: Preparation for two legs half circle aikido (WaterDance)

Below are some observations that can be seen when the emotions of fear or *uncertainty* are present and clients are presenting in a destabilizing sympathetic state during a WATSU session, with methods to stabilize back to a parasympathetic response from the role as practitioner. Again, these destabilizing responses will be channeled through the eyes, facial expressions/grimaces, voice, holding patterns, breath, skin, reflexes and heart rate.

Client cues to look for
Destabilizing sympathetic state (of the client)

- An inability to maintain eye contact during the initial session on land or in water during the medical intake process.
- A low voice or rapid speech during the intake process.
- Rigid holding patterns while being moved into flexor and extensor planes of movement.
- Rapid or shallow breathing and no increase in depth of respiration as the session continues.
- Flushed skin color on neck or face or other parts of the body.
- Opening eyes during a session.
- A startle reflex may be present even if a practitioner is being very sensitive with the head and its position.
- Rapid heart rate.

Stabilizing to a parasympathetic response (by the practitioner)

- Connect back to the breath.
- Readjust movements and support of the body in the water as needed.
- Slow down the movements.
- Make sure that you have thoroughly explained what will happen before the session begins as well as what positioning you may place your client in as the session ends.
- Make sure your client knows that they can stop the session at any time.
- Initiate linear movements that can be very calming to the central nervous system.

Practical somatic tips for ending a session
- Provide a sense of somatic grounding from the element of water to the element of earth for your client. As an example, the wall is an ideal place to end a session by planting your client's feet and having them feel the surface of the wall at their back as they begin to open their eyes.

- Some therapists choose to be positioned outside of the gaze of their client's direct visual field if their eyes are not yet opened after a session so their client has privacy and personal space to process what just transpired in the water. You might consider being off to the left or the right side of your client's midline at the completion of a session. This may also be an ideal time to energetically utilize any rituals or movements that may remind you as a practitioner of the boundary that is between you and the client.
- Give pause to wait for your client to speak first and give feedback about their water experience before you provide your feedback. This strategy honors what was experienced and felt and gives them agency to freely have an opportunity to express their "felt" somatic experience.
- Let your client have space to not judge them or know what has transpired.
- Always refer to mental health professional(s) if you feel the client's emotional or psychological needs are moving out of your scope and provide the necessary resources as needed.
- Align yourself with other healthcare practitioners that you would trust your client receiving physical, spiritual, emotional or psychological services from as needed.

Childhood trauma

Research suggests that childhood trauma or early life adversity (ELA) may cause disturbances in body-brain signaling accuracy within the mechanism of interoceptive processing and is a major determiner of mental health. "Early life adversity (ELA) may cause permanent disturbances in brain–body signaling. These disturbances are thought to contribute to physical symptoms and emotional dysregulation in adulthood" (Schaan *et al.* 2019). The current study investigated the effects of childhood trauma on young adults' interoceptive accuracy as an indicator of brain–body communication that may be dysregulated by ELA. Sixty-six participants completed an online questionnaire followed by a laboratory session including the socially evaluated cold pressor stress test during which ECG, salivary cortisol, and interoceptive accuracy were assessed. Childhood trauma was negatively related to interoceptive accuracy (IAc) after the stressor.

The conclusion of this study reveals that childhood trauma is associated with lower IAc after an acute stressor, which may be explained by higher trait unpleasantness. The findings support current models of chronic stress induced malfunctions of neural circuits underlying successful brain–body communication. This finding may facilitate the development of prevention strategies targeting children who experienced childhood trauma with the aim to raise awareness to stress-induced bodily changes over time and thereby enabling them to better differentiate cardiac signals from the stream of ascending bodily signals. This may have helped them to "(a) better differentiate emotions from bodily changes and thereby to (b) better perceive and regulate their emotions" (Schaan *et al.* 2019).

This study reveals that the more trauma a person experiences in childhood, the less accurate that person will be in perceiving and understanding their interoceptive processes. This is worth noting since clients will most likely be coming into the water environment with a host of past experiences and likely traumas from across the lifespan or possibly childhood traumas that we or they may not fully understand in the moment. Our ability to recognize these aspects of sensory processing and the many spectrums of trauma will strengthen our compassion and equally our professional boundaries and clinical awareness. Somatic listening does not just happen with the auditory input and subjective information and health history that our clients tell us alone, it comes from tracking the body from the moment they first walk through our doors and into our pools. As we float our clients we watch their expression, breath patterns, movement tendencies and state of calm or even state of distress, becoming a witness is one of our primary objectives. Sometimes our client's experiences can be explicit and obvious, but other times what lies beneath can be quite subtle, but the magnitude just as profound. Trauma can occlude our client from fully feeling grounded and inside their body and these traumatic experiences present in a variety of ways. One may deeply feel the weight of the world while others may feel numb, shut out, or disconnected from the life around them. Ultimately, trauma detracts from the present context of self and the client's interaction with everyday life. The compensatory patterns that exist may be more internal or external, but often a tapestry of both elements can appear in sessions. Tapping into self-perception, introspection and organizing one's own internal and external triggers is key for practitioners to fully understand where clients may be on the continuum of interoceptive awareness and processing.

WATSU and aquatic bodywork benefits for post-traumatic stress disorder

PTSD can present itself in a variety of forms that can include childhood trauma or combine with other life adversities. A mixed-methods study that was done by Healing Wave Aquatic (formerly known as The Wave Academy) with Johns Hopkins University (Corcoran *et al.* 2016) found that aquatic bodywork was helpful in decreasing the wounds of trauma. A total of 15 participants who experienced a traumatic event related to military duty and who were being treated for PTSD participated in a one-hour aquatic therapy session for eight weeks. A variety of assessments were used to track PTSD symptoms including a Life Events Checklist (LEC), Post Traumatic Growth Inventory (PTGI), PTSD Checklist-Military

(PCL-M), Profile of Mood States (POMS) and Functional Assessment of Chronic Illness Therapy-Spiritual (FACIT-SP). PTSD symptoms measured by the PCL-M changed significantly ($p \leq 0.1$) over the eight-week period, but symptoms were not significant when compared to the other assessments. There were also significant changes in participants' POMS scores when baseline and week eight results were compared. What is most interesting, and also in alignment with the essence of WATSU, is the qualitative feedback from this same study. After clients' feedback was analyzed, the four most prominent themes, relaxation, self-reflection, body-awareness and reduction of symptoms, underscore the signature phenomenological and embodied experience of the practice. WATSU practitioners contributed to the qualitative segment of the study as well, and findings confirm the experience of witnessing and noting changes related to clients' sense of self as described in this chapter. The notion that WATSU facilitates reflection and self-awareness was supported by providers who shared: "Client was very relaxed and at ease in the water. Seemed to be able to drop into a space of deep relaxation. Very comfortable to work with" (relaxation); "She has had consistent shifts, healing and releasing in each session has been amazing to witness and hold[ing] space for her in the warm water therapy pool" (client progress). Other clients added: "[I was] able to be more aware, and clear on how my body felt"; "The water session helped a lot to bring calmness...the water help[ed] bring out a physical pain...I couldn't pinpoint, but now I can." Overall, these comments illuminate the transformative aspect of the practice, revealing the ways in which clients are able to drop deeper into awareness as facilitated by the witnessing gaze of the observant practitioner.

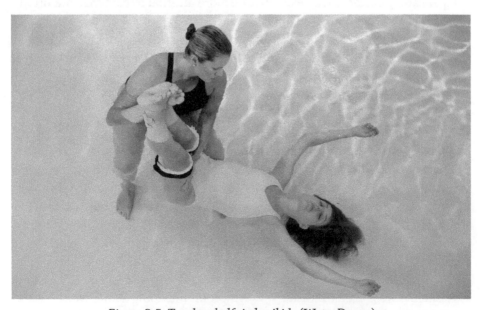

Figure 3.5: Two legs half circle aikido (WaterDance)

The historian (*client*) and the narrative listener (*therapist*) within embodied practice

In the water, clients have the ability to become better historians, or to deepen their ability to frame their past trauma experience by gradually decreasing their triggers and sympathetic response within the present moment of their lives. These positive improvements toward self-regulation can also be mirrored by our ability as practitioners to not only witness but listen to their narrative after a session has ended. Hippocrates articulated one of the founding principles of narrative medicine and listening, stating, "It is more important to know what sort of person has a disease than to know what sort of disease a person has" (Hippocrates Health Institute 2014). In order for practitioners to truly be effective with their clients, they must listen. A client's "felt" sense of being heard is paramount in the healing process not only within their water experience but how their collective somatic experiences are integrated and better understood between water sessions. It is about understanding the meaning of the client's experience and their storyline, not just what symptoms preclude them from obtaining optimal well-being but acknowledging their health story. In order to deliver compassionate care, practitioners must be equipped with strong verbal and non-verbal communication skills to navigate the waters of narrative listening. This reflects yet another qualitative element while using approaches like WATSU and other aquatic forms of therapy.

Clients are able to access memories and experiences in a safe manner through the therapeutic benefits of water, and process these through their many stages. Sometimes, individuals cannot see the depth of their flight, fight, freeze, fawn or "sensory overload," and "disconnection" since they have been functioning in a hypervigilant or disassociative state with a compensatory strategy for some time. We also must take note that when these first compensatory strategies were devised when a trauma occurred in a client's experience this is what kept them from avoiding pain, danger and obtaining some sense of safety. We must be sensitive to the pervasive nature and progression of these strategies and just witness them in the many states of self-preservation. However, when they experience a state of calm, we might observe that they are able to look at their trauma with a softened eye, mind and heart while a new neural pathway grows to better process the wounds of trauma and separation. Getting back in the body requires a proper safety net from the practitioner as witnessing and acknowledgement can awaken and deepen a therapeutic state or "healing crisis." A new and healthier perception can grow within the client's mind, body and heart when the imminent threat that no longer exists is acknowledged in the context of a client's present environment. As a client continues to have more of these states of calm or parasympathetic activation, with time they learn tools to better process trauma and narrate their trauma story in a safe and lasting way that helps to provide healing on a very deep level which extends outside the confines of a therapy pool. As practitioners, one way to think of this process of homeostasis that begins to re-regulate within this ocean of self in the context of a safe environment is to ask a question: *Within the client's somatic experience, is the action (stimulus) from the current outside world with no imminent danger equal to the current reaction (response) within the context of the present moment?* This homeostasis, re-regulation or therapeutic integration process should also be addressed outside the confines of the pool to further determine how the CNS is re-regulated and responding to proprioceptive and environmental inputs. Partnering up with other integrative medicine team members who specialize in cognitive behavioral therapies and psychological and somatic services is essential. We dive deeper into how the presentation of trauma permeates birth, childhood, attachment, PTSD and family constellations within a client's somatic experience in Chapter 4.

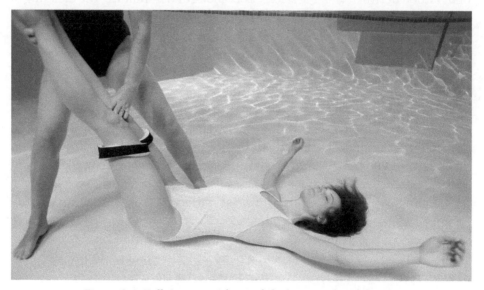

Figure 3.6: Full immersion (toward the bottom of pool, letting the hips touch before the head) (WaterDance)

Non-ordinary states or altered states of consciousness

As mentioned previously, non-ordinary states or altered states of consciousness may be reached by clients during WATSU/Sub-Aquatic or other related aquatic sessions. Some of these states may include but are not limited to:

- re-living past experiences and memories
- mystical experiences

- a lapse in the sense of space and time
- theta brainwave activating meditative states
- optical cortex colors or images
- emotional release during or after a session
- increasing depth of respiration
- a sense of catharsis
- a sense of oneness
- a deeper felt sense of self.

These experiences with non-ordinary states of consciousness can help clients examine new pathways toward self-actualization, flexible thinking, a sense of oneness and an opening of the mind and heart toward new perceptions of self-healing. These new and altered experiences can penetrate or alter old mind-sets or compensatory patterns that were once created and executed during a traumatic experience to help them feel safe but are now maladaptive and ineffective in the present context of their healing journey.

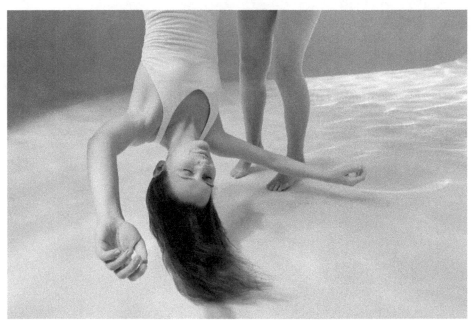

Figure 3.7: Two legs half aikido (with both legs out of the water, bringing client into total inversion) (WaterDance)

Therapeutic integration: A multimodal approach to embodied practice

A constellation of archetypes within altered states of consciousness can intertwine with the interoceptive experiences in a profound manner during an aquatic session. Images may flood the mind and emotions may flood the body. A deeper sense of keeping in alignment with WATSU practitioners' scope of practice, it is key to seek other ways clients can digest and process these experiences outside the container of the aquatic environment. Utilizing a multimodal approach to therapeutically integrate may help a client to further understand and express their experience between sessions. It is imperative for practitioners to provide these resources that provide mutual reinforcement and embodiment with aquatic bodywork treatment and improve interoceptive awareness and processing by enhancing integration through nervous system and emotional regulation. These are just some of the clinical services and self-regulation practices that clients can or may be already engaging in when they begin their treatment with aquatic practitioners. These modalities and practices can be utilized to further enhance a client's ability to integrate their experiences during, after, and between water sessions:

- cognitive behavioral therapies
- psychotherapy
- Pranayama practices
- psychedelic-assisted therapies
- EMDR
- talk therapy
- trauma sensitive or informed somatic yoga
- art therapy
- meditation
- acupuncture and Chinese Medicine
- journaling
- music therapy
- equine-assisted psychotherapy
- spiritual practices
- prayer
- forest bathing
- Somatic Experiencing
- tapping.

We emphasize that WATSU is not always a stand-alone therapy. Psychological, physiological, humanistic, mind-body and spiritual approaches can intersect and reinforce improved self-regulation, quality of life and the continuum of care toward positive therapeutic response for our clients. What we see in practice is that clients may need other resources outside the pool that bridge the gap in their care. Communicating with other allied health professionals with consent from your client can also build a team approach that is integrative, interdisciplinary, patient-centered and compassion-driven. Investigating and creating relationships with other practitioners with varying scopes is key to effective and successful somatic aquatic practice.

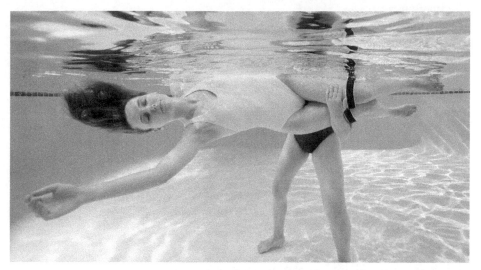

Figure 3.8: Knee snake facing away (WaterDance)

Summary

In the deepest waters of somatic aquatic practice, aquatic practitioners must hone their craft to provide a viable trajectory toward a client's deepest interoceptive examination and knowing of their body's internal "felt" sense. A centeredness that is steeped and embodied in appropriate modulation of the senses for each client's unique needs, medical history and life experiences. WATSU, and its related aquatic bodywork forms, is indeed a somatic aquatic tool for deepened interoceptive embodiment within the ocean of self that flows from the container of somatic practice. The call to the water awaits, for our clients to intimately commune with their interoceptive sense of self and align with the deepest depths of oneness. Our primary intention as practitioners is to be observers and net holders while our clients engage in this ritual or act of completion and union with wholeness. Lastly, we would like to give gratitude and thanks to Dr. Theresa Silow, PhD, LPCC, Somatic Psychologist and Professor of Somatic Psychology at the California Institute of Integral Studies in San Francisco, California, for her many inspiring insights during this chapter's creation.

References

Chen, W. (2021). *Interoception and Health: New Journal Article and Funding Opportunity*. National Center for Complementary and Integrative Health. Blog, January 22, 2021. www.nccih.nih.gov/research/blog/interoception-and-health-new-journal-article-and-funding-opportunity?nav=govd.

Ceunen, E., Vlaeyen, J.W. & Van Diest, I. (2016). On the Origin of Interoception. *Frontiers in Psychology*, 7, 743.

Conrad, E. (1998). *Life on Land*. Santa Monica: Continuum.

Corcoran, R., O'Flaherty, J., Morrissey, L., Ross, S.M. & Cheung, A.C.K. (2016). An evaluation of the Wave Academy approach to reducing post-traumatic stress disorder. *Journal of Education & Social Policy*, 3(4): 36–42.

Feinstein, J.S., Khalsa, S.S., Yeh, H., Al Zoubi, O. *et al.* (2018). The elicitation of relaxation and interoceptive awareness using floatation therapy in individuals with high anxiety sensitivity. *Biological Psychiatry: Cognitive Neuroscience and Neuroimaging*, 3(6): 555–562.

Gintis, B. (2007) *Engaging the Movement of Life*. Berkeley: North Atlantic Books.

Hanna, T. (1986). What is somatics? *Somatics: Magazine-Journal of the Bodily Arts and Sciences*. Accessed November 17, 2014.

Hippocrates Health Institute (2014). Treating the Person. Accessed July 16, 2014.

National Institutes of Health (n.d.). *Interoception Research*. www.nccih.nih.gov/about/nccih-strategic-plan-2021-2025/top-scientific-priorities/interoception-research.

Silow, T. (2010). *Integral Theory in Action: Applied, Theoretical, and Constructive Perspectives on the AQAL Model*. New York, NY: State University of New York.

Stern, D.N. (1990). *The Diary of a Baby*. New York: Basic Books..

Chapter 4

The Imprint of Trauma

How the Body Shows the Story

KAREN DAVID AND MARY SEAMSTER

We would like to place a stipulation for those reading this chapter on trauma and somatic therapy in water. Please note this is not a how-to chapter that allows you to go out and practice outside your scope of practice (SOP). Please remain inside your professional scope and get additional training when needed. The persons involved in this chapter have extensive training in both body-centered psychotherapy and working with emotional trauma in water. Clients are primarily referred by therapists and an agreement is signed between all parties allowing practitioners to share clients' information. Finding a referring therapist is of the upmost importance in being able to facilitate these very complex circumstances.

Imprints description from the teachings from Anna and John Chitty[1]

Description of trauma

When a person experiences deeply distressing events, their ability to cope may be overwhelmed. Such trauma may result in feelings of helplessness, diminishing their sense of self and creating blocks that inhibit human potential. They may experience symptoms of fear, denial or shame, leading to nightmares, emotional outbursts, insomnia, depression, anxiety, dissociative disorders or substance abuse problems, which are hallmarks of post-traumatic stress disorder (PTSD). Fragments of memories from the earlier traumatic events can surface, causing the person to become disorganized and dysregulated in

---

1   Anna and John Chitty are the co-founders of the Colorado School of Energy Studies, a school for somatic and energy therapies.

their daily lives. Not everyone who experiences trauma develops PTSD. Our primitive brain, or limbic system, holds the memories that we don't consciously recall (implicit memories) as well as those that we do remember and that continue to cause us pain (explicit memories). PTSD can disrupt the autonomic nervous system (ANS) by constantly activating the limbic system as if the person were still in the trauma. The ANS may get stuck in constant alert or in constant shutdown, affecting body systems of the blood, liver, kidneys, spleen, hormones, immune system, skin and joints.

Dysregulation of the ANS and PTSD are believed to be the cause of illness, according to Maté (2003) and Levine (2010). Examples of trauma capable of ANS dysregulation include but are not limited to: stress in utero, physical or emotional injury, natural disaster, bullying, childhood maltreatment, epigenetics, war and environmental stressors. Underlying resentment and anger are a part of suppressed emotions, which Gabor Maté (2003) believes are the root of many illnesses. One can ask, "What did we have to do to stay alive?" Maté believes the strategies employed to stay alive contribute to illnesses or addictions later in life. We have stored the emotions and kept the strategies—the depression, self-medication, isolation and anxiety.

Jiang *et al.* (2019), in their article "Epigenetic modifications in stress response genes associated with childhood trauma," talk about adverse childhood experiences (ACEs). We recommend you visit the website of the American Society for the Positive Care of Children (American SPCC) and look at/take the quiz.[2] The quiz covers questions such as: "Did a parent or other adult in the household often or very often... a) Swear at you, insult you, put you down, or humiliate you? or b) Act in a way that made you afraid that you might be physically hurt?" It goes on to ask whether you had enough to eat, or whether your parents were too drunk or high that you were neglected. Caveat, it does not take into consideration community violence, racism, discrimination and housing insecurity, issues which are presently at the forefront of our society. After taking the quiz, if you responded yes to two or more of the questions, it is posited that you are more likely to be unable to face challenges in your daily life. To further elucidate this, it adds, "Most studies have shown that unrelated to the traumatic event, additional risk factors for developing PTSD include younger age at the time of the trauma, female gender, lower social economic status, lack of social support, and premorbid personality characteristics (personality traits existing prior to illness and or injury)." Clients who come under these risk factors are likely to develop a subsequent PTSD in the wake of a new trauma.

When trauma is inflicted in circumstances where we cannot fight back—being raped or spanked, or even having medical/dental work—the ability to escape gets trapped inside, resulting in excessive tension. Peter Levine (2010)

2   https://americanspcc.org/take-the-aces-quiz

has explored this in his work, tailoring therapy at just such tension—allowing the client to move in ways that they might have used to escape at the time of the trauma. Traumatic implicit memories can be experienced as overwhelming emotions such as despair, shame, self-loathing, helplessness rage and chronic hypervigilance.

Please refer to our chapter on AMNION as it is inexorably intertwined with this chapter.

Epigenetics: Ancestral trauma

Aristotle noted, "One who sees things from the beginning will have the finest view of them."

When studying with Ray Castellino,[3] we learned that when our grand-mothers were in their fifth month of pregnancy with our mothers, the precursor cell of the egg that we developed from was already present in our mothers' ovaries. Therefore, it is theorized that three generations of genetic memory are stored in each and every one of us.

In his book *It Didn't Start with You*, Mark Wolynn (2016, p.19) states, "Scientists are now able to identify biological markers evidence that traumas can and do pass down from one generation to the next." Here's how: trauma can leave a chemical mark on a person's genes, which can then be passed down to future generations. This mark doesn't cause a genetic mutation, but it does alter the mechanism by which the gene is expressed. This alteration is not genetic, but *epigenetic*. He talks about Rachel Yehuda's research on the effects of intergenerational PTSD. Yehuda, a professor of psychiatry at Mount Sinai School of Medicine in New York, has done numerous studies examining the neurobiology of PTSD in Holocaust survivors and their children (Yehuda & Seckl 2011). The researchers were able to trace hormonal levels (cortisol, the stress hormone) in the Holocaust survivors and found that "children of Holocaust survivors who had PTSD were born with low cortisol levels similar to their parents'; predisposing them to relive the PTSD symptoms of the previous generation" (Yehuda & Seckl 2011).

I (Mary) have been extremely lucky to have clients referred to me from several well-respected therapists. Each time I meet a client for the first time and conduct an intake, I'm intrigued by how the themes of the long-deceased great-grandparents or living grandparents are showing up in the physical structure and emotional bodies. Most times the body just is showing signs of chronic physical ailments such as irritable bowel syndrome, autoimmune disorders, headaches, joint pain and the like. The primary reason they have come these last few years during the pandemic is for chronic anxiety and systemic overload/overwhelm.

---

3   www.castellinotraining.com/foundation

Recently, a client came complaining that they had a lack of compass or orientation and were having difficulty moving forward through a challenging transitional portion of their life. They found themselves lost in their daily lives, knowing they were in a transition, but they weren't able to find a way to move forward. Themes of annihilation, despair, collapse and abandonment kept the client from finding their own resources and potency to take action. The puzzle piece that gave us the biggest clue was when the client told the story about how their grandmother had called her daughter (the client's mother) to let her know she had just killed her husband (grandfather). While still on the phone with the client's mother, the grandmother proceeded to kill herself. *Pause to take this in.* From this story, it's easy to trace the epigenetics of her ancestral trauma. The client was conceived in the pre-embryogenetic soup of her mother's trauma. As we commenced to work in the pool, the trauma tension field began to have less impact on the client. By the end of the two-hour session, she stood up and said, "I now know I'm strong enough to face whatever is coming my way. I am not my mother's trauma. I am differentiated and am able to find a new way forward. I feel stronger and more capable to carry forth the tasks of transition."

This is not the only client who has suffered debilitating trauma, but it's different when it's passed down epigenetically. Clients often speak of having had no actual trauma in this lifetime's memory, no incest, no medical interventions at an early age, no physical or emotional abuse and no war experience. Their bodies tell a different story. The woven matrix of their ancestors permeates the structure in their adult bodies. When they walk into the pool, they bring with them the hurts and also joys of their respective family members.

When clients show up at our pools

When a client shows up for the first time in our pool, we assess their readiness to receive a session. Not everyone is ready to give up the control of their body to the water, let alone to a stranger. Going from a vertical stance, feet on the ground, lying supine can be a daunting undertaking. In these sessions, a client can remain vertical throughout, or at most just be floated in head cradle and noodle, with no contact, just presence and attunement. As practitioners, we look for clues which tell us whether they are in a sympathetic response or a parasympathetic response. Most common responses to trauma are fight, flight or freeze. During a fight-flight-freeze response, many physiological changes occur. The reaction begins in the amygdala, the part of the brain responsible for perceived fear. The amygdala responds by sending signals to the hypothalamus, which stimulates the autonomic nervous system. The ANS consists of the sympathetic and parasympathetic nervous systems. The sympathetic nervous system drives the fight or flight response, while the parasympathetic nervous system drives the freeze response. How you react to the perceived threat depends on which system dominates the response at the time.

What should we look for in our clients? Do they arrive agitated, speedy or dysregulated? Do they have difficulty stringing clear, coherent sentences concerning a sequence of events? Do they come speaking about their anger, their annihilative rage, with their jaws tight, and are they wanting to take on a fight? This is evidence of the client being in a sympathetic response. A fight response is self-preservation no matter who you hurt in the process. The client has the perceived threat that they are in imminent danger and the situation is life threatening. Their body braces for an oncoming perceived blow and they quickly respond with a counter jab. With these kinds of clients, we have to take care that we do not become the focus of the perceived attack. Finding a neutral tone of voice, kind eyes and a warm welcoming demeanor can often lessen the fight response.

Do we recognize when our client arrives with a flight response? They complain of having restless legs at night, and their eyes dart furtively around the pool as if looking for the threat. They circumambulate around us in a large swath, sometimes making us feel slightly dizzy trying to follow them. Are they prone to doing excessive exercise routines and always on the go? With these clients we would use a more soothing touch, and do more cranial sacral-like contact. We want to quieten not stimulate the nervous system.

Commonly, our clients come in a freeze response; they complain of feeling stuck in their lives, and in their bodies. Their skin looks pale and lifeless, their breath is shallow, they have the experience of being cold, frozen and numb. They undergo times in the session and in their lives where they become dissociative, disappear and become helpless. It's important to track this in our clients as being dissociative can lead to recapitulation of the original insult. Make sure prior to ending the session that you have brought them back to the present day and time.

Neck-hold information

A common characteristic of trauma held in the body is a frozen startle reflex. A frozen startle reflex is where the neck and head are slightly thrust backwards. Babies are born with an involuntary startle reflex. The majority of babies lose their startle response, also known as Moro reflex, at about three to six months. The startle reflex can remain in adults and mimic the classic flight, fight or freeze response. In a 2009 study, Jovanovic *et al.* found that early childhood trauma can have an increased risk for adult psychopathology: "Increased startle may be a biomarker of stress responsiveness that can be a persevering consequence of early trauma exposure during childhood."

The necks of our clients "bear the burden." Robert Scaer (2001), in his book *The Body Bears the Burden*, talks about how clients will come in with repeated traumatic vehicular accidents. When he sees that each accident recapitulates the same pattern of a previous event, he questions what the original wound was that the client is attempting to recreate. In his book, he mentions the use of WATSU as being beneficial for unearthing the original held impact—the impact that keeps being played out until it's recognized and seen. Water is an excellent medium for unraveling the trauma from the tissue. Early on one client stated, "The experience of it (trauma) releasing from my tissue, and the freedom for the physical and the emotional bodies to re-organize, is very profound."

Neck structure often tells their birth story; were there complications at birth? Was the baby born with an umbilical cord wound tightly around the neck? Did mom have to have an emergency c-section? Was there mishandling or mis-attunement by the medical professionals? We often hear about clients as babies being dropped by distracted caregivers. Since these are all pre-verbal experiences, there are no words, just memories embedded in the nervous system. The skilled handling of the practitioner helps dissolve the freeze and move the stuck energy out, discharging through the limbs. As freedom is more fully embodied, the client can be seen kicking their feet. We often see what looks like the ability to run away from imminent danger. They come out of their sessions more alive, more potent and more seen.

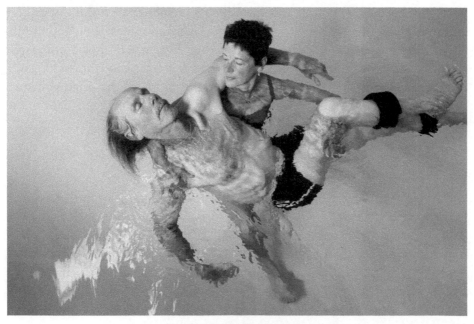

Figure 4.1: Parkinson client

Holding a boundary

When we first start working with a client, we assess their ability to hold a boundary. Boundaries that keep us safe can be affected by early trauma. Most trauma clients need to be made aware of the sphere around them, their personal space. Personal space is where their edge meets "other." If a client is able to establish themselves within their comfortable boundary, they are more likely not to disassociate, hide or disintegrate. They will find a way to stay present and in real time.

For example, let the client choose where they wish to be in the pool. Find just the right place that makes them orient to safety and trust you as a practitioner. Circumambulate the client with a distance of two arm lengths. You will note where the boundary of the client pulls you in and where the boundary pushes you away. This exploration is done at a snail's pace, with the practitioner keeping a close eye to changes in breathing, skin color and facial expressions. Do not move not too close, nor too far away.

Having the client drop inside into their felt sense of the space around them can be an exciting first step to creating ease in the system. This is a great way to come into relationship with the client and also to palpate where the original breaches to the protective boundary occurred.

As practitioners, we have seen breaches in a client's boundary that originated in utero. There can be a myriad of reasons why this illusive boundary is ruptured. Fetus/client can have the recollection of when Dad beat Mom while she was pregnant. As a client unfolds their personal gestures in the water, we see them turn away from the violence and they try to hide. At times, the one in the womb wants to protect Mom from inside. All attempts to save Mom or other family members from imminent violence are futile as they are not able to move. Some of the words they use to express this is "It's like waking up from an extremely long dream...like those dreams when there's danger but you can't run or can only run in slow motion."

Overview of somatic psychology literature
Definition

Somatic psychology is the psychology "of" the body (rather than "about" or "at" the body), focusing on the living experience of embodiment as human beings. This new approach to a vision of the psyche concerning the human experience may indicate a profound change in our understanding of what it means to be human. In application, somatic therapies rely on the vital exchange between psychological and physical states and symptoms, based on how the mind and body interact. Proponents of this therapy believe a person's beliefs, feelings, thoughts and attitudes can have an impact on how their body functions.

Diet and exercise and some traumatic events are external physical factors which may also impact a person's mental and emotional state. According to somatic therapy theory, the sensations associated with past trauma may become lodged within the body and reflected in a person's expressions, pain, postures or other forms of body language. Talk therapy can help address trauma, but in some cases therapeutic body techniques can provide a more holistic healing approach, resulting in increased self-awareness, and the resolution of psychological concerns without the need for resolving deep-rooted mental health issues.

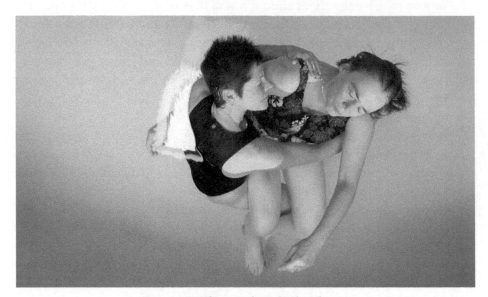

Figure 4.2: Client with Multiple Sclerosis

History of somatic therapies

While somatic psychotherapies are not yet a well-integrated discipline, they are founded on ancient sources. Asian philosophies tend to offer a more holistic view of the body, with yoga, Tai Chi and Qigong practices cultivating awareness and use of the breath to awaken the senses and obtain the free flow of spiritual and emotional energies. Indigenous cultures worldwide impart notions that "the entire universe exists within the energetic composition of every human body" and "the subtle energies of our embodiment impact the entire universe" (Barratt 2010, p.113). Western development and establishment of somatic psychotherapy occurred in the early 1900s with the work of Wilhelm Reich (Hinchley 2010), a former student of Sigmund Freud. Reich believed repressed emotions and even an individual's personality are reflected in muscular tension, posture and physical movement. He believed the use of physical pressure was needed as a therapeutic method for a person to achieve emotional release. Others built on his work, incorporating the connection of mind and body to facilitate a more holistic approach to the treatment of trauma. (Often, psychology systems tended to treat the body as a mute "thing" whose chaotic impulses had to be managed by the organized structures of the brain, rather than recognized as a source of wisdom to which we might listen.) Currently, somatic psychotherapy has expanded significantly as the theory of body-mind connections has become more popular and mainstream. Some of these approaches include Hakomi, Somatic Experiencing, EMDR, biodynamics, Feldenkrais, Alexander technique, Continuum and AMNION aquatics to name a few. (You can review the website of the European Association for Body Psychotherapy[4] or of the United States Association for Body Psychotherapy[5] to get a sense of the scope of the practitioners and training organizations in this field.)

There is often an inherent bias against the efficacy of somatic therapies within a scientific community that values only "evidence-based" findings that are externally observable and measurable and appear to be the result of a unilateral manipulation. However, qualitative studies should be defended. Anecdotal evidence may not meet the narrow standards of evidence, but they do provide a valuable sense of processes involved that are neither public nor readily measurable. The personal value to the patient is often just as important as a measured outcome. The case study included in Chapter 14, is an example of how qualitative findings can impact quality of life measures. Such case studies are necessary to ascertain some sense of what is involved in processes that are neither public nor readily measurable.

Implicit memories and neurobiology

Implicit memories are those we don't consciously recall; they exist just below the level of conscious awareness and are difficult to identify. Explicit memories have a beginning, middle and end, and we are aware they have happened. Implicit memories include conditioning of autonomic responses, procedural memory derived from skills and habits, and reflex pathways. More primitive brain areas contain implicit memories including behavioral, protective and emotional components (Siegel 2015). These memories appear, for example, when our heart begins to race when in a setting similar to where some trauma occurred, even before we are consciously aware of the similarity of the setting. This is the primitive response of the limbic system of the brain. We may not remember the actual event, but our body contains the story and will respond with a movement toward or away from a cue, and our emotions will tell us if we feel safe or not. Our body responds to what is unconscious in implicit memory and can induce feelings and sensations

---

4   https://eabp.org
5   https://usabp.org

that have more to do with the memory than the current situation (Cappuzzi & Gross 2010). Bringing to light physical representations of implicit memories which existed in shadow can give patients greater freedom to think, feel and act in the present (van der Kolk *et al.* 2014). The human neocortex can integrate a great variety of information, to attach meaning to the input and to apply logical thought. When a person physically acts out an implicit memory, they have the chance to integrate this experience by recognizing what happened in the past, and what is happening now, and the choices they have. This integration allows people to discover new ways of modifying their responses based on the information they discover. Neuroimaging studies of veterans who experienced PTSD following multiple deployments showed hyperarousal in the primitive, reactive areas of the brain and hypoactivity in their neocortex activity (Weber *et al.* 2005). They have difficulty being fully engaged in the present. Implicit memories or past traumas can disrupt the ANS by constantly activating the limbic system as if the person were still in the trauma, causing chronic stress that manifests as physical symptoms (Schore 2003). Somatic therapy may help the ANS to begin working more optimally by dampening the more defensive systems of the ANS and facilitating more social behavior (Porges 2015).

Perception

Perception is part of the implicit memory and categorized as a pleasant or unpleasant experience. When we remember a pleasant event, the implicit memory is felt in our body with warmth and happiness. Pleasant experiences may become a resource for future relationships: an experience to tap into to feel warmth and happiness time and again. In the case of unpleasant experiences, it is the wash of shame or the fear that our body remembers and experiences that causes us pain, rather than the actual event itself. Effective therapy helps a client seek relief from the body memory when the intellectual mind knows that the real threat is no longer there. With implicit memories, it is important to encourage the client to recognize that it is their neurobiology that isn't supporting a life that pleases them, rather than something being wrong with them. Once a client can be lifted out of shame, a connection can begin. Bonnie Badenoch (2008) speaks of how a practitioner can meet a client empathically; that is, meet them where their need is at the moment. The technique is not to teach them, but to meet them where the pain is.

Polyvagal theory

Polyvagal theory describes neurobiologically why "meeting a client" is so critical. The ANS regulates fight and flight (as we have been traditionally taught), but also connection with others (social nervous system through the vagus nerve). Connections between people and the role of the vagus nerve is an important basis for mind-body medicine.

Stephen Porges (2007) has described how polyvagal theory explains what is happening physiologically in the different parts of the vagus nerve and how people respond to connection. The vagus nerve acts bi-directionally by giving and receiving information about safety and connection (Porges & Furman 2011). The nerve is comprised of 20 percent motor neurons and 80 percent sensory neurons, providing us with continual information about what is happening in the body as well as controlling body functions. The more ancient branch of the vagus nerve enervates the regions below the diaphragm and comes into play with sympathetic nervous system activation. A myelinated, more modern branch of the vagus nerve system innervates the striated muscles of the face, heart, ears and throat (voice). It is these features of the autonomic nervous system that allows us to receive cues from others about safety and connection. One can activate the parasympathetic nervous system to freeze (primitive, unmyelinated portion), but also to connect with others (modern, myelinated portion of the vagus nerve). People need each other. When something unexpected or threatening happens, people will look around and see how other people are responding to the potential threat. Babies do this all the time, and if the caregiver is calm, the baby will learn to be calm too. This regulation happens by using the neuro-regulation of the face and other structures at and above the heart in response to a threat. A person will turn to social interactions to monitor stress and transition to calmness or action. If a person is left alone or overpowered, their nervous system turns to more primitive methods of reaction, and either flees or shuts down. This primitive system comes online only when the modern system (social nervous system) is not present or perceives a threat. Connecting socially with others is a neurological response that helps humans manage stressors and supports resilience. Listening and witnessing is a part of reciprocal behavior. When a person feels safe, they are accessing parts of the brain not available when activated in fight, flight or freeze. A person can then be creative and bold. This state of having the social nervous system engaged and being connected to others becomes a resource because a person knows they can use social behavior to calm themselves. When a person is in this state, they are receptive to kindness and understanding in the eyes, faces and speech of others.

Attachment

People develop their social behaviors initially with their primary caregiver as they form their early attachment relationships. The state of the primary caregiver's nervous system and brain has a powerful imprint on the child's brain patterning. If a parent is responsive and emotionally attuned at least 30 percent of the time, the baby will likely develop a *secure attachment* (Ainsworth 1969). If a parent is indifferent, absent or critical, the child will likely have an *insecure-avoidant attachment style*, withdrawing from personal interactions and being uncomfortable with intimacy. If a parent is inconsistent or unpredict- able, the child is likely to have an *insecure-anxious/ambivalent attachment style*, fearing abandonment, feeling anxiety or being constantly vigilant (on high alert). Finally, if a parenting style is abusive, frightening or unpredictable, the child can have a *disorganized attachment style*, exhibiting difficulties regulating emotions and acting in an odd or ambivalent way in stressful situations.

Early attachment can also affect how a child will begin to self-regulate (Schore 2003).

Because attachment and implicit memories are linked, regulatory patterns of various types of bonding become etched in our bodies and brains. If a child's mother experiences anxiety, the child will be biased toward anxiety even from birth. This early wiring is the foundation for how we all learn and adapt to this human life. Temperament and environment relate to future outcomes of a child's personality; yet when a child looks into the eyes of an anxious mother, the resonance circuitry seen there will preclude the child from responding to stressful stimuli in an anxious manner. When a child (or any person) is present with someone, they are taking in a great deal of information through mirror neurons and resonance circuitry (Rizzolatti 2005; Iacoboni 2009). A person will hear the tone of voice, see a face, notice body language—all senses that assist a person in internalizing another. A person will do whatever they need to stay connected, as humans are designed for mutual relationship, not independence. This concept becomes crucial when clinicians are working with clients. In the area of mind-body work, a practitioner must be conscious of the ability of the client's body to reflect self-knowledge and regulation of health and well-being. If a client has no memory of a safe person in their past, it will be difficult for them to get better without experiencing a safe, trusting relationship (van der Kolk 2002). A goal of therapy becomes providing kind, compassionate care that helps rewire implicit regulatory patterns. When a practitioner provides calm attunement, the client has a chance of rewiring old neurobiology and creating new stories and perceptions.

Neuroplasticity of brain responses is an encouraging factor in the treatment of trauma and somatic disorders (Doidge 2007). Rick Hanson (2009) believes we can change unwanted behaviors and feelings in our lives by simply focusing on positive thoughts for a few minutes each day. New learning always creates new neural circuits, but it is when new learning also unwires old learning that transformational change occurs (Ecker 2015). The therapeutic reconsolida- tion process can be fulfilled by a broad range of techniques, and the goal is transformational change, as distinct from ongoing symptom management (Ecker 2015). Daniel Siegel (2015) suggests that the creation of new neural circuits happens through a variety of types of psychotherapy and the ANS has an inherent capacity to self-regulate.

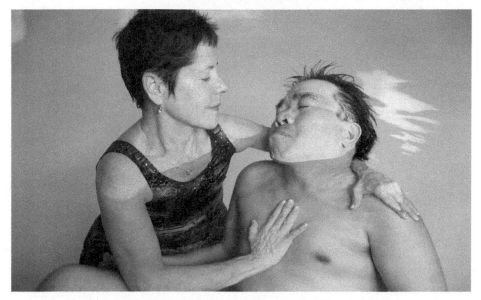

Figure 4.3: Client with Cerebral Palsy

Interoception and exteroception

The major strategy of somatic psychotherapies involves a "bottom-up" process of directing the client's attention to internal sensations, both visceral (interoception) and musculoskeletal (proprioception and kinesthesis). This is different from the more traditional therapy treatments which are "top down" or more cognitive in nature, often invoking trauma memories.

In our aquatic work, we specifically avoid re-evoking traumatic memories. Instead, we approach the charged memories indirectly and slowly. We facilitate the generation of new corrective interoceptive experiences that physically contradict those of overwhelm and helplessness. *We are all born with a blueprint of health that is obscured by the imprint of our trauma. Somatic therapies introduce a formula for retrieving the original blueprint.*

References

Ainsworth, M. (1969). Object relations, dependency, and attachment: A theoretical review of infant-mother relationship. *Journal of Child Development*, 40: 969–1025. Accessed December 18, 2014 at www.psychology.sunysb.edu/attachment/online/attach_depend.pdf.

Badenoch, B. (2008). *Being a Brain-Wise Therapist: A Practical Guide to Interpersonal Neurobiology*. New York, NY: W.W. Norton & Company.

Barratt, B.B. (2010). *Emergence of Somatic Psychology*. London: Palgrave Macmillan.

Cappuzzi, D. & Gross, D.R. (2010). *Counseling and Psychotherapy: Theories and Interventions*. Alexandria, VA: American Counseling Association.

Doidge, N. (2007). *The Brain That Changes Itself*. New York, NY: Penguin.

Ecker, B. (2015). Memory reconsolidation understood and misunderstood. *International Journal of Neuropsychotherapy*, 3(1): 2–46.

Hanson, R. (2009). *Buddha's Brain: The Practical Neuroscience of Happiness, Love and Wisdom*. Oakland, CA: New Harbinger Publications.

Hinchey, K. (2010). *The Legacy of Wilhelm Reich, M.D.* Retrieved from www.wilhelmreichtrust. org/legacy_of_wilhelm_reich-2010_10_30.pdf (link no longer valid).

Iacoboni, M. (2009). Imitation, empathy, and mirror neurons. *Annual Review of Psychology*, 60: 653–670. doi:10.1146/annurev.psych.60.110707.163604.

Jovanovic, T., Blanding, N.Q., Norrholm, S.D., Duncan, E., Bradley, B. & Ressler, K.J. (2009). Childhood abuse is associated with increased startle reactivity in adulthood. *Depression and Anxiety*, 26(11): 1018–1026.

Jiang, S., Potovit, L., Cattaneo, A., Binder, E.B. & Aitchison, K. (2019). Epigenetic modifications in stress response genes associated with childhood trauma (ACEs). *Frontiers in Psychiatry*, November 8, 2019. https://doi.org/10.3389/fpsyt.2019.00808.

Levine, P. (2010). *In an Unspoken Voice: How the Body Releases Trauma and Restores Goodness*. Berkeley, CA: North Atlantic Books.

Maté, G. (2003). *When the Body Says No*. Hoboken, NJ: John Wiley.

Porges, S.W. (2007). The polyvagal perspective. *Biological Psychology*, 74(2): 116–143. doi:10.1016/j.biopsycho.2006.06.009.

Porges, S.W. (2015). *The Polyvagal Theory for Treating Trauma*. Teleseminar Session with Stephen Porges and Ruth Buczynski. Retrieved from http://stephenporges.com/images/stephen porges interview nicabm.pdf (link no longer valid).

Porges, S.W. & Furman, S.A. (2011). The early development of the autonomic nervous system provides a neural platform for social behavior: A polyvagal perspective. *Infant and Child Development*, 20(1): 106–118.

Rizzolatti, G. (2005). The mirror neuron system and its function in humans. *Anatomy and Embryology*, 210(5–6): 419–421. doi:10.1007/s00429-005-0039-z.

Scaer, R. (2001). *The Body Bears the Burden: Trauma, Dissociation, and Disease*. Binghamton, NY: Haworth Medical Press.

Schore, A. (2003). *Affect Dysregulation and Disorders of the Self*. New York, NY: W.W. Norton & Company.

Siegel, D. (2015). *The Developing Mind* (second edition). New York, NY: The Guilford Press.

van der Kolk, B.A. (2002). Beyond the Talking Cure: Somatic Experience, Subcortical Imprints and the Treatment of PTSD. In F. Shapiro (ed.), *EMDR as an Integrative Psychotherapy Approach: Experts of Diverse Orientations Explore the Paradigm Prism* (pp.57–83). Washington, DC: American Psychological Association.

van der Kolk, B.A., Stone, L., West, J. *et al.* (2014). Yoga as an adjunctive treatment for post-traumatic stress disorder: A randomized controlled trial. *Journal of Clinical Psychiatry*, 75(6): e559–e565. doi:10.4088/JCP.13m08561.

Weber, D.L., Clark, C.R., McFarlane, A.C., Moores, K., Morris, P. & Egan, G.F. (2005). Abnormal frontal and parietal activity during working memory updating in post-traumatic stress disorder. *Psychiatry Research*, 140(1): 27–44. doi:10.1016/j.pscychresns.2005.07.003.

Wolynn, M. (2016). *It Didn't Start with You*. New York, NY: Viking.

Yehuda, R. & Seckl, J. (2011). Mini review: Stress-related psychiatric disorders with low cortisol levels: A metabolic hypothesis. *Endocrinology*, 152(12): 4496–4503.

Chapter 5

Ethics with the Right Use of Power in WATSU® Practice

DR. CEDAR BARSTOW

WATSU, as a healing modality, needs to be grounded in and guided by an ethic of care and sensitivity. The dictionary definition of ethics is the study of what is right and wrong and of duty and moral obligation. In the context of this chapter, *ethics is a set of values, attitudes and skills intended to have benevolent effects when applied through professional behavioral guidelines, decision-making processes and the practice of compassion.*

The central ethical question is: Is what I am doing or how I am being in the best interests of my client? Ethics is therefore about being in benevolent relationship. Often, we think of ethics as simply a list of rules and guidelines to memorize and follow. Rules and guidelines are important, but even more important is the quality of the professional relationship.

WATSU, like other professional relationships, takes place in the context of a power difference. This power difference has both healing purpose and multiple relational impacts and dynamics that actually are the reason and foundation for the need for professional ethics. I have come to understand that the biggest and proper context for *ethics* is the *right use of power*. Here I am using the dictionary definition of power: *the ability to have an effect or to have influence.* Power is not static, not a monolithic thing, not force, manipulation or exploitation. Like ethics, it is relational. It is how power is used that makes it harmful or benevolent.

Some 25 years ago, when I heard this phrase—ethics is the right use of power—I got excited and inspired. Ethics, in one phrase, shifted from an onerous and scary set of rules, to a larger and life-long exploration of power and how to use it wisely and well in relationships.

A student in one of my classes once said, "I don't need to take an ethics class. I have good intentions." As I delved more deeply into the study of power in relationship, it became abundantly clear that good intentions, while necessary, aren't sufficient. Right use of power needs to be learned. There are relational dynamics, concepts and skills involved. Further, learning these skills and concepts can best be accomplished by learning them from the inside out compared to the rule-side in what we could call embodied ethics—or ethics with wisdom and power with heart.

This chapter will be an introduction to *ethics with the right use of power*, and will cover some essentials that are important for WATSU practitioners:

1. Power differential: its nature, its value, its impacts and its responsibilities.
2. Ethics of touch: what to pay attention to and what to watch out for.
3. Self-care: as an ethical issue.
4. Dual role relationships: what they are and how to manage them when appropriate.
5. Scope of practice: making referrals, and completing both sessions and treatment.
6. Additional relational challenges for using power ethically.

Power differential

"I'm trying to imagine ethics without an awareness of power. That would be like trying not to step on anyone's toes, without an awareness of one's feet." (Susan Mickesic)

The power differential is the inherently greater or enhanced power and influence that WATSU practitioners (and other helping professionals) have compared to their clients. Understanding both the value and the many complex impacts of the power differential is the core of ethical awareness. Written codes for behavior are based on the strong positive and negative impacts of this power differential.

Clients are in a position in which they must trust in the knowledge and guidance of their caregiver. This difference results in a greater than ordinary possibility of vulnerability on the part of the client. Consequently, clients are unusually susceptible to harm and confusion through misuses (either underuse or overuse) of power and influence.

Value of the power differential
The power differential has great value. Used wisely and appropriately, it creates a safe, well-boundaried, professional context for growth and healing. In brief,

your role as a WATSU practitioner is to create a safe space, empower your client, protect your client's spirit, and see a wider perspective.

More specifically, when used ethically, the power differential offers clients some very important assurances:

- Confidence in their caregiver's knowledge, training and expertise. *You provide information about your training and demonstrate your competence.*
- Security and safety. *You assure your clients and earn their trust. Your actions support their experience of safety.*
- Direction and support. *You provide guidance, respect and kindness. You assist your clients in getting the most from their sessions.*
- Role boundary clarification. *You set and maintain clear and appropriate boundaries.*
- Allocated responsibilities. *You assist your clients in understanding what your professional responsibilities are and what is expected of them.*

Two kinds of power: Personal power and role power

In talking about the power differential, it is necessary to clearly describe and distinguish between two kinds of power. This distinction is important because it makes clear that the increased power that accompanies a position of authority is role based and not the same as personal power.

- *Personal power* is our birthright ability to have an effect and to have influence.
- *Role power* is the add-on additional power (and responsibility and opportunity) that accompanies a positional role.

I like to show the difference between these two powers with scarves. When I am a therapist, I have my personal power, of course, but I wear my added-on role power as if it were a scarf around my shoulders. When I leave my office, I take my role-power scarf off. My personal power stays with me. As a metaphor, I could imagine that my scarf has access to and stores information and awareness embedded in my role power. For you, as WATSU practitioners, wearing a scarf is not practical, but in the water, your role power is more than symbolically clear in that you are the one standing and holding and moving your client, while your client is lying and being moved in the water. Perhaps you would like to think of a special thing to wear when you are in your up-power role as a reminder that your increased power comes from your role.

Here's a little chart that illustrates the differences between personal and role power.

Table 5.1: The difference between personal power and role power

PERSONAL POWER (PP)	ROLE POWER (RP)
• PP is our birthright. It is our individual ability to have an effect or to have influence.	• RP, or positional power, is earned, awarded, elected or assigned. It is a power add-on.
• It is accompanied by the inherent human right to be treated with dignity, respect and fairness.	• RP is separate from our PP and is thus mutable. It automatically accompanies any position of authority.
• Although PP is always present, we can be more or less aware of it and have more or less access to it.	• RP carries an increased or expanded amount of power and responsibility.
• Our PP can be limited by ourselves and by the misuse of power by others, but in most situations, we can retain some PP through positive attitudes and self-respect.	• It is integrated with PP. Status power (SP, enhanced personal power and influence that is culturally conferred) often accompanies RP.
• We can learn to use our PP better in both up-power and down-power roles.	• Up- and down-power dynamics create the need for ethical guidelines since those who are down-power are more vulnerable and at risk of harm.
• PP comes in many forms, including the power of communication (articulateness), presence (charisma) and creativity.	• Some assigned roles carry greater increased power and responsibility than others and thus will have a greater negative or positive impact on others.
• PP can be developed.	• Examples: WATSU practitioner, doctor/nurse, teacher/principal, coach, employer, clergy, chairperson, therapist/ social worker, supervisor, elected official, chief executive officer, parent, director, bodyworker, police officer.

Two kinds of positions: Up-power and down-power

I refer to those in positions of increased role power as having "up-power" and those in the corresponding positions of lesser power as having "down-power." These are simple and directional terms not intended to indicate disrespect, disempowerment, exploitation or manipulation, better or worse, or power over or power under. Instead, these terms are intended to denote role differences in responsibility and in vulnerability.

Up-power and down-power positions have cognitive, emotional and somatic differences. As an exercise, I ask my students to walk around the room imagining walking with someone who has up-power compared to them. My students notice a variety of things: feeling smaller, more cautious, protective, turned inward (or, for some, feeling relaxed, eager, relieved). Next, when imagining walking with someone with whom they have up-power, they notice feeling more spacious, focused on the other, taller, kind and caring, alert. It is very clear to them that the two roles are experienced differently. For most, this is a surprise. A student described the difference in this way: "When I'm a practitioner, my personal needs and 'stuff' are behind me resting against my shoulders, and when I'm a client, my personal needs and 'stuff' are sitting right there in a huge ball on my lap, visible and available."

In our everyday lives, we move back and forth daily between being in up-power positions and down-power positions. (You could explore these shifts by consciously putting on a scarf or other item when in role and taking it off when leaving the role for a couple of days. For example, in a day you might move from being with an equal-power intimate partner to being an up-power parent to being a down-power patient in a dentist's office to being an up-power WATSU practitioner and then home to being an equal-power partner.) We are usually unaware of the shift. This unconscious shifting of roles makes it more difficult to clearly understand the dynamics and impacts. Some up-power roles carry a stronger differential than others and therefore a stronger risk of harm. For example, the President of the World Bank or a policeman or a therapist or a WATSU practitioner has a greater power difference than the chair of a committee or a clerk in a store. But all up-power roles have impacts and dynamics.

Power differential responsibilities

As a practitioner, your wise and sensitive handling of the responsibilities that belong with your caregiver role is what earns you the needed trust of your client. Table 5.2 is a chart of these responsibilities that you can use to self-assess.

Table 5.2: Power differential responsibilities

Scale	Please self-reflect on a 1–10 scale (10 being high)
	• Setting and maintaining appropriate boundaries
	– environmental (the safety or privacy of the setting)
	– emotional (focus on their emotions)
	– physical/sexual (non-sexual contact)
	– financial (you are the one being paid)
	– time
	– role (staying in up-power role)

cont.

Scale	Please self-reflect on a 1–10 scale (10 being high)
	• Earning trust and being trustworthy
	• Creating needed safety
	• Staying in charge
	• Holding the larger container of wholeness and hope
	• Being sensitive to your impact
	• Inviting and being non-defensively responsive to feedback
	• Keeping your own personal life in the background
	• Tracking and attending to the relationship and resolving difficulties (150% principle)
	• Making assessments of results
	• Keeping appropriate records

Power differential vulnerabilities

The up-power role is weighted toward responsibility. However, the down-power role is weighted toward vulnerability. Here's how.

By agreeing to and taking on the down-power position (which will allow them to receive the healing, caregiving or help they seek), your clients become more vulnerable. They may be vulnerable in any or all of the following ways, where they:

- are asked or required to reveal information which may be painful, private or delicate
- have a role-related increased desire and need to be respected, liked and accepted and so may be reluctant to question, object, say "no," offer critical feedback, or reveal embarrassment or shame
- may, when feeling disrespected, unacknowledged or wronged, exaggerate or escalate the situation
- may idealize and/or devalue the caregiver
- may transfer feelings or relationships from their past onto their caregiver
- may not know what kinds of behavior are unethical
- may not be clear about touch, like saying "yes" when meaning "no"
- may think or experience down-power as no power and disempower themselves
- are more susceptible to being rejected, shamed, disrespected, taken advantage of, unduly influenced, or manipulated

- may have unrealistic expectations of the up-power practitioner
- can be too easily and strongly influenced by the words and actions of their up-power caregiver especially when in an altered state, as can happen in a WATSU session
- may need assistance in learning how to use their down-power position well.

Understanding and owning your power and influence

Because the power differential is role-dependent, it is easy to over-identify (get inflated or addicted) with this increased or enhanced power. It is just as easy to misuse this increased power by under-identifying with it. The central idea is the necessity to understand and *own* your role power so that you can be conscious and informed.

Here are several misunderstandings that illustrate the multiplicity of the impact of the power differential for both helping professionals and clients:

- Believing in equality, you may find it difficult to accept that your role creates a power inequality, and that this inequality is actually essential to your effectiveness.
- Rushed for time, you may underestimate the power differential and over-focus on technique or useful information. Effective use of your role power involves balancing technique with the essential need for relationship connection and repair when needed.
- In fear of manipulative and wounding abuses of power, you may find it difficult to understand that you must own the power that you have, to be able to use it for good. Underuse of power is also a misuse of power.
- Misunderstanding your elevated role power as confirmation of your wisdom and even your infallibility, you may inadvertently disempower, disregard or disrespect your clients.
- Motivated by a desire to be of service, you may find it difficult to comprehend that your impact may be different from your intention, and that it may be experienced as confusing or harmful.

150 percent principle

This principle is not an exact equation, but a memorable image. While both parties are 100 percent responsible for the quality and integrity of the relationship, the practitioner, as the one in the role of greater power, is 150 percent responsible for the health of the relationship. The caregiver has more responsibility for making sure both parties are using their power consciously and skillfully, being accountable, and resolving situations when difficulties arise. While this greater responsibility can feel like an unfair burden, it is actually an important counter-balance to the potential vulnerability of your client. Many misuses of power occur because of what I would call power-blindness. Practitioners blame clients for not speaking up about a problem, forgetting that there is a risk of rejection or humiliation for clients to give challenging feedback, for example.

Some clients are more easily harmed. Clients who are most susceptible to misuses of power:

- lack personal awareness
- are not relationally skilled
- are impaired by pain, anxiety, trauma or shame
- have low self-esteem.

These clients will need special attention and extra 150 percent principle awareness.

Here's a summary of some attitudes with skills attached to cultivate in working wisely and well with the dynamics set up by a power difference:

- Own your role power: self-reflect and self-correct.
- Be guided by the 150 percent principle: see apology as leadership.
- Respond to and use feedback: track, resolve and repair.
- Set and maintain good boundaries: integrate strength and heart.
- Stay present and connected: consult often.

Clients just want to know that you can be trusted, no sleight of hand, no deception, no grandiose technique is needed. (Mary Seamster, WATSU practitioner)

Relational dynamics and challenges

As you can see and surmise, the nature of the power differential brings with it some challenges and some opportunities.

Let's start with the opportunities. Empowering and refining yourself in using your up-power role offers a chance to do some deep personal development work. In order to use your power sensitively and effectively to support your client's growth through taking your responsibilities to heart, you will also be working on your own personal growth. This is extremely important work. Over time, through mistakes, regrets and apologies, you will become more and more able to own your power, be both strong and compassionate and respond to criticism non-defensively and with accountability.

Good leadership is not easy, but it is worthy and can bring much satisfaction. Two qualities that are universally valued in leaders may surprise you. One is humility. Cultivate humility in your up-power relationships. Humility can be confused with disowning your power, but it is very different. It involves owning your power and then experiencing yourself as a vehicle for bringing out the best for those in your care.

> There is guidance for each of us, and by lowly listening we shall hear the right word... Place yourself in the middle of the stream of power and wisdom that flows into your life. (Ralph Waldo Emerson 1841)

The second is the ability to use your power both as strength and as heart. I call it standing in your strength while staying in your heart. We often think of power just as strength or force. But the heart or compassion side of power is at least as powerful as the strength side of power. We don't need to separate these two. It's challenging, but we can learn to take charge and do it with the energy of empathy and compassion. When the generativity and responsiveness of our power is guided by loving concern for the well-being of all, we will have an ethical and sustainable world. Power directed by heart. Heart infused with power. This is key to the right use of power.

Table 5.3: The differences between up-power and down-power positions

WATSU practitioner: UP-POWER ROLE	WATSU practitioner: DOWN-POWER ROLE
Is in service	Is served
Has increased power and influence	Is more dependent and easily influenced
Is paid for time and expertise	Pays for service
Sets and maintains appropriate boundaries	Accepts and may challenge boundaries
Own needs and personal process are not focused on	Own needs and personal processes are known and focused on—self-revelation is important
Has less vulnerability	Has greater vulnerability to rejection, criticism, undue influence, being taken advantage of, disrespect
Is depended on for trustworthiness, need to earn trust	Needs to trust
Is 150% responsible for tracking and repairing relationship differences	Is 100% responsible for naming and working with difficulties

cont.

WATSU practitioner: UP-POWER ROLE	WATSU practitioner: DOWN-POWER ROLE
May be idealized and/or devalued	Is more susceptible to idealizing and devaluing
Makes assessments and evaluates results	Collaborates with or responds to assessments

Now let's talk about the challenges that may arise from the dynamics of the relationship summarized in Table 5.3.

Interestingly, in terms of fully owning your power, it seems that "the more powerful we feel, the better we use our power...and conversely, the less powerful we feel, the greater the chance we'll misuse power. The gap between our self-perceived sense of power and our objective power accounts for a great deal of power misuses" (Diamond 2016, p.79). How do you personally relate to this? Identify a time when your lack of feeling powerful caused some harm by you making a mistake and misusing your power.

Challenge: Overuse of role power

Harms caused by the overuse of power are common on the news and in law suits. Many people in up-power roles fail to understand that their role power is an embedded add-on to their personal power and become convinced, therefore, that their personal and role power are one and the same. When this happens, they self-identify with their role power and get inflated or addicted to this mis-perceived power. Severe power inflation and addiction lead to exploitation, over-control, force, manipulation, and even seeing those down-power to them as objects to serve them. These cases make the news. Less severe overuse of power also causes harm and looks like the caregiver becoming over-directive, overbearing and over-confident. The virtue of humility is all but lost. Even for conscious people, it is easy to over-identify with role power and cause unintended harm. It requires conscious awareness that whatever you say or do will have a much deeper and stronger impact than you intend. I remember suggesting to a client that she might want to journal about her experience. I was shocked when she returned the next week very angry with me: "You're just like all the others. You ordered me to journal. You think that journaling is going to solve everything. I want to be treated as ME. I don't want to be just another chess piece that you can move around and get paid for. And I hate journaling." Whew. I had not realized my suggestion would be taken as an order. I had not yet earned her trust. I was glad to discover that I could recover from this mistake and go on to earn her trust.

Challenge: Underuse of role power

Underuse of role power is also a misuse of power. This statement comes as a big "aha" to many caregivers and leaders. Recognizing, valuing and owning role power and influence are essential aspects of good care. The inherent increased power of a role is not the problem. Caregivers tend to have a force-and-exploitation understanding of power and tend to be oversensitive to abusive and manipulative use of power and thus often dismiss or deny their inherent increased role power. I hear things like: "I refuse to act as if I have power over my clients." "I trust my clients to know what is best for them." "I'm very sensitive to issues of diversity and white privilege. I just won't go there. Those words up- and down-power trigger me." "The minute I heard the word down-power, I just collapsed. I never want to cause my clients to feel disempowered by my being up-power." Do you personally recognize any of these thoughts?

Story: One of my students, when role-playing being in an up-power role and wearing a scarf to symbolize the additional power of her role, simply took off her scarf and handed it to her partner who was playing the role of client. She didn't want to own her role power. Rather than feeling good about being given the scarf, her client described feeling quite uneasy, even frightened when her partner took off the scarf. She was truly concerned that her therapist would not be capable of providing her with the care and support she needed. We can treat our clients as equal human beings deserving of respect and dignity while still valuing, owning and using our role power.

Self-reflection: On a continuum, where would you put yourself in the range of over- to underuse of your power? Is there a place you tend to be or do you move along that continuum with a wide range? Can you think of a time when you overused your power? What happened? If you could do it again, what would you do differently? Can you identify a time when you have underused your power? What would you do differently if you could do it again?

Challenge: Responding to expectations, saying goodbye to being "just me"

When in your up-power role, you automatically become a projection screen for expectations. These projections will come from each client's personal history in relation to people in authority. They may be positive expectations. They may be negative expectations. They may be expectations of perfection. They may be expectations of disappointment, betrayal of trust or disapproval. Here are some examples of expectations that most likely would be unexpressed or unconscious. Notice what it would be like to hear these from a client. *"I expect you to care for me unconditionally. I expect you to know what I need even when I don't know. I expect you to be impeccable. I expect you to be totally trustworthy. I expect you to be 100 percent fully present. I expect you to always understand me. I expect you to hold good boundaries even when I challenge them. I expect you not to hurt me in any way."*

Your role power changes how you see yourself (for example, inflating or deflating yourself), how others see you (full of projections), and how you see others (from a responsibility frame). If you are a priest, you can't be "just me" with your parishioners. As a WATSU practitioner, if you meet your clients in the grocery store, you can't expect to be "just you" even though your role power doesn't create as much of a power difference as it does for a priest.

Self-reflection: What's it like to know that when in your up-power role you can't be "just me"?

Feeling these expectations can be overwhelming. "Why would I want to put myself in a position to receive all these expectations! No wonder I feel tense or nervous. I've felt every single one of these." Naming them can bring relieving objectivity and the opportunity to differentiate and work with unrealistic expectations directly.

As noted above, clients tend to both idealize and devalue those in an up-power role with them. Here are a few appreciations that could also be idealizations. *"You are just amazing! I don't know anyone else with so much skill. You have changed my life. I wish I had the kind of presence you have. I can't believe you figured that out so quickly. You have healed me."*

On the other side, you will receive feedback that could be devaluation such as: *"You should have known. I can't believe you said that to me. How could you be so insensitive and abrupt? I expected you to live up to your principles. You totally missed what I said. How could you be so wrong?"*

The idealizing spectrum covers a continuum of expressions that call for different responses. On one end, there are genuine expressions of appreciation, such as: *"I'm so grateful for your help and support."* Receiving and being nourished by these statements is good for the relationship and empowering for your clients. On the other end are the idealized expressions that come from a disempowered place, such as: *"You're the best. I wish I had it all together, like you do."* These deserve reflective attention: "I'd like to know more. Can you tell me more about your wish?"

Empowered appreciation ←→ *Disempowered appreciation*

Likewise, the devaluing spectrum calls for discernment in response. On one side of the spectrum are genuine expressions of difficulty, misunderstanding or hurt; for example: *"I don't understand why you said that. I thought you understood me."* Attention to the relationship and maybe also to relationship repair is what's needed. On the other end of the spectrum are indications of distress that call for attention to and addressing a personal issue; for example, *"You're just like all the others. You just tell me I shouldn't do this and expect it to solve the problem. I'm not a formula."*

Relationship difficulty ←⟶ *Personal issue*

Both positive and negative expectations and projections can be uncomfortable to receive. Likewise, both idealization and devaluation can be uncomfortable and often problematic. However, it is freeing and relieving to know that these responses from clients are part of the power differential dynamic.

Challenge: Getting your needs met elsewhere

We all have ordinary needs for friendship, sex, appreciation, control, respect, financial well-being. Self-reflect on which, if any, of these needs are not being met well enough in your current life. When any of these ordinary human needs are unmet in our personal lives, it is all too easy to try to meet them, usually unconsciously, through our up-power roles where our felt-sense of power is increased. Getting up-power inappropriate needs met through your role causes much harm, for example when practitioners establish inappropriate friendships and/or sexual relationships with clients. Or they keep clients longer than needed to make more money. Or they are agreeable when challenge is needed, in order to keep their client's affection.

From another angle, here is another self-reflection. Make a list of the things that you get from your up-power role that feel rewarding and satisfying and that you would miss if you didn't have them. What are they? Appreciate them! Get curious. Ask yourself where else you could find these satisfying experiences if you had to give up your role.

Challenge: Feedback—don't take all of it personally, and don't take none of it personally

Feedback is any response, negative or positive, that is given to someone else about the impact of their behavior. For example, feedback could be about skillfulness, ideas, presentation, style or impact. Feedback is a specific form of communication that is deliberate, considerate, specific and somewhat detached. Feedback provides an opportunity to learn how others perceive your behavior and to let others know how they are perceived. It is aimed at fostering more awareness rather than getting another to change in accordance with your wishes or perceptions.

The feedback challenge in relationships in which there is a power difference is that your clients will be unlikely to offer feedback that could be experienced as critical or challenging. There are three reasons for this. 1) Your clients are usually invested in you liking them, and therefore won't want to be critical because it could negatively affect your feelings about them. 2) Your clients need to trust you and may not want to question your responses or techniques. 3) Your clients are vulnerable to being hurt by your response to their feedback. For example, they may fear that your response would be defensive, or shaming or blaming.

Being collaborative with your clients may seem obvious as a right use of power, but collaboration depends on your clients knowing that their feedback, whether negative or positive, will be well received by you. They need to know you have heard them and that you will respectfully consider what they are telling you.

There are two factors that can inhibit your response. One is being defensive instead of receptive. The other has to do with the normal feedback loop that helps us understand and refine our relationships. In power differential relationships, like the one you have with your clients, the feedback loop gets skewed on the positive side. Your clients keep telling you what's good and keep not telling you anything challenging. You, therefore, get a very inflated view of yourself and your impact. This feeds into the tendency to over-identify with your role power.

Unrealistic or overblown idealizing and devaluing feedback, of course, further complicates your discernment about how to respond respectfully and authentically. Refer to the discussion of the idealizing/devaluing challenge in a previous paragraph.

Right use of power is a life-long engagement with understanding more about your impact on others. Be proactive and ask for and encourage all kinds of feedback. Often, when I have a gut feeling that the relationship needs attention, I specifically ask for challenging feedback. For example, "I know you appreciate what we're doing together, and I'm wondering if there is anything that's not going so well. I welcome all kinds of feedback. Your honesty will help us collaborate better." I find that negative feedback always has an element of truth and perceptiveness in it, even if it is small or minor. So, I advise—don't take all of it personally, and don't take none of it personally. Taking all feedback personally can cause you harm in that you are taking things that might be projections as personal to you. Taking none of it personally can cause harm to your client when they feel that their feedback offering is dismissed as irrelevant to the relationship.

Challenge: Dual role relationships
A dual role relationship is any additional relationship with a client or student occurring simultaneously with the therapy or educational relationship, or with a previous therapy or educational relationship. The impact of the power differential is what makes these relationships problematic and challenging.

Ordinary, everyday boundary crossings such as a chance meeting in the grocery store, attendance at a church service, being at the same party and seeing a client at a concert are not considered dual role relationships because they do not involve new roles and they are not ongoing relationships. These meetings can be simply managed by a practical protocol of acknowledging each other and leaving it to your client to name your professional relationship if they choose.

Multiple role relationships are prohibited or discouraged in ethical codes. However, in small and/or interwoven communities, some dual roles are often unavoidable. The 1993 American Psychological Association Code of Ethics recognizes that when consciously managed and not exploitative, they are not necessarily harmful (with the exception of sexual relationships and offering a commission or reward to clients for referring other clients to you).

A different term, "undue influence," replaces the category "dual role relationship" in the Colorado Association of Psychotherapists Code of Ethics. Recognizing that dual role relationships occur in any size community, this terminology appropriately focuses attention toward the *potential client harm from undue influence* rather than on prohibiting multiple role relationships. This code says simply: "Members shall not enter into a therapeutic relationship with a client where there is undue influence to the detriment of the client. Members shall be especially sensitive to conflicts of interest that may arise from dual relationships during or immediately before or after a therapeutic relationship." When a dual role relationship is determined to have low risk of undue influence, there are guidelines (some listed here) for consciously, honestly, openly and attentively managing this relationship.

Types of dual role relationships

The following would be considered multiple role relationships:

- Friendship
- Business or financial
- Barter
- Serving together on a committee
- Being an administrator or supervisor to your client
- Being a colleague, supervisor or student of your client in another arena
- Being in a staff group or professional peer group
- Sexual (current or previous)
- Rewarding clients to solicit other clients
- Consistent activities in political, social or religious groups

- Loaning money
- Attending workshops and trainings.

Dual role factors and considerations

Dual role relationships can be the source of serious ethical and relationship problems. In the state of Colorado, grievances about dual relationships are in the top third of those filed. You will need to be impeccably clear about boundaries and ongoing communication in managing a multiple role relationship.

Here are some factors to consider in deciding if a possible dual relationship could become problematic as a WATSU practitioner:

- Whether the practitioner has any kind of evaluative function, such as grading, assessing performance, hiring or firing.
- The length of time between the WATSU relationship and any other relationship, if the dual role would not be concurrent.
- Whether the exchange of goods and/or services would be contraindicated or exploitative.
- The nature and frequency of the dual function or role.
- The degree of intimacy involved in the WATSU relationship (generally the greater the intimacy, the greater the need for caution).
- The nature and seriousness of the client's problem and kind of therapy used.
- The stage in the therapeutic process: beginning, middle or end (generally, the earlier the stage, the greater the need for caution).
- The ability to keep the two relationships separate—client's ability, practitioner's ability and the capacity for the practitioner/client system to handle the two relationships.
- The level of maturity and communication skills of both parties.

Reasons to discourage dual role relationships

Here are some reasons to not enter into a dual role relationship:

- It is considered undue influence when the practitioner has any kind of evaluative function. Thus, dual role relationships where there is an evaluative function are generally unmanageable.
- The client can be more easily and deeply hurt by an unintended gesture or comment.
- The client may be consciously or unconsciously afraid of being judged or evaluated.
- The practitioner may not be as confronting with the clients they see

in other roles. The caregiver's own need to be liked and accepted may lead them to be less challenging.

- Dual relationships tend to impair the practitioner/therapist's judgment.
- The possibility of exploiting the client is more likely when the relationship takes on social dimensions.
- There is potential for conflict of interest.
- The client may become inhibited due to fear of losing the relationship. The client may fear losing respect, or being excluded by the therapist, and thus may censor disclosures and find it difficult to be honest about their feelings (especially negative ones) in the relationship.
- Blurred boundaries can distort the professional nature of the therapeutic relationship.
- The therapist may have the adulation of the client. When there is a dual relationship, a "fall from grace" may be especially confusing, difficult and personal, instead of primarily role-related.
- The client may have unconscious expectations that the (former) therapeutic contract takes precedence over the new relationship.

Safeguards

These are some safeguard choices that could be used when entering into and managing a dual role relationship:

- Contemplate and sense what the additional relationship might be like. Try it on in your mind and see how it feels.
- Secure the client's informed consent.
- Discuss the potential risks and benefits of a dual relationship.
- Continue to assess and discuss the impact throughout the course of the relationship.
- Consult with other professionals to resolve dilemmas.
- Get supervision when the risk for harm is high.
- Document the dual relationship in case notes.
- Carefully examine and re-examine the motives of both parties.
- Create a personal process for roling and de-roling.
- Delineate boundaries on time, space, payment and purpose very clearly.
- Be available and non-defensive if or when the client brings up a problem. Take the initiative to talk about concerns that arise.
- Remember that, although you are both equally responsible (100%), you, as the one with the greater original role power, are more responsible (150%).

Successful managing of dual role relationships that are necessary or deemed to have less risk of undue influence seem to depend on three things: clarity of the boundaries, mutual understanding of the risks, and ease and skillfulness of communication between both people.

Increased influence of all-power/no-power misperception

The impact of the increased power and responsibility that accompanies any up-power role is most clearly seen and felt through the tendency of the up-power person to see themselves or be perceived by their client as having "all-power." The traditional hierarchical view and experience was that the doctor knew all and the patient knew nothing, the therapist knew all and the client knew nothing. We now know and honor the fact that clients are the experts on their experience and the therapist or practitioner is the expert on the methods they use. Both inside and outside information is needed for effectiveness. For the most part, at least in the helping professions, the power differential has been reduced; however, many clients are only familiar with the idea that their therapist has all-power and they have no-power. Nothing could be further from the truth. Sometimes, as a WATSU practitioner, you may need to help your client understand that you will need to work together—that you don't have all the power and they don't have no power.

It is important that I also mention here, when talking about increased power and influence, that the context and water process for WATSU is one which tends to create a non-ordinary state of consciousness for your clients. A non-ordinary state of consciousness is a "mild to deep trance in which awareness is focused in a different way than in ordinary life" (Taylor 1995, p.102). When in this non-ordinary state, the impact of your words and actions are even stronger. As a student says: "I'm amazed! It never occurred to me that my clients are often in a non-ordinary, mindful state of consciousness that needs even more sensitivity than usual. Thanks for pointing this out. This will translate immediately into more skillfulness and likely more effectiveness with my clients."

Non-ordinary consciousness

We all have experiences of non-ordinary states of consciousness, some very pleasurable and some traumatic. Non-ordinary states of consciousness engender special concerns about the right use of power because the impact of the power differential is heightened and expanded when clients are in a non-ordinary state. Thus, greater sensitivity and skillfulness in understanding and using your increased role power and influence for promoting well-being is needed.

As caregivers, we work with clients on a continuum of states of consciousness. This continuum moves from ordinary everyday states to mild reverie in which our clients are relaxed, thoughtful, focused internally and able to respond to questions. Clients may move fluidly along this continuum or make sudden shifts requiring attentive tracking.

Self-reflection: Here's a list of some of the qualities and effects of non-ordinary experience. Which ones do you recognize?

- Time distortion
- Increased intensity of feeling and sensation
- Greater need or capacity for faith and trust
- Increased sensitivity and awareness through all senses
- Consciousness expansion
- Relaxation or diffusion of boundaries
- Increased felt sense of the "truth"
- Increased sensitivity to authenticity.

Some of the most effective, profound and long-lasting change and healing happens in a non-ordinary state. A colleague of mine, Anna Cox, says, "I truly believe that deep healing happens primarily in non-ordinary states and that a therapist must be able to enter and relate comfortably to clients in these states with facility. Sometimes the non-ordinary state is the depth of the connection, and sometimes it is meditative, and sometimes it comes from intensity of feeling."

Since psychotherapy, body therapy, massage and WATSU are designed, for the most part, to help people focus their awareness in an altered, internal state, clients may be in non-ordinary states more often than we think. In non-ordinary states, heightened and expanded sensory, emotional and spiritual experiences provide a context for very profound healing and self-discovery, and also require special sensitivity.

Impact and intention

Another simple dynamic that is magnified by increased role power is the difference between impact and intention. The most effective and skillful use of power is made possible by being aware of and responsive to your impact on others. When your goal is to be of the best possible service to your clients, it is imperative to be interested in and attentive to their responses to your use of your self, your role power and your expertise. The best training and the best modalities will ultimately be compromised if you are not paying attention and then adjusting to how your clients are responding.

You may say one thing—for example, "I'd like to suggest you try…"—but your impact may cause unexpected and unintended pain if your client takes this suggestion as an order to obey or as a put down or manipulation. There need be no argument or defensiveness when this occurs. You and your client are *both right*. Your intention was good. Your client's experience (probably based on their past history) was of feeling misunderstood, judged or disrespected. In other words, they felt harm.

Impact is the effect your behavior has on others. Intention is the effect you want to have. In professional relationships, the power differential increases the potential for difference between impact and intention. Cultural, sexual, religious and class differences strongly influence discrepancies between intention and impact.

A lack of understanding of this very simple concept of intention and impact accounts for a surprisingly large percentage of relationship difficulties. When you know your intention to be good, it can be challenging to shift your perspective to understand that your client experiences these actions and words as painful, critical, disrespectful or confusing. When you understand that both of you are "right" in being true to your experience of a set of words or a behavior, resolution no longer needs to be focused on who's wrong, but rather on clarifying how you understand each other.

Understanding the difference between intention and impact can help you shift your focus from defending your position to being curious; from who is right or wrong to clarifying intentions; from anger to compassion; and from giving up to resolution and relationship repair.

Keep in mind that your client may have a hard time standing up for themselves because of the impact of the power differential. Your client may withdraw, swallow feelings, take their distress elsewhere, or their feelings may come out in other ways. It may be challenging to learn how to handle misunderstandings with grace, immediacy and non-defensiveness.

Five keys
You may find these keys useful for unlocking impact and intention discrepancies. In resolving and getting reconnected, what's most important is not what you meant but understanding how it was received.

Sensitize yourself to the possibility that your impact was different from your intention.

Listen to your client's experience (*i.e., "Please tell me about your experience just now"*).

Validate your client's experience (*i.e., "I can understand how you could feel [hurt]"*).

Explain your intention in a simple way—no need for paragraphs (*i.e., "It wasn't my intention to hurt you. My intention was…"*).

Ask what else is needed (*i.e., "How are you feeling now?" Or, "Is there anything else you need around this?" Or, "How are we doing now? Is there anything needed for relationship repair?" Or, "What I wish I had done/said is...and what I'll do next time is..."*).

Tracking and contacting impact can help the relationship self-correct quickly and successfully. Like navigating a sailboat, the person at the helm keeps the goal in sight but uses the wind to tack and then correct. The journey seldom takes one straight line to the dot on the horizon, but the more frequently you self-correct, the smoother and quicker your arrival. A big self-correction takes a lot more effort than a little one, but too many tiny corrections can slow the process to a snail's pace.

Touch that doesn't cause harm

Touch, of course, is essential in the WATSU system. And yet, the use of touch is considered unethical in most therapeutic modalities. It is a tender and sensitive subject. Whole communities have exploded when teachers have had emotional affairs, been sexually involved with students or used touch inappropriately. Years of cultural, theoretical and ethical controversy surround the use of touch in the helping professions.

Touch is necessary to both physical health and emotional well-being. Babies who aren't touched enough fail to thrive. My colleague, Greg Johanson, is willing to go so far as to say that not to use the power of touch (therapeutically and appropriately initiated) is itself unethical. Restoring a satisfying and healthy relationship to touch may indeed be considered a worthy goal in therapy. The body is a rich source of wisdom. The use of body information and informed and conscious touch is a powerful tool for healing, self-awareness, establishing good boundaries and cultivating more satisfying connections.

Controversy arises from the following factors:

1. It is never ethical to use sexual touch with a client or to engage in or imply sexual intimacy or the future possibility of such. The very strong healing power of touch is matched by the equally strong harm caused by sexual intimacy in a relationship of trust. The prohibition by organizations of even non-sexual touch in helping relationships is intended to prevent the egregious harm caused by inappropriate touch.

2. Human beings automatically and uniquely assign meaning to touch. Thus, therapeutic touch is easily misinterpreted by clients as sexual, forceful, caregiver-serving or controlling. Touch is deeply longed for

and a source of deep vulnerability. The use of therapeutic touch is ethically and relationally complex and requires assessment, sensitivity, good tracking and clarity of intention on the part of caregivers.

As WATSU practitioners, you know and have experienced the profound value of non-sexual touch for growth and healing. The following information is based on work by my colleague Jaffy Phillips.

Assessing for the use of touch

When you touch someone, everything changes. Touch is a physical and relational experience that is generally imbued with layers of historical, cultural and psychological meaning. The meanings evoked by touch are often unconscious or non-verbal, and they can manifest somatically and/or relationally before the client is able to articulate anything about them. Boundary violation, transference and counter-transference are the most common examples of this kind of response. Unaddressed, these issues can wreak havoc in the therapeutic relationship and ultimately harm the client. When using touch in WATSU, the following categories are important considerations. It is assumed that when introducing clients to the WATSU process, the use of touch is discussed and you obtain informed consent.

Boundaries and intimacy

Touching is an intimate act and one that carries the potential to invade the client's boundaries and/or trigger strong transferential reactions. It can also be a confusing and overwhelming experience for a client with poor boundaries or a poorly developed sense of self.

Variability of meaning

The same kind of touch will be experienced by different clients in different ways, depending on the circumstances, the client's personal history and cultural background, the personal qualities of the therapist, and the quality and duration of the therapeutic relationship. It is important that the therapist avoids re-enacting negative aspects of the client's interpersonal or touch history and reinforcing any of the client's negative associations to touch.

History of abuse

Clients for whom touch is a central issue include those who have been sexually or physically abused and those who have a history of intimacy issues. In working with these clients, practitioners should proceed with extra care, tracking and discretion in order to avoid reinforcing the client's negative associations with touch.

Potential for risk of sexual interpretation

Touch may be interpreted by a client as sexual contact. Minimize this risk by some or all of the following:

- The presence of a clear contract about the use of touch.
- Clarity about one's own intentions and motivations for touching a particular client at a particular time.
- Clarity about one's own sexual boundaries.
- Scrupulous use of supervision.
- Making sure the client has tracking and reporting ability.
- The ability of client and therapist to stay in truth.
- The presence of the client's partner, a co-therapist or group members in the setting.

Risk that touch will be used to gratify the needs of the therapist

Touch can be used to gratify other (non-sexual) needs, including the therapist's need for intimacy and closeness, the need to be experienced as a nurturer by the client, and the need for physical contact. Therapists can minimize the risk of this type of exploitation by becoming familiar with their own needs through personal therapy and self-awareness practices, establishing outside sources for their gratification, and regular use of supervision.

Signs of danger for helping professional

- Different quality or use of touch with different gendered clients.
- Touch used in an unexamined way in response to a client's request.
- Touch that occurs in secret, or with reluctance of the therapist to discuss their use of touch with colleagues or a supervisor.
- Touch that occurs in the context of sexual attraction, by either therapist or client.

Summary of therapeutic touch

To summarize the guidelines, therapeutic touch should be:

- non-sexual
- mindful
- appropriate
- with permission
- conscious
- cautious
- well-boundaried

- uncontaminated by the caregiver's personal needs
- in the service of the client
- carefully tracked and contacted
- adjusted as needed.

WATSU is an elegant and healing form for the therapeutic use of touch.

Challenge: Managing trigger and shadow behaviors

One of the most important gifts you can give yourself and your clients is to do the inner work of understanding how and when you get triggered by another's behavior. This is a very personal process. Knowing your triggers and shadow behaviors can allow you to grow yourself as a practitioner and prevent unnecessary harm and misuses of power. You will acquire some choices. Over time, starting with recognizing that you got triggered, and apologizing instead of denying, blaming or defending, you will be able to catch yourself before you get triggered.

Self-reflect for a moment. Can you name two or three situations in which you habitually get triggered? Do you notice any warning signs that could help you be proactive and preventative?

Challenge: Self-care—do your job and know your limits

Self-reflect: Look back over a couple of weeks and note times when you felt you reached your energy limit but pushed yourself to go on. What are you afraid would have happened had you allowed yourself to stop? Think of three benefits you would have had if you had allowed yourself to stop or pause.

Sitting in my seat with my seat belt fastened on dozens of airplanes, I have half-heard the flight attendant say, "Put your oxygen mask on yourself first before putting it on your child." On my last flight, I pondered this. Of course, when you are in the service role, you need literally to make sure you are breathing or you will be of no help to your clients. Helping professionals tend to focus their energies and attention on the service and care of others to the detriment of their own care. So committed to service and healing, they frequently forget that when they are "burned out," their clients won't be getting the level of professional care that the caregivers are capable of offering.

Self-care, rather than being a luxury, is a significant ethical issue. In fact, I consider it an ethical imperative!

Results of inadequate self-care

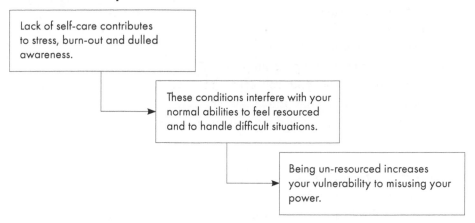

Lack of self-care contributes to stress, burn-out and dulled awareness.

These conditions interfere with your normal abilities to feel resourced and to handle difficult situations.

Being un-resourced increases your vulnerability to misusing your power.

Note: the term resourced means being connected to and supported by personal resources, for example centeredness, confidence, compassion, education and training, supervision, empowerment, social network.

I'd like to point out that although we focus on misusing our power with others, we also misuse power with ourselves. There are several subtle and not so subtle ways that we cause harm to ourselves.

- *Failing to prevent or reduce harm to ourselves:* for example, getting so overwhelmed or over-worked that we develop debilitating symptoms of caregiver burn-out.
- *Failing to repair harm to ourselves:* for example, being overly self-critical, having unreasonable expectations, lacking self-compassion, feeling ashamed and not attending to healing these.
- *Failing to promote our own well-being:* Undervaluing our work and effectiveness, not finding nourishment in our work, and not confidently owning our role power.

Self-care and the 150 percent principle

"Yikes! How do you adequately take care of yourself when your job requires you to bear 150 percent responsibility for those in your care? I'm overworked already!" I am often asked about this by students and readers. So, in one of my programs, we addressed this question and came up with a list of ways to take care of yourself at the same time that you are staying in the role of greater responsibility:

- Know you can't fix people.
- Apologize.

- Accurately assess the 150 percent.
- Let yourself grieve.
- Forgive.
- Take down-time.
- Use supervision and peer support.
- Remember to take your role off when you transition from work mode.
- Be careful about what phone calls you take.
- Discern when you have done enough and then let go.

Challenge: Knowing your limitations

Before offering some resources for self-care, here is a self-care challenge—knowing your limitations. There are two kinds of limitations to pay attention to. One is personal limitations. It seems that leaders who are aware of and even mindfully transparent about their strengths and their growing edges and places where they need help are more successful, empowering, well liked and respected than leaders who either believe they can do everything, or think they need to pretend they, as a leader, are capable of all things. Not many of us helping professionals are competent at doing everything. Working with clients, yes, that's what we are trained for, but we aren't necessarily good at marketing, writing, teaching, lecturing, producing webinars and handling finances. It is good to know what you need help with.

The other kind of limitation has to do with being clear about what kinds of healing modalities you have training and competence in. The next skill is to be able to track when you are getting in over your head or starting to go beyond your level of competence. This is not as easy as ethical codes and guidelines would have it. Although, it is ethically important and simple to let your clients know your training and areas of expertise in advance so that they can make an educated choice to work with you and your WATSU skills and clinical scope. However, it is not always possible to accurately assess the issues your client will bring to your sessions, or, particularly in WATSU, what deep patterns or traumatic experiences might come up in a session.

"Providing services outside area of competence" is the second most frequently filed grievance, and "failure to terminate" and "failure to refer" are in the top ten most frequent complaints. As a member of ethics committees, I can attest to how important it is to 1.) be clear up front about your education and training, 2.) assess as soon as possible when you are over your head and 3.) make referrals in a supportive and compassionate way so that your client does not feel that you don't like them or that this is their fault.

Sensitively and clearly referring or completing

Here are some examples:

"I'm feeling that what I have to offer isn't what you need right now for your healing. I'd like to recommend that you make an appointment with…"

"I notice a lot of intense feelings and memories are arising during your WATSU sessions. I think it would be really helpful for you to see a psychotherapist for processing and additional support."

"I'll be going on vacation starting in two months. I'll be gone for three months. I would like to refer you to a colleague of mine with whom I think you would be a good match. When I return, you can stay with her, or return to working with me."

"Something pretty strong is happening right now. I'd like to help you slow down and reconnect with your body and the water and me."

Often completing or referring is that simple and direct. However, the impact of the power differential on clients creates an increase in their vulnerability to rejection and criticism. Clients both need and want you to like them and be impressed by their progress. They want and need to be valued and respected.

From their increased vulnerability, any of the above kind, rational and direct sentences can be misunderstood as rejection, disapproval or abandonment. Termination that is not mutual or only partially mutual can cause great pain that can resurface even months after the actual termination. Clients may be working on issues of attachment and self-esteem that may get triggered by termination that is not of their choosing. Even professional reasons like changing job, going on sabbatical, being out of your area of expertise or sexual attraction don't matter when clients interpret the termination as rejection. Tracking for indicators from your client that they may have felt rejected or criticized can help you take these feelings seriously and address them even though these responses may not seem reasonable to you.

Challenge: Self-care resource: Developing more resilience

Resilience is the ability to bounce back from adversity. Nature has plenty of resilience when we don't interfere. We need our resilience now too, and we will need more of it in the future. Resilience has a repeating cycle most easily felt in the seasons, but also operating in tropical zones where these seasons are more subtle.

The Resiliency Cycle (adapted from Gestalt and Hakomi models) has some simple lessons to teach us about using our considerable powers to work with nature for mutual resilience and health.

There are four stations on the Resiliency Cycle: Clarity, Effectiveness, Satisfaction and Relaxation. All four experiences are needed for resilience.

Clarity: Sensing of purpose or vision, gaining insight, gathering relevant information, feeling fresh and open.

Effectiveness: Being energized, focused and effective; responding appropriately; being willing to invest time and energy.

Satisfaction: Opening to nourishment, feeling gratitude, sensing being in the flow, reflecting and integrating.

Relaxation: Completing and letting go, slowing down and resting, having a sense of emptiness, making space for something new to form and grow.

Western culture in particular seems to have become stuck in the path of acquisition, urgent creativity and the cultivation of individuality. We are busy and productive. We move back and forth between *Clarity* and *Effectiveness*—back and forth between getting an idea and making it happen. We don't take enough time to reflect. We don't relax and let go, except when we get sick. We seem to miss the essential stations of *Satisfaction* and *Relaxation*. These two are so important that most spiritual traditions honor them as prayer, meditation, gratitude, surrender and letting go.

In my personal life, I notice that I feel almost compelled to take immediate action on any good idea I have. My ideas are unburnished by reflection and integration of the action that went before. My actions are unmediated by letting go and emptying out so that a new idea or action can have space to be nurtured. My speed also gets in the way of my intuition and with being in tune with the people I work and live with.

Self-reflection: I invite you now to take a look at the cycle and notice how you go around the cycle in your life. Where do you start? Are there aspects that you omit or keep repeating?

In nature, the leaves fall allowing the tree to be empty and resting. New leaf buds form in the emptiness, waiting until the time is ripe for them to emerge into full-leaf abundance and glory. And then, after they have fulfilled their purpose and flow, they let go to rest and make space for the next buds to form.

Self-care package

Good self-care is a rich package involving more than just getting enough sleep. Self-care involves taking care of yourself both within the context of your helping relationships and in your life outside your work.

Practitioner self-care assessment chart

The primary question is: What does it take for me to show up for my clients in a way I feel good about? Give yourself an opportunity to look at your self-care personally and within the therapeutic relationship. Rate yourself on a scale of 1–10, with 10 meaning that you are very good at this aspect of self-care.

Balance

1. Maintaining an appropriate workload	1 ←——————→ 10
2. Creating diversity of expressive, recreational and spiritual activities	1 ←——————→ 10
3. Developing the ability to both savor and serve	1 ←——————→ 10
4. Setting a high priority for self-care	1 ←——————→ 10
5. Attending to your inner balance	1 ←——————→ 10

Rest

6. Getting enough rest and retreat time	1 ←——————→ 10
7. Planning ahead for times of renewal	1 ←——————→ 10
8. Allowing for goof-off time	1 ←——————→ 10
9. Getting adequate physical exercise	1 ←——————→ 10
10. Being kind and compassionate toward yourself	1 ←——————→ 10

Satisfaction

11. Approaching clients with an attitude of curiosity—savoring and being nourished by their essential qualities; feeling gratitude	1 ←——————→ 10
12. Appreciating the value and importance of your professional offerings	1 ←——————→ 10
13. Finding novelty in daily routine and resting in the ease of familiar skillfulness	1 ←——————→ 10
14. Feeling a sense of inner satisfaction and pleasure in your work	1 ←——————→ 10
15. Staying in touch with your desire and vision for service	1 ←——————→ 10

Support		
16. Using supervision and personal support	1 ←——————→ 10	
17. Keeping appropriate records, disclosure forms and malpractice insurance	1 ←——————→ 10	
18. Knowing, accepting and accommodating for your limitations	1 ←——————→ 10	
19. Seeking and using feedback	1 ←——————→ 10	
20. Accessing continuing education that is inspiring, informative and stimulating	1 ←——————→ 10	

Challenge: Variety is the spice of life—cultivate role and status power differentiation

The greater the percentage of time you spend in your up-power role, the more difficult it becomes to separate your personal power from your role power and the more identified you will become with your up-power persona. You may also lose your capacity to shift the focus onto yourself and the useful vulnerability that is required to be able to make the best use of your down-power experiences as a student, patient or employee. The remedy? Take a class in something that interests you and is new to you. Be mindful of your down-power position when you visit the doctor. Join a choir or play on a team with a director or coach. Serve on a committee as a member, not the chairperson. Keep noticing when you are moving around the complex network of up- and down-power roles and situations. Cultivate a variety of up- and down-power positions in your daily life so that you can be empathetic in each position and not get stuck in up or down.

I'd like to close this chapter with a review.

Twelve ways to use your power wisely and well

1. Understand that you have and will continue to misuse your power. Give up the idea that you will never cause harm by having an impact different from your intention, being tired or distracted or making a hurtful mistake. You, like everyone else, are human and subject to the deteriorating effects of increased power. You, like everyone else, are continually learning about power. Good intentions are simply not enough.
2. Stay connected to those down-power from you in both aspects of your power: strength and heart. Actively maintain and nurture

connectedness and universal compassion along with appropriate boundaries. Stand in your power while staying in your heart.

3. Own your status and role powers. Saying yes to them enables you to be able to use them wisely and well.

4. Elicit accurate and authentic feedback. Refine your ability to self-reflect and self-correct. Don't take feedback too personally or not at all personally.

5. Learn how to track for and attend to situational difficulties and relationship conflicts. Most can be resolved and even repaired with skill, humility, non-defensiveness and a rapid response time. Develop confidence in your ability to resolve and repair.

6. Cultivate a variety of up- and down-power roles so you can keep a felt sense of the shine and shadow of each side of the power differential and, in addition, stay role-fluid.

7. Remember that when you are in role, you are never just yourself. You are, on the one hand, a projection screen for the expectations and fears of others, and on the other hand, in your role you have a distorted view of others and of reality.

8. Keep in mind the 150 percent principle: while everyone has 100 percent responsibility for maintaining the health of the relationship, the person in the up-power role has greater responsibility (150%).

9. Embrace your limitations as well as your strengths. Be willing and learn how to apologize and forgive when needed. Amplify the gifts of leadership and mitigate the perils.

10. Choose to know, understand and handle your shadow temptations and habits and the pull to be self-serving. Get your personal needs met, but get them met outside your role and rank.

11. Avoid burn-out with proactive self-care and resilience.

12. Value and appreciate the good you can do with your personal, role and status powers. Deepen your ethical center pole and commitment to well-being and the good of all.

Further reading

Barstow, C. (2005). *Right Use of Power: The Heart of Ethics: A Guide and Resource for Professional Relationships* (tenth edition). Boulder, CO: Many Realms Publishing.

Colorado Association of Psychotherapists (n.d.). Code of Ethics. https://coloradopsychotherapists. org/code-of-ethics.

Diamond, J. (2016). *Power: A User's Guide*. Santa Fe, NM: Belly Song Press.

Emerson, R.W. (1841). *Essays: First Series, 4. Spiritual Laws*.

Taylor, K. (1995). *The Ethics of Caring*. Santa Cruz, CA: Hanford Mead Publishers.

Chapter 6

Palliative Aquatic Programs™

Serving Medically Fragile Infants, Children and Adolescents

SHEILA PYATT AND DR. DAVID M. STEINHORN

Introduction

In 2004, Sheila received a letter attached to a newspaper article describing George Mark Children's House (GMCH), located in San Leandro, California. GMCH is a unique facility that provides palliative care to children who are medically fragile or approaching end of life. Patients receive "around-the-clock" skilled nursing care from experienced pediatric nurses and the entire family is included in a dimension of care that supports the needs of body, mind, spirit and emotions of child and family. The House had only been open for two months and was the first of its kind in the entire country.

When she saw a photo of a small pool with a Hoyer lift located close to the nurses' station, Sheila immediately felt it was an opportunity she could not resist! In this holistic environment, Sheila saw an opportunity to provide gentle warm water sessions for medically fragile children diagnosed with a variety of challenging health conditions. With a position on staff secured at GMCH, as a holistic nurse, she developed a robust pediatric palliative aquatic program which has provided several thousand medically fragile and dying children with palliative aquatic sessions. The most sacred and poignant sessions were those provided to children approaching end of life or who were actively dying and these incorporated parents and family members whenever possible. Families were deeply grateful to be able to hold and caress their beloved child in the supporting element of warm water. The sessions enhanced the intimacy of the parent-child bond and allowed non-verbal, intimate communication through touch as Sheila gently directed their movements in the water. Over time, nurses, volunteers, medical students and clinical Residents and Fellows from the University of California have joined Sheila in the water as she worked with the children to relieve their discomfort and pain. Approximately 4000 sessions later, this program has become a favorite with the families served by GMCH. The medical staff at GMCH also recognize the benefits provided to patients, such as improved sleep and reduced spasticity. Sheila has presented the Pediatric Palliative Aquatic Program at conferences in the United States as well as in South America, Canada, Europe, Israel and Mexico. Little did she know in 2004 that she was embarking on one of the most challenging and rewarding journeys of her life!

Over the past three decades, the concepts of *palliative care* and *hospice care* have become better known and understood within the medical community and, ultimately, among the general public in the United States. Diverse palliative care services are now available along the entire life continuum for adults and children diagnosed with "life-shortening and life-limiting illness" (Hughes & Smith 2014). However, in 2004, the field of pediatric palliative and hospice care was still in its infancy in most areas of the United States. Established as an homage to her late brothers George and Mark, GMCH's visionary founder, Dr. Kathleen Hull, created a beacon of healing and care for medically fragile children. It has served as a model for similar facilities developed elsewhere in the United States and in other countries.

The World Health Organization describes palliative care as:

...an approach that improves the quality of life of patients and their families facing the problem associated with life-threatening illness, through the prevention and relief of suffering by means of early identification and impeccable assessment and treatment of pain and other problems, physical, psychosocial and spiritual. (Benini *et al.* 2008)

Palliative care as it applies to children includes some further unique characteristics:

- Palliative care for children is the active total care of the child's body, mind and spirit, and also involves giving support to the family.
- It begins when illness is diagnosed and continues regardless of whether or not a child receives treatment directed at the disease.
- Health providers must evaluate and alleviate a child's physical, psychological and social distress. Effective palliative care requires a broad multidisciplinary approach that includes the family and makes use of available community resources; it can be successfully implemented even if resources are limited.
- It can be provided in tertiary care facilities, in community health center and even in children's home. The principles apply to other pediatric chronic disorders. (Benini *et al.* 2008)

Eventually, infant, pediatric and adolescent patients who receive palliative care will transition to hospice care, which is:

> ...a special kind of care that focuses on the quality of life for people and their caregivers who are experiencing an advanced, life-limiting illness. Hospice care provides compassionate care for people in the last phases of incurable disease, so that they may live as fully and comfortably as possible. (American Cancer Society 2019)

This is referred to as end-of-life care in contemporary hospice care for patients of all ages and extends into the final phase when patients are actively dying.

To illustrate the role of pediatric palliative aquatics in the context of caring for medically fragile children, we will share some of the actual aquatic sessions provided to these patients.

Palliative Aquatic Program origins

The Palliative Aquatic Program grew out of Sheila's ten years of experience in special needs aquatics for children with chronic medical diagnoses. She began to provide individual aquatic sessions to patients at GMCH after her shift ended. Night staff noted that children who received a session slept better and required less pain medication. In 2005, at the request of the leadership/management at GMCH, Sheila designed the Pediatric Palliative Aquatic Program (PPAP) utilizing the small on-site pool at GMCH.

Children who had been admitted for end-of-life care and their parents were invited to participate in the PPAP. Parents realized they could float their fragile child safely and comfortably in warm water with less concern about causing pain. They recognized the benefits of the program and frequently requested sessions for their children during their respite care visits at GMCH. The PPAP became part of the services offered to children and their families and continues at GMCH.

Palliative aquatics embodies a heart-centered, intuitive approach in a supportive and nurturing environment. It is *holistic* in its essence and inclusive of all patients' cultures and beliefs, and sensitive to the challenges of each patient's illness. In this way, palliative aquatics represents an important integrative medicine modality, designed for that unique patient population.

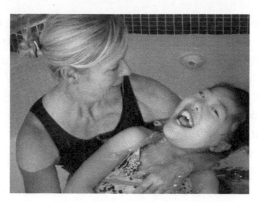

Figure 6.1: A child experiences joy in the pool

Based on her training in both land and aquatic modalities, Sheila noted consistent patient responses to sessions across various age and diagnostic categories. During these warm water sessions, patients' respirations routinely changed from tense, labored and shallow upper chest breathing, to slower, deeper and more relaxed respirations. The most consistent patient responses were observed by nurses on the night shift. They noted that children who had received a session required less pain medication and slept better, often through the entire night. They experienced fewer muscle spasms and seizures, and less neural irritability.

Ultimately, palliative aquatic care embarks on a path to optimize the quality of life of medically fragile children as they journey toward a spiritually profound end-of-life transition.

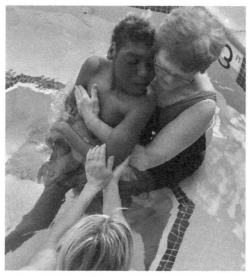

Figure 6.2: A child with a tracheostomy tube is brought gently into the pool

The influence of the Special Needs Aquatic Program Water Magic™ on the development of the Palliative Aquatic Program

The community-based Special Needs Aquatic Program, fondly referred to as SNAP, provides children with special health challenges with a place for their abilities to shine, as they exercise, play and have fun being in warm water. This unique aquatic program was developed and implemented in 1991 by Dori Maxon, a physical therapist and educator. It continues to thrive today in the San Francisco Bay area.

SNAP profoundly influenced the development of the Pediatric Palliative Aquatic Program at GMCH. During their work in SNAP, volunteers learned multiple ways of holding and supporting children with special needs in an aquatic environment. They developed insights and increased sensitivity relating to the challenges faced by families of children with special needs. It was Dori Maxon who suggested that Sheila looked at GMCH in 2004 with the brief comment: "You need to work here." The lessons learned in SNAP provided Sheila with a solid foundation for the subsequent development of the PPAP. As often happens in the mysterious circle of life, she was granted the further privilege of caring for some of these SNAP kids when they came to GMCH for respite and end-of-life continuum of care. Sheila is grateful to have witnessed and been an active team member guiding those individuals beyond this earthly existence.

The influence of WATSU in palliative aquatic programs

Harold Dull's WATSU, specifically *Water Breath Dance*, profoundly influenced the breath when floating a receiver (patient) at heart level. Being aware of our breathing patterns and learning to connect with those of the patient is the first step in creating a meditative (mindful) state during a session and really one of the foundations of our palliative aquatic programming. Harold's teachings emphasized that "the deeper you drop into the emptiness of the bottom of the breath, the more it will feel as if your client is drawing you out of the void as the breath comes back in and the water lifts you without effort" (Dull 2004, p.22). What Harold continued to further highlight in his text is that connecting the breath with movement was an invitation to the receiver (client) to free the body and mind from physical and mental stressors. In addition, gentle movements and dynamic holding that is the staple of WATSU provided the client with an opportunity to feel the embrace and support of the water. Harold's expertise in Zen Shiatsu allows us to comfortably stretch and apply pressure to the energy meridians of the body. The beauty and grace of the *Water Breath Dance* over the last 30 years has given the palliative care population countless hours of respite from pain, anxiety and isolation. Gentle movements, touch and this foundational move continue to bring comfort and relaxation to children and adults suffering from life-limiting and life-shortening illnesses.

We have incorporated the *Water Breath Dance* in our work with children as well as other simple, gentle WATSU moves to illicit rotational movements with the spine and trunk that enhance a full body experience while buoying the spine. When practitioners are fully present, we pay close attention to the rise and fall of the patient's chest, observing in detail the patient's degree of tension, facial expressions, respiratory effort and breathing patterns. In practice, the respiratory pattern is one of the keys to understanding the non-verbal child's state of being and connecting with the patient one-to-one, which is an essential element of presence. Palliative aquatics is not simply a technique that can be studied, learned and applied. It requires a concerted effort to be present to the patient and their needs in the moment.

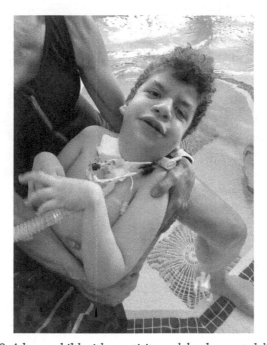

Figure 6.3: A larger child with spasticity and developmental disabilities

The provision of continuous oxygen during a session or a child with a tracheostomy does require us to emphasize our focus on the child's breathing and respiratory effort. We observe the depth and rate of respiratory effort and whether it is indicative of congestion, pain or muscle spasms. The *Water Breath Dance* required us to "fine tune" these assessment skills, especially during sessions for those approaching end of life. The movements of WATSU were modified to meet the needs of those receiving palliative care. For example, we found that slower linear movements reduced nausea and provided time for the practitioner to observe the patient's responses more closely and in greater detail.

An indigenous healing perspective for medically fragile children nearing end of life

In 2005, shortly after starting the Pediatric Palliative Aquatic Program at GMCH, Sheila met Larry Swimmer and his wife, Sandy. Both Larry and Sandy are originally from the Pine Ridge Indian Reservation (Lakota Nation) in South Dakota. In addition to their many community activities, the Swimmers were foster parents to several children who had been born addicted to cocaine, and they understood the needs of medically fragile children.

Larry expressed genuine interest in Sheila's work in pediatric palliative care, especially with the aquatic program at GMCH. He was very interested in the spiritual aspect of this work, and what he saw as the healing power of water during a session for the child, family and clinicians. Larry noted the importance of the nurses who facilitated both the preparation of the child prior to the aquatic session and the child's care after the session. He recognized that the nurses formed an integral part through the pre- and post-session care of the children and the families, during which the staff themselves also experienced a process of healing and completion. The nurses knew they were part of a ceremony. From his indigenous background, Larry recognized that "any ceremony [the aquatic therapy session] has a process, a rhythm. Part of the ceremony is to restore balance and harmony. [As] the patient releases pain or anguish, harmony and balance go back to staff [in sacred reciprocity]. Then this process starts over with the next patient. The pool is a focus and a reminder to staff [that] a child is being prepared [for what will come]."

It is important for the reader to recognize that water therapy is a *process* and not a technique to be applied *mechanically*. Everything works in synergy: the patient, the family, the staff, the physical setting (pool facility) and the water, each contributing to the whole process. The clinician's spirit bears witness to this process, helping patients and their families shift or grow at a deep inner level to prepare to leave with dignity. One of our goals is to help the patient and family achieve an understanding of the fullness of life, then to release and let go, a process that must take place whether the life is short or long. The palliative aquatic practitioner's role is to help develop the process for staff, patient and family one case at a time. Bearing witness to a patient's suffering and life journey is something healthcare providers are frequently called on to do. By standing for and with the patient in the water and bearing witness to the process they are going through, the aquatic therapist or clinician facilitates a process of inner enlightenment through engaging the spirit of the person and allowing it to come full circle. In Larry Swimmer's words, "All we can do is to start the process of a new beginning. We give the body and the earth spirit back to the earth."

The aquatic therapist's role as a sacred witness

One of the most important roles of the palliative aquatic therapist during an aquatic session is that of a "sacred witness." Larry Swimmer described this role: "In my awareness, I know Spirit is holding the child. When the parent is holding their child, they too are witnesses. The parents know (often at an unconscious level) they need to release their child. In standing for someone in the water, there is a connection, a synergy, and an understanding that parents feel and come to accept through the process. It is important for the child and parents to come full circle, by releasing the pain and coming to joy, peace and light. Patients sense through the aquatic experience where they come from as they complete their circle of life. Parents connect with their fragile child and come full circle as well."

Sensing when the person was on the edge of life, Larry would play his flute and chant to prepare the patient. He pitched his voice and his flute to find where the person was in the end-of-life journey until he felt a "tug." He continued to play until the person reached a joyous place. During this process, the patient's relatives were also elevated to the same place, a process that could be enhanced by chanting or drumming. In our experience, patients often achieve a reduction of pain, which causes happiness and a sense of pure joy, as the body comes into synergy at all levels.

Larry Swimmer's thoughts and observations, presented in the Lakota manner of explanation, deserve deep reflection. Over the years, we have acquired a more universal understanding of the multiple layers at play during palliative aquatic sessions. Larry's understanding of the physical, cognitive, emotional and spiritual aspects of the program have provided a depth and richness to the program, reflecting the essence of his being, his life and his work in service to others within his Lakota community and our aquatic one as well. Being a former Catholic nun through the Society of Helpers, Sheila is drawn to the deep spiritual transformations and nuances that occur in the end-of-life transitions for children. She sees great value in sacred witnessing through this indigenous lens and would like to see its ability recognized in best palliative and hospice practice models. Providing spiritual solace, closure and comfort to patients and family members alike is a shared vison within palliative care and holistic nursing paradigms that can be seen within an indigenous model similarly.

The essence of our work: Presence and intention

Our relationship with our patients, and, by extension, with their families, requires that we work with *presence* and *intention*. *Presence* is a manifestation of the practitioner's connection with the patient. It requires the use of one's whole *being*. The patient's affect, facial expressions, respiration, movements and response to touch and sound are influenced by our focused presence. This element is essential, especially during those moments when a patient is hovering between life and death, when our presence serves as a sacred witness to the process unfolding before us.

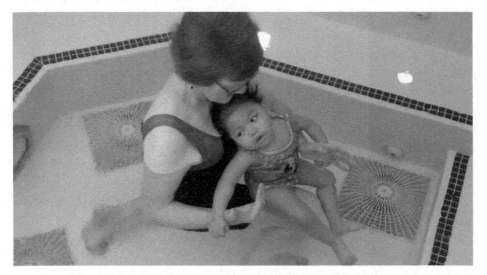

Figure 6.4: A practitioner provides support for an infant in the water

Intention is a critical component of our care. It is something that is usually assumed in medical care—that we intend to comfort our patients and ease their suffering—but it is rarely expressed consciously, even to ourselves. Our *intention* is to fulfill the goals of palliative care during an aquatic session, which are to alleviate suffering in all its forms, improve the client's quality of life and enhance the relationship between parent and child. In the case of dying patients, our intention is to ease the transition and allow the pain and suffering of this lifetime to end with the death of the body, and that only joyous and meaningful experiences are carried forward by the human spirit as it moves to whatever comes next. To achieve these goals, practitioners use the remarkable properties of water: its buoyancy, viscosity, flow and warmth, and its intrinsic cleansing nature to facilitate the patient responses. With great sensitivity to the child's cues, we "follow the lead" of the client, who determines how still or how active a session will be. Holistic modalities such as gentle massage and appropriate music are integrated into each session. When appropriate, parents and family members may join their child in the water during a session. Some children become deeply silent, then fall asleep in the water while tenderly being held in the arms of a parent or practitioner. On other occasions, the client is more active and engaged during the entire session. These warm water sessions foster an intimacy and joy among family members at a time that can be stressful and uncertain for both patients and families.

Practitioners have noticed similar responses among patients of different ages and diagnoses. Some of the most notable features include more relaxed respiratory effort and reduced muscle spasticity, because the child is weightless and no longer fighting gravity through proprioceptive reflexes. In these conditions, a sense of peace and calm arises as a child falls asleep in the practitioner's arms. Palliative aquatic practitioners experience this work as *holistic* in its essence and intention. The practitioner attends to the needs of the *whole* child—body, mind, emotions, spirit—and, when present, the needs of family members. When we as staff can support the child's reality, we affirm the child's life as they experience it and rejoice in everything that gives the patient pleasure, meaning, comfort and joy.

To understand what an end-of-life session looks like, we will describe an actual aquatic session provided to a teenager approaching the end of her life. Annie is 16 years old and has been diagnosed with brain cancer. Try to imagine what she may experience. How does it feel to be gently submerged in near body-temperature water while being supported in the arms of an aquatic practitioner or family member? The following description is provided with the permission of Annie's family.

ANNIE'S STORY

Annie had been diagnosed with brain cancer at age 12. Four years later, she was admitted to George Mark Children's House. There were no more treatments available that would cure or palliate her cancer. The staff knew that one of Annie's last wishes was "to have a bubble bath." Roberta, the night nurse, asked if Sheila could take Annie in the water. Sheila felt honored to give this child a palliative session in the warm pool on site.

The nursing staff discussed how to move Annie from her bed to the pool without increasing her pain. Her father and grandfather purchased some camping mats so she could be transferred more easily from her bed to a gurney. Staff timed the administration of Annie's medication to alleviate pain caused by movement. Annie was carefully lifted onto the gurney and transported to the pool area. Gently, her father and grandfather placed her on the pool deck. Sheila stood in the pool and received her as the men slid Annie and the mat into the water.

The session

The family had gathered on deck, seven people representing four generations of relatives. Sheila remembers catching a glimpse of Annie's little brother, huddled on deck near the stairs. He appeared lonely and stunned. (A child's illness impacts the entire family, but often the healthy siblings are lost in all the activity surrounding the ill child.) The silence in the room was palpable as the family waited for the session to begin.

A few minutes later, Sheila slid Annie off the mat, and submerged her gently into the warm water. She held Annie in her arms with her head precisely supported at the crook of her elbow. Sheila placed a small floatation device under Annie's knees to support her low back. Annie's dad positioned himself opposite Sheila, ready to help as needed. Slowly, Sheila moved Annie in a circle, moving her "head first," while observing her face for any indication of pain.

As Sheila moved Annie through the water, family members kneeling at the edge of the pool would touch her head or kiss her and say, "I love you, Annie." Both their sadness and joy were palpable. "She looks so beautiful," someone whispered. "She looks so peaceful." "This is fantastic." "She is trying to speak."

Sheila asked the family to guide her since they could understand Annie's facial expressions. Sheila explained to them, "The water is a powerful medium for healing. Annie can feel your presence and your energy." Sheila could sense they were surprised by her words. Knowing that each person needed to absorb this entire event, Sheila said no more. The silence was punctuated with an occasional comment, a memory or a soft chuckle. Sheila believes that everyone experienced the sacredness of the moment. She felt they were saying goodbye to their precious child in a very special way.

Sheila placed Annie in her father's arms so he could hold her. He cradled her head with one hand and held the floater with the other, while Sheila provided extra support. He, too, kissed Annie and told her how much he loved her.

When it was time to take Annie out of the water she began to cry. Sheila surmised it was the abrupt return to gravity from a weightless state that caused her discomfort. Or was it the withdrawal from a "safe" place of peace, love and tranquility that she was crying for? She was gently rinsed, quickly patted dry, then placed on the gurney. Annie was covered with a blanket and transported to her room. As she passed the nurses' station, someone exclaimed, "Look! She is smiling."

After drying off, Sheila went to Annie's room to check in on her. Her dad, still in his wetsuit, hugged Sheila and said, "I never would have dreamed…"

Her grandfather formally shook hands with Sheila and said, "It gives a whole new perspective…" They left their sentences unfinished, as if to ponder this event more fully.

Annie died early the following morning.

In all her years of working in the water, Sheila recognizes that she had never experienced moments like these until she began the work at GMCH. No words can fully describe the feeling of trust she sensed from this family as she held their dying child in her arms. In a sacred, silent manner, their beloved child said "goodbye" to each of them.

Water has a special place in all the world's religious traditions. We gestate and are born through amniotic water, we are hydrated and cleansed through water, and we receive our final purification through water in many traditions, even if only a ritual bathing after death. Is it any wonder that the experience with Annie felt like a sacred and mystical experience for her on her last day of this lifetime?

Qualities and skills of a palliative aquatic practitioner

The training and experience of the aquatic practitioner is critically important in maintaining the safety and success of the Pediatric Palliative Aquatic Program.

There is currently no accepted standard nor certification process for palliative aquatic practitioners. The following information is based on over 15 years of providing palliative aquatic sessions for adults and children as well as training practitioners in this method who come from varied backgrounds. As already mentioned, palliative aquatics is more than a technique that can be replicated given enough hours of training. In addition, the palliative aquatic practitioner must possess personal integrity, intelligence and interpersonal skills to attend to the needs of the body, mind, emotions and spirit of medically fragile and dying children. Because of the dire conditions patients experience, Sheila maintains that professional, in-depth training from trained practitioners is of utmost importance.

To assure safe and effective sessions with children and adults, the palliative aquatic practitioner must have:

- education in human development
- a license to touch
- an understanding of medical terminology and basic physiology
- the ability to work within a team and to respect input from others
- experience of working with medically fragile children and adults in conventional hospice and palliative care settings.

Training and certification in WATSU can also be a helpful foundation and precursor for palliative aquatic specialties.

New aquatic practitioners are paired with an experienced nurse aquatic specialist who often has given sessions to the child during previous visits. An indispensable quality for a palliative aquatic therapist is the ability to focus on the subtle cues and needs of each patient, so they may respond to their unique needs in the moments before, during and after the session. At any given time, if any practitioner does not feel safe in giving a session to a child, or if they do not feel well, they should cancel the session.

If the practitioner providing the aquatic session is not a nurse and if the medical situations listed below are present, then it is very important to have an experienced registered nurse or licensed vocational nurse on deck, or preferably in the water, to respond appropriately in case of emergency. If neither a registered nurse nor a licensed vocational nurse is available, the session should be postponed until sufficient staffing can be assured.

The presence of a registered nurse, either on deck or in the water, is required if the patient:

- is seizure prone
- needs continuous oxygen, usually via nasal cannula
- has a tracheostomy that will require suctioning and protection
- is large or heavy with poor control of body movements, for example flailing in the water.

Palliative aquatic practitioner requirements
Physical abilities

- Average strength, coordination and flexibility.
- Able to swim a short distance to respond quickly during an emergency situation.
- Able to assist with patient transfers during entering and exiting pool via a Hoyer lift or two-person lift.
- Able to maintain the safety of a patient who may become agitated and move erratically.
- Able to respond quickly to emergency situations, such as seizures and respiratory distress that require suctioning of tracheostomies, or provide urgent medical intervention.
- Acceptance of own physical limitations and judicious adherence to safe practices which constitute personal integrity.

Cognitive skills

- Good patient assessment skills, ability to prioritize, and problem-solve "in the moment" issues.
- Adaptability to ever-changing situations and demands.
- Collaborative skills and a non-judgmental attitude.
- Respect for the experience and insights of others.
- Understanding of cultural differences and needs of families.
- Understanding that continuing education is a priority.

Emotional qualities

- Steadiness and a calm demeanor when working in an emotionally charged situation, such as providing a session in collaboration with family members whose relative is dying.
- Ability to separate one's own emotions from those of family members.
- Flexibility and a good sense of humor when schedules and sessions do not go according to plans.
- Commitment to self-care and reflection.
- Heightened sensitivity to another person's needs (emotional intelligence).

Assuring a safe environment during family aquatic sessions

In the palliative care facility where this program was piloted, parents and siblings frequently join their child in the water for a family session. If the child is strong enough to tolerate sounds and activity, these sessions provide families with opportunities to bond and enjoy a family activity together. Families experience a sense of "normalization" in their lives, however brief.

When parents and family members participate in a session with a very fragile or dying child, staff ask parents to seat themselves comfortably on the pool bench before we place the infant or child in their arms. There is no compromise on this issue of safety and security in the palliative aquatic therapy environment. Responsibilities for safety and liability rest on the shoulders of staff and the facility.

During the first few moments of a session, the staff assess how "water savvy" the parents are. Usually, the level of comfort can be observed in an adult's body language and facial expressions as they enter the pool. Some parents and family members are "naturals" in an aquatic environment. They intuitively know how to hold their child and where to support the child's body for maximum comfort and safety. Other parents may be dealing with both the unfamiliarity of being in water and their anticipation of the imminent death of their child. In this latter instance, staff take responsibility for directing the entire session and in maintaining the safety and comfort of all participants.

Some parents feel confident enough to take their child into the water by themselves without the presence of the aquatic practitioner. If parents are comfortable and *have demonstrated safe behavior in the water*, there is usually no safety issue. However, if parents are not at ease or skilled in the water, the aquatic practitioner will ask them if they would be willing to have one or two training sessions with a member of the aquatic staff before working alone with their child. In addition, parents may need a "spotter" on deck to ensure that the child is safe at all times. The spotter can pay attention to the child's cues, respiratory effort, airway support devices and physical safety without the additional task of positioning and holding the child in the water. The GMCH handbook for parents describes the conditions under which parents may take their well children into the pool for sessions.

Some parents have requested training so they can work with their child at home. Several have requested "spa-size" pools for their child from Make a Wish and similar foundations so they may provide these soothing sessions for their child. These responses speak to the value of our work and its importance as a component of palliative care services. Funding for training of parents and family members needs to be made available to ensure the efficacy and safety of these programs in a home environment.

A palliative care pediatrician's view of the Pediatric Palliative Aquatic Program

The families of children facing incurable illness are confronted with tasks that most parents never have to face. In addition to the medical needs of their child's condition, often entailing prolonged hospitalization and family separation, our families must navigate the needs of healthy siblings, the loss of normal family routines and the impact on employment and social relations. While every child offers their parents new lessons and opportunities to grow as fathers and mothers, children with chronic health challenges bring unique opportunities to their families. We have seen parents and siblings mature and grow enormously as emotional, caring human beings over the course of a child's incurable illness. While no parent would have knowingly signed up for such a life assignment, we regularly hear from parents who would do it all over again, if they needed to. While some parents recognize that the last intensive care unit admission to prolong life may have been one step too far, our families cherish the additional moments they have with the beloved children, regardless of the personal cost.

As described so well in the preceding material, the Palliative Aquatic Program can offer families and their health-challenged child opportunities for more normal interactions than are typically seen in the medical setting. The most dramatic effect is the deep, intimate connection between parent and child. During these moments of intimate connection, we have the feeling that the parent and child are in a sacred communion, heart-to-heart, soul-to-soul. These are moments when deep processing of emotions occurs in a non-verbal fashion, which the parent is often unaware of until afterwards. Life-closure work is a central goal of palliative and hospice care and focuses on processing feelings, thoughts and memories accumulated over a long or short lifetime. When patients are too young, weak or debilitated to engage in verbal processing, integrative modalities such as palliative aquatics can provide an avenue for non-verbal processing of life's experiences, sometimes more effectively than words can. In so doing, Sheila believes the Palliative Aquatic Program offers families an opportunity to maintain and deepen the parent-child bond that is an essential element of the "contract" that exists between parent and child.

Summary

The Pediatric Palliative Aquatic Program is a unique modality that addresses the needs of a child receiving respite or end-of-life care. When appropriate and safe, family members may join their child or sibling during an aquatic session. These moments together in a warm pool provide families with an opportunity to be together in an enjoyable setting during a respite care visit. The warm water enhances relaxation as siblings or parents play with their child. Siblings enjoy an experience with their brother or sister in a happy setting, knowing their brother or sister is well cared for.

During sessions with children approaching end of life, parents have an opportunity to safely hold their beloved child in warm water while seated comfortably. Or they may prefer to simply be present on deck while the aquatic practitioner provides the session. This gentle, sacred time provides parents with moments and memories they will forever cherish long after their child has died.

References

American Cancer Society (2019). What is palliative care? www.cancer.org/treatment/treatments-and-side-effects/palliative-care/what-is-palliative-care.html.

Benini, F., Spizzichino, M., Trapanotto, M. & Ferrante, A. (2008). Pediatric palliative care. *Italian Journal of Pediatrics*, 34(1): 4. doi: 10.1186/1824-7288-34-4.

Dull, H. (2004). *Watsu: Freeing the Body in the Water.* Middletown, CA: Watsu Publishing.

Hughes, M.T. & Smith, T.J. (2014). The growth of palliative care in the United States. *Annual Review of Public Health*, 35: 459–475. www.annualreviews.org/doi/full/10.1146/annurev-publhealth-032013-182406.

Further reading

Adams, J. & Garcia, C. (2005). Palliative care among Chumash People. *Evidence-Based Complementary and Alternative Medicine*, 2(2): 143–147. doi: 10.1093/ecam/neh090.

"A Midwife to the Dying" (2013). Krista Tippett in conversation with Joan Halifax.

Becker, B.E. (2009). Aquatic therapy: Scientific foundations and clinical rehabilitation applications. *American Academy of Physical Medicine and Rehabilitation*, 1: 859–872.

Becker, B.E., Kasee, H. & Whitcomb, R. (2007). *Autonomic Nervous System, Cardiovascular and Circulatory Effects of Cool, Neutral and Warm Water Immersion.* Pullman, WA: Washington State University.

Becker, B.E., Kasee, H., Whitcomb, R. & Sanders, J.P. (2009). Biophysiologic effects of warm water immersion. *International Journal of Aquatic Research and Education*, 3: 24–37.

Gaab, E. (2015). Families' perspectives of quality of life in pediatric palliative care patients. *Children*, 2(1): 131–145. doi: 10.3390/children2010131.

Gaab, E. & Steinhorn, D. (2015). Families' views of pediatric palliative aquatics: A qualitative study. *Journal of Pain Management Nursing*, 6(4): 526–533.

Hufford, D.J. (1997). Integrating complementary and alternative medicine into conventional medical practice. *Alternative Therapies*, 3(3): 81–83.

Kerr, C.E., Wasserman, R.H. & Moore, C.I. (2007). Cortical dynamics as a therapeutic mechanism for touch healing. *Journal of Complementary and Alternative Medicine*, 13(1): 59–66. doi: 10.1089/acm.2006.5245.

Park, C.L. & Halifax, R.J. (2011). Religion and Spirituality in Adjusting to Bereavement: Grief as Burden, Grief as Gift. In R.A. Neimeyer, D.L. Harris, H.R. Winokuer & G.F. Thornton (eds), *Grief and Bereavement in Contemporary Society: Bridging Research and Practice* (pp.355–363). New York, NY: Routledge.

Sandelowski, M. (1991). Telling stories: Narrative approaches in qualitative research. *IMAGE: Journal of Nursing Scholarship*, 23(3): 161–166.

Weeks, J. (2014). *Chronicles of Health Creation: Joint Commission Issues New Pain Standards in Response to Integrative Medicine Team.* HuffPost, http://huffingtonpost.com/john-weeks/integrative-medicine-and-_b_6213662.html.

Chapter 7

Speech Therapy in an Aquatic Setting

CALIAS DULL, SUSAN NACHIMSON AND DR. RITA ALEGRIA

There is emerging evidence of the benefits of conducting speech and language therapy in warm water and incorporating elements of WATSU into clinical practice. Speech-language pathologists (SLPs) assess the disorders of speech and language in individuals from birth through to geriatrics. All ages, regardless of diagnosis, have the potential to benefit from WATSU. Conducting sessions in warm water has the added benefits of assisting with muscle relaxation and providing additional whole-body sensory support, and may facilitate engagement with younger clients. Warm water creates a safe and relaxing space for clients to "open up" and speak about their individual and therapeutic needs. The proprioceptive input from the hydrostatic pressure also facilitates speech production. Within pediatrics, conducting therapeutic sessions in warm water may increase engagements and opportunities for play, which is a child's primary occupation.

SLPs develop treatment modules following formal and dynamic assessments based on each individual's needs. Elements of both dynamic assessment and treatment may be conducted in warm water. Therapy in an aquatic setting can provide an optimal environment for diagnostic therapy because of the informal atmosphere, warmth, physical support and basis for fun.

The practice of speech pathology includes a vast array of systems, involving feeding, speech and all aspects of communication. It is the interaction among these systems that produces effective and efficient eating, speaking and communication throughout one's life span.

Communication involves the interplay of numerous areas, including pre-speech, speech, hearing and language. All of our systems are connected and the interaction among systems is vital for effective communication. It is important to look at the whole-body function in relation to hearing, speech and communication. This includes both hyper- and hyposensory functions. Touch, hearing, sight, smell and taste all have bearing on the human system (Oetter 1995). Sensory limitations may dramatically interfere with appropriate function of pre-feeding, oral-sensory motor, hearing, speech, and receptive and expressive language function.

Pre-speech covers respiratory integrity, phonatory integrity, oral-motor integrity and feeding. Respiratory integrity includes breathing from first breath after birth throughout one's lifetime in relation to swallowing, speaking, moving and interactive communicating. Phonatory integrity refers to an individual's ability to hear and imitate sounds to create meaningful words and speech. Oral-motor integrity refers to how an individual uses their mouth, lips, tongue, jaw and breath to eat efficiently and produce sounds. Feeding refers to the newborn suckling on the breast or bottle through infant/toddler first foods to mature eating patterns. All of these systems interact to produce efficient eating and speaking patterns.

Motor speech involves the development and function of oral-motor integrity for the production and sequencing of sounds and ability to incorporate changes in pitch and intonation. Pitch refers to the relative highness or lowness of a tone as perceived by the ear, which depends on the number of vibrations per second produced by the vocal cords. Intonation refers to the variation in spoken pitch when used, not for distinguishing words as tone, but rather for a range of other functions such as indicating the attitudes and emotions of the speaker, signaling the difference between statements and questions, and between different types of questions.

Language is a system of communicating. Cognitive development encompasses general intelligibility, comprehension and using one's understanding in communication. SLPs also work on pragmatic language (i.e., the social rules and conventions for language), communicative intent (i.e., a desire to convey and to receive information between individuals) and symbolic language development (i.e., associating symbols with meaning). Alternative communication systems refer to the use of pictures, recorded words, and so on, by individuals who may not be able to develop typical functional speech or language.

Whole-body benefits in water

All of our systems are connected and the interaction among systems is vital for effective communication. It is important to look at the whole-body function in relation to hearing, speech and communication. This includes both hyper- and hyposensory functions. Touch, hearing, sight, smell and taste all have bearing on the human system. Clients with autism spectrum disorder (ASD), cerebral palsy, Down syndrome, seizures, and so on, often experience sensory resistance to specific stimuli (touch, taste, smell, etc.). Sensory limitations may dramatically interfere with appropriate function of pre-feeding, oral-sensory motor, hearing, speech and receptive and/or expressive language function. Speech therapy in an aquatic setting facilitates a whole-body approach and incorporates sensory integration. WATSU provides additional sensory input and may dramatically benefit speech sessions.

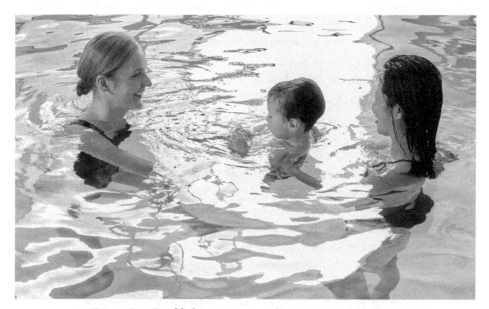

Figure 7.1: Establishing rapport and joint attention in water

The following illustrate specific ways that warm water facilitates systems of speech production. It is vital to complete all appropriate aquatic training before bringing clients into the water, and to remain cognizant of professional ethics and scope of practice.

Respiration: Respiration is the foundation for efficient feeding/eating and general voicing. The steady pressure of water on the ribcage facilitates increased ribcage expansion and oxygen into the lungs. General playing and floating in the water provide this support. Toys which require a child to blow may also improve vital capacity. A therapist with the appropriate training can keep the body immersed to nipple or clavicle level as medically indicated. Watch and listen to the changes that spontaneously occur. Note the quality of inhalation and exhalation with respiratory depth changes. It may be beneficial to bounce a young child up and down. Additionally, ramps, steps and seats may be incorporated so the client can develop increased confidence and independence in the water.

Phonation, articulation, speech: All verbal attempts are counted! Lip closure and awareness of specific sounds can all be done with water play (i.e., blowing bubbles, blowing whistles, utilizing pipe connectors, toys and balls of differing weights that provide different levels of resistance).

Oral-sensory: Hyper/hyposensitivity can dramatically interfere with respiration, feeding and phonation. Incorporating splash toys into pediatric therapy can increase a child's ability to tolerate sensations. For children with hyposensitivity, this can also increase their overall awareness and identification of sensations. The therapist may opt to use a ramp, steps, a long seat or a small island where the child can be independent in the water to allow accidental falling which splashes the face and body. This causes the child to be more attuned to their environment and increases sensory awareness. Multiple materials may be used, including washcloths, PVC pipe connectors, squeeze toys, balls, pool basketball and other toys that splash water towards children's faces while they are making choices and having fun. In contrast, on land, these children may fight, run away, cry or resist facial sensory preparation.

Joint attention and pragmatic language: Rhythmical, sing-song vocalizations, rhyming and singing appeal to many clients. Rhymes and songs with refrains paired with splashes or other movements will increase anticipation, delight and active vocalizing (even if the response is "No!"). Any toys or games that facilitate interaction and a back-and-forth exchange may be utilized to support pragmatic language. The child may be prompted to request specific toys and engage in turn-talking with their caregiver or therapist. Always use strategies that reflect the goals and objectives developed from informal and formal assessment.

Vocabulary and language development: Always create opportunities for the child to name objects, activities, friends, areas in the pool, and so on. Use language for pointing to and labeling different areas in the pool, saying new words or calling to a friend to practice using speech and vocabulary and syntax. Use *all* opportunities for expanding descriptive language, adding newer concepts as often as possible.

After a client is medically cleared for participation in water the following things may be considered along with knowledge and skills for treating in a water-based setting:

- It is expected that SLPs who use the water-based setting as a modality receive basic training in water-based therapy and are proficient in appropriate handling techniques. They would also benefit from consultation and collaboration with other trained professionals such as other SLPs, physical therapists or occupational therapists who are trained in sensory integration and motor function.

- Develop ideas through the clients' likes and dislikes—they are the best teachers!
- If a client is resistant to one approach, try another, and follow the client's lead when possible.
- Always have dry towels or washcloths nearby. Allow clients the opportunity to wipe and dry their own face for improved sensory awareness and independence. This can be incorporated into their "sensory diet" and "sensory preparation."
- Whenever possible, use an aquatic setting that provides a place where a child can get around independently (e.g., ramps, pool stairs, benches, floating platforms with water flowing over). Adults can be supported either in floating, holding or leaning on the side of the pool.
- Adapt all aquatic practices based on the client's individual medical case history and therapeutic needs.
- Remember that the recommended temperature is 93–96° Fahrenheit/33.9–35.6° Celsius.

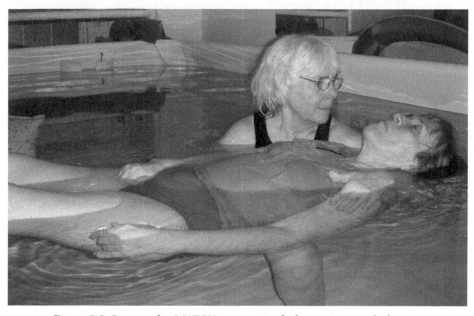

Figure 7.2: Post stroke: WATSU preparation before active speech therapy

CASE STUDIES

Case study 1

A four-year-old male was referred to an SLP for assessment and treatment. He presented with schizencephaly, spastic quadriplegia, dysphagia, cortical blindness, ASD, oral-motor feeding limitations, speech delay and an expressive/receptive communication disorder. The client was ambulatory but unstable on his feet. Due to his physical limitations, it was extremely important to monitor the water level. The client enjoyed water more than any other play. Therapy sessions were held twice a week for a year and alternated between land and water sessions.

SLP goals:

1. Become safe in water, including normalizing facial and chest hypersensitivity; appropriate breathing; independent movement with no risk of aspiration.
2. Develop normal facial sensory input, oral-motor function for eating and speech.
3. Support appropriate voicing for phonation and speaking (breath control and function for speech).
4. Develop receptive and expressive vocabulary related to spa play and items relating to spa.
5. Develop enjoyment during each speech therapy session!

The SLP floated the client in a supine position, allowing buoyancy to assist in support of his body. In addition, touch was applied to pressure points to support spinal elongation, head support, pelvic positioning and facilitation of fuller inhalation and exhalation. The child enjoyed the bubbles in the spa and, while being floated in a supine position, learned to accept splashing into his face with responses starting with total startle, to giggling, to acceptance without any response. The SLP used position changes (NDT) to do face-to-face play in the water with lips touching the water. The child was able to keep his mouth closed while his lips were submerged with no hypersensory reaction.

Blowing toys were utilized to facilitate increased lip rounding and opening of the mouth for vowel variety (NDT). Due to the age of the child, therapy was primarily play-based. Play consisted of sitting on a ledge in the spa with SLP supporting the child in sitting, followed by the child getting up and moving independently in the spa, occasionally slipping and falling into the water with his head and face submerged. Success was measured by the child's ability to do this with no sputtering or coughing. The SLP supported the child by demonstrating Touch Cue strategies and practicing safe water-in-mouth positions if the child demonstrated signs or symptoms of aspiration. When the child demonstrated putting his mouth in the water with closed lips, independently, while sitting on the SLP's lap, he was released for an independent trial to jump into the water to retrieve a preferred toy. The child eventually learned to jump up and down in the water after tossing and retrieving a preferred toy. He appeared unbalanced but was able to recover with no more than one coughing episode per session and attained no coughing per session for five consecutive sessions by the end of the year, becoming water safe for play with very little need for adult handling.

Feeding sessions yielded some active chewing with his preferred food texture. No noticeable oral hypersensitivity was observed when a spoon was presented or during chewing or swallowing. Drinking thin liquids and smoothies was uneventful, including consecutive sips and swallows of water.

Signing and verbal stimulation for receptive and expressive vocabulary: *bubbles* (jets in spa), *more, stop, yes, no, big cup, little cup, all done,* and so on. The child did not relate to using signs or specific vocalizations for individual words. Instead, he preferred gestures by going up to the bubbles, laughing and raising his arm to make a request "time for bubbles." He laughed and became visibly excited when the bubbles were presented.

Case study 2

A 47-year-old female was referred to the SLP following a severe closed head trauma. Treatment areas included breath support, vocalizing and audibility. The client presented with limitations in her ability to utilize optimum breath support for speaking. She presented with restricted diaphragmatic movement during breathing for relaxation and would speak beyond her available residual air supply. An evaluation of her speech demonstrated strain, decreased loudness corresponding to limited air supply, and fluctuating intelligibility. Mild oral dysarthria (i.e., limited oral muscle control) was noted secondary to her traumatic brain injury.

The client attended three diagnostic therapy sessions. During her initial assessment, the client presented with limited diaphragmatic moving during easy, relaxed breathing. She had a tendency to speak with her head pulled into capital extension (i.e., head back, chin tilted upwards) which resulted in a stiffening of the muscles supporting her neck. She spoke with a deep monotone vocal quality. During her initial sessions, the client was uneasy in a supine position. When she was placed in this position, she reported ear sensitivity and demonstrated increased muscular tension. However, she enjoyed walking in the water and was comfortable in an upright saddle position. From the saddle position, she was able to increase her inhalations and exhalations and engage in voicing practice. Practicing voicing (mmm) and doing blowing activities in the water helped decrease facial muscle stiffness and increase intelligibility of sound production. Increased loudness was observed on land after the session.

During subsequent sessions, the client was placed in a full saddle WATSU position. She practiced combining breath and arm movements. She attempted to increase right-sided upper extremity movement in the water in order to provide fuller breath support for voicing. The client experienced difficulty following complex directions and responded to a slower pace with fewer words and demonstrated adequate control of her breathing patterns. Facial brushing with a soft, dry terry cloth facilitated better lip closure and a softer facial mask during speaking. Practice with soft vowels increased some activity at the temporomandibular joint where the upper and lower jaws meet. When the client continued to talk while walking out of the pool her jaw appeared less tense, demonstrating good carry-over of skills for speech practice in the water.

Case study 3

This is a detailed observational description of a ten-year-old female child with spastic cerebral palsy who received speech therapy intervention in an aquatic setting for a one-year period.

The objectives were to verify whether the intervention of a speech therapist in an aquatic setting promotes the improvement of communication in a case of cerebral palsy. At the beginning of treatment, M. was able to say "mama," "papa" and "ahh" with no complete lip closure, and vocalized with decreased breath support and volume. She required maximal assistance for all movements and was only able to maintain lip closure and sustain a sound for two to three seconds. When her face neared the water, she demonstrated a strong startle response, which frequently caused bouts of coughing as small amounts of water were inhaled. When attempting to vocalize, she would produce full body extension and could not disassociate speaking and these movements.

After one year of speech therapy in an aquatic setting, she produced more sounds, such as /m/, /b/, /p/, /w/. She exhibited increased coordination, strength and range in her ability to blow bubbles for five to six seconds. When she lost her balance from standing or sitting and her face went into the water, she now blew bubbles and required only minimal to moderate assistance to recover. She initiated putting her face in the water with lips closed and held her breath for about five seconds. She was able to roll in both directions, using controlled flexion of her neck and trunk while maintaining lip closure. She demonstrated increased ease at reaching, grasping and releasing and gained new skills through play and social activities that promoted functional movement, communication, balance and independence.

M.'s case is one of many stories that we have encountered in which we noted the benefits of aquatic therapy. The type of methodologies and strategies such as the one presented suggest positive qualitative results. However, in order to allow significant conclusions, additional research and comparison between subjects, therapists and even between institutions, a larger sample size is needed.

Case study 4

Observation of a hands-on case: evidence of speech therapy sessions in an aquatic setting on a patient with communicative dysfunction and secondary feeding issues.

The child was evaluated in September 2013 when he was two years and five months old. The parents attended the SLP appointment as they had heard about speech therapy in water and wanted an opinion regarding communication, language and, most importantly, feeding. They asked if their current SLP could also attend the meeting.

G.'s previous "land" intervention from early intervention included two-and-a-half hours of speech therapy between the ages of 1.10 and 2.5 years old. During this time, G. was very reluctant regarding chewing and was eating mainly soft foods like soup, yogurts, gelatin and purees. Cereals would take time, but he would eat them. When asked if he liked to bathe, his mom reported that he loved it but didn't like to wash his hair because he couldn't stand water on his face.

In the evaluation, it was observed that G. established contact with a stranger, not requiring any security by an adult. He would participate in social routine activities, knowing how to anticipate them. When he pointed at pictures, he expected that someone would respond (Sandbank et al. 2017). His joint attention was inconsistent and poorly developed. He had a tendency to focus his attention on objects or events. When he looked at the therapist or his parents, it was normally only to observe or imitate. He tried to resolve his own problems in an autonomous way. When he was not able to, he would ask for help by pulling the hand or arm of an available adult. After evaluation and an explanation from the therapist, therapy in water was begun by mutual agreement. It was established that G. would continue to have the same format of speech therapy sessions on land and this would be supplemented with 45 minutes per week in water. The SLP colleague and therapist established a plan with the same goals. They were already using visual aids, and likewise initiated the use of the same supports and added more for pool toys, objects and materials. The parents were always in the pool too. The transition to water was slow and with no stress. The first sessions began with G. inside a big bucket with a warmer temperature than the pool and slowly he made the transition of the bucket to the pool. Without even noticing, G. was already in the water in the therapist's arms, facing his mother. With time, the child developed greater adaptation to water, increasing his self-confidence that many times he demonstrated with a happy facial expression. He enjoyed being in the water as long as he was not moved too quickly or unexpectedly, and the water did not touch his face. When this occurred G. moaned for a towel to dry his face off before continuing any activity. When in an aquatic setting, G. showed great motivation and enthusiasm, not wanting to finish the session—behavior not evidenced in early interventions in room sessions. His parents reported that during land sessions, as soon as a signal was made to "end the session," G. would rapidly run to the exit door and quickly put on his coat ready to leave for home. In water, G. would willingly stay over the time if this was allowed.

By the tenth water session, G. was slowly moved into deeper water, as one of the speech goals with this boy was to use the water as a medium to decrease oral hypersensitivity (it is a major factor for children with feeding issues) (Campion 2000). Splashing can challenge a sensitive body to accept sensations of water over the body, face and head. Washcloths, PVC pipe connectors, squeeze toys, balls and other toys that splashed water up into G.'s face were used. The therapist played with him in an up-and-down movement, while going underwater blowing bubbles through her mouth. The little boy caught on immediately and pushed his head under even before the adults in the pool were ready. He came up quickly, laughing and repeating the activity again and again. He was supported so that he wouldn't go under unexpectedly. Then Mom was asked to get ready to catch him. The therapist and Mom faced each other, nearly touching. G. loved doing this, and when asked if he wanted to go under the water, he did this immediately. Mom moved backward a step, G. was released, and he independently dived under with his whole body and reached her, and she pulled him out while he laughed, squealed, breathed in, and turned back to the therapist for more.

In his next two visits, G. enjoyed splashing in the water, being "thrown" into the air and caught again, and spinning. This allowed him to be suspended with a foam noodle under his arms and around his chest. While being supported in water at body temperature, G. was consistently comfortable and free from the challenge of gravity pull. This reduced stress environment facilitated more normalized patterns that could then be brought into focus for better land function. It is thought that a client's memory of successful integration of sensory awareness, upper and lower extremity movement, vocalizing and oral-motor function can go on to facilitate successful function on land (Melo & Pires 2018). At this point, Mom reported that showering/bathtime had become a fun part of the day.

In the following sessions, the child used both hands to start and play the proposed game. He started to verbalize "more," "toy," "up" and "no" and looked for interaction with the therapist. Slowly, his vocabulary began to increase and out of the blue he started to say the names of all the animal toys in the pool. Verbal requests started to be more frequent, and G. also started to accept more chewing toys like robbers with different diameters, floatable chewing fruits (banana), gummy bears, straws and soft animals that he would put in his mouth and chew.

The water sessions established better body contact and greater interaction between G., his parents and therapist, and also more verbalizations. First-session fear was transformed over time to a willingness to participate, have fun and enjoy himself. After eight months of intervention, G. could eat more variable consistencies of food, and although he still rejected meat, he ate a full piece of bread, biting and chewing it. He initiated communication and showed an improvement in his interaction with his peers at school. The child started to be more open to different exercises proposed, asking for (sometimes choosing) exercises at session time and interacting with greater communicative intention.

Adult with cerebral palsy testimonial:

Doing WATSU with Susan Nachimson was an innovative treat, nothing like I have experienced or seen before. In the water, I could assume positions that I can't assume on a mat due to gravity and the two-dimensionality of the mat. The water supports me in any position. My body is more flexible than ever. I think WATSU is like yoga, which is impossible for me, with my spasticity, to do in any other environment. Also, the heat of the water allows me to be more flexible. I could have stretches done to my hips with ease that are painful when my therapists do them on a mat. The stretches to the hips done in water felt invigorating and released much tension throughout my body. I especially liked the pressure applied to my lower back. The movement that accompanied poses like the "dolphin" and the "seaweed" helped me gather my breath and get it rhythmic, the goal of techniques like WATSU. The water helped regulate the pace that my body was moving in these poses and this prompted me to pace my breath.

Summary
WATSU strategies and principles provide numerous potential benefits to clients of all ages and diagnoses receiving speech-language therapy. Conducting therapy in warm water provides a unique opportunity for connection and sensory support. It facilitates the whole body and the interplay between all systems of speech production, as opposed to isolating specific areas. There is emerging research into the benefits of speech therapy in an aquatic setting and further research is warranted.

References

Campion, M.R. (2000). *Hidroterapia: Princípios e Prática*. Sao Paulo, Brazil: Editora Manole.

Melo, P. & Pires, C. (2018). *Interação Terapêutica Em Contexto de Meio Aquático e Contexto de Sala Em Crianças Com Perturbação Do Espetro Do Autismo Em Idade Escolar*. Universidade de Évora.

Oetter, P., Richter, E.W. & Frick, S.M. (1995). *MORE: Integrating the Mouth with Sensory and Postural Functions*. Stillwater, MN: PDP Press.

Sandbank, M., Woynaroski, T., Watson, L.R., Gardner, E., Keçeli Kaysili, B. & Yoder, P. (2017). Predicting intentional communication in preverbal preschoolers with autism spectrum disorder. *Journal of Autism and Developmental Disorders*, 47(6): 1581–1594.

Chapter 8

WATSU® in Sports Medicine

TOMASZ ZAGORSKI

Introduction

WATSU was developed by Harold Dull in 1980 in Harbin Hot Springs, originally as a form of new, non-verbal communication using warm water and the connection of two people performing bodywork, Shiatsu and stretching meridians. Breath connection, heart-to-heart connection and unconditional acceptance of whatever rises up in the session according to the Zen Shiatsu non-doing approach were additional tools in this new communication, but also signature qualities of this concept (Zagorski 2008).

Harold, being a genius creator himself, also gave space for the contribution of others, which allowed WATSU to grow beyond Harbin and spread around the world as a recognized bodywork approach. Physiotherapists have discovered useful practical applications for neurological and orthopedic patients, and there are many applications in psychotherapy. With years of development and many new specialists involved, we have more and more new, very specific applications of WATSU in rehabilitation (Schoedinger 2008; Kulik *et al.* 2016). The spa industry has discovered that WATSU benefits match very well with their clients' demands of relaxation, bliss and the need for separation from everyday stress. The healing through water nature of WATSU corresponds perfectly with the sanus per aqua (spa) philosophy. In addition, the Zen Shiatsu oriental roots of WATSU are a powerful marketing tool for selling it as a spa treatment. WATSU is being offered by an increasing number of spas, some of which have dedicated pools for WATSU sessions, and some five-star resorts are considering including it in their offerings (Orzel-Zagorska & Zagorski 2010).

Roots of WATSU for athletes

WATSU sessions have been applied to athletes from time to time by many practitioners who have access to such types of clients. It was a coincidental event that was not incorporated into standard training and recovery programs. As a former competitive runner, having a background as an athletic coach and sports therapist, and working with top-level athletes, I found WATSU a great tool for improving athletes' recovery process. I had a unique opportunity to experience the effects of a WATSU session while being in intense, professional training, when the body experiences extreme loads. I could compare this with the feeling of WATSU effects when training at a recreational level and with no training at all. In each case, the results were different. Bringing together the perspectives of an athlete, a coach, a sports therapist and a WATSU practitioner gave me new insight into WATSU and its potential new applications in sports medicine. In this way, WATSU for Athletes was born in 2008, when the first article was published at www.watsu.com. The aim was to provide customized WATSU sessions for athletes as a means of supporting their athletic recovery and training (Zagorski 2016).

The concept is based on training and therapeutic knowledge and many years of work with the best athletes in the world, supported by analysis of the newest scientific research. In my work with athletes, I applied cutting-edge knowledge as well as innovative and intuitive tools and methods.

The principles of the WATSU for athletes concept and specific means applied in my work have been verified in practical work with athletes of various levels (Zagorski 2018). The newest trends in the development of athletic training and sports therapy, including fascial therapy, have been taken into consideration and I have consulted with distinguished practitioners and scientists. What's more, hundreds of hours of exploration in the water had a big influence on me.

The current shape of the concept and the teaching materials result from several years of work and provide a solid amount of knowledge, useful for candidates aiming at working with athletes in the water and using WATSU. Since WATSU and training constantly develop, so too does the work in the new field of practical WATSU application in sports medicine.

Benefits of WATSU in sports medicine

When we analyze the physiological effects of WATSU on the body in the context of sports medicine the main benefit of WATSU sessions seems to be a relaxation response as a means for improving recovery after training and competitions. More effective recovery, in conjunction with specific movements and bodywork in gravity-reduced conditions, plays an important role in load compensation and injury prevention (Zagorski 2018). Also, some of the psychological benefits of WATSU sessions, such as stress reduction and anxiety reduction, improving body awareness through relaxation, and improved sleep quality, are significant contributions to sports medicine.

Athlete benefits

An athlete during a WATSU session is in warm water, with no pressure, no action-reaction response, no expectation setting, in the supporting hands of someone who is giving 100 percent of their attention and care. This situation and feelings are very different and often contradictory to what they encounter in their typical competitive training lifestyle, which is full of stress, pressure and expectations. This contrast is a very powerful tool for the body and mind in healing and recovery. From a physiological point of view, warm water immersion, together with repeated gentle WATSU movements in water, decreases activation of the central nervous system (CNS) and increases activation of the parasympathetic autonomic nervous system (ANS), which results in a relaxation response (Becker 2010; Cameron 2013). Skeletal muscles have no demand for work because of reduced gravity. Nice surroundings and good support provide a feeling of safety and pleasure, which promotes a parasympathetic response seen as a decrease in heart rate (HR) and blood pressure (BP) and changes in heart rate variability (HRV) typical for relaxation and recovery (Tufekcioglu & Çotuk 2009). These are the ideal circumstances for the recovery and healing processes to begin. If we compare this situation to traditional recovery conditions described briefly as a part of train, eat, sleep, repeat, where an athlete lies down in the bed and thinks about the training done, about how it was hard, about how far they are from the optimal form, how others performed better, and so on, we can clearly see why WATSU promotes recovery faster and improves its quality.

Typical recovery procedures require some effort (foam rolling, stretching, compensatory exercises) and are time consuming or sometimes boring (spending an hour attached to or inside a specific machine). A recovery massage, which is supposed to be nice and relaxing, is usually painful because of muscle soreness. After very hard effort during training, we experience another kind of work during recovery. WATSU gives the opposite feeling. During a WATSU session, you don't have to do anything; simply lie down and enjoy the gentle movements, with a progressive feeling of calm, and the worst part to worry about is the session's end. If you are sleepy after the session, which is a marker of the parasympathetic shift of the ANS, you can go to bed and sleep without unnecessary and energy-consuming thinking. The sleep quality itself is much better after the WATSU session. Gentle, repeated movements, done in warm water, help with blood circulation in the limbs and promote the removal of exercise metabolites from the muscles, and the water pressure helps to move the lymph from the limbs. WATSU's gentle stretches help to restore myofascial elasticity, which is decreased by higher post-exercise muscular tonus. Specific myofascial release in water (MRW) techniques, in addition to WATSU sequences, can restore tissue mobility and release restrictions caused by tissue overload and compensatory adaptations (Zagorski 2014). According to the healing principles of Traditional Chinese Medicine (TCM), the application of specific Shiatsu points may also improve the recovery process. Because of relaxation, athletes can feel their bodies better. They may learn to recognize a subtle difference between tension and release and develop it in very small parts of the body or in an antagonist group of muscles. This interplay between tension and release recognition will aid them in stressful competitive situations where proper body control is key. Athletes can also benefit from interpersonal relationships during a session when they are truly connected in a one-on-one situation, rather than focusing on hard effort, which is common in most training and competition situations. It gives feelings of appreciation, acceptance and unconditional love—a gift from Harold through WATSU.

Benefits for therapists and coaches

Therapists can also benefit from learning WATSU. For many practitioners, it is a life-changing experience and a paradigm shift in thinking about healing and therapy. The philosophy of being here and now with other people with no agenda is diametrically opposed to the pragmatic, task-oriented approach of most therapists, particularly in sport, which is by definition a result-oriented activity. Surprisingly, this philosophy broadens their horizons and improves the effectiveness of the traditional therapy they have been practicing for years (Zagorski & Kulik 2014). Sports therapists have an additional powerful tool for increasing recovery and, at the same time, a tool for offloading their physical work, because, in water, they get less tired when they use water principles and work ergonomically. Those who use hydrotherapy are already expanding their therapeutic repertoire, and those who are new to water treatments can discover its incredible healing potential.

Coaches are constantly on the lookout for small things which can improve training and recovery, and as a result give even a small advantage in the competitions. With WATSU, they get quite big and powerful things. They know they need to cooperate with wise, skilled and well-trained therapists in order to be on the same page and be supported by the therapist's work. They know how new things can be beneficial for their athletes, and usually they encourage their therapists to learn. Because knowledge about WATSU in sport is not common among coaches and it comes mostly from therapists, it is recommended to educate coaches not only with explanations and presentations, but also by giving them the opportunity to receive a session, so that they can learn from their own experience.

Contraindications for warm water hydrotherapy in sport—how much, when and when not to?

These are the fundamental questions that all practitioners need to answer in order to work with athletes in a safe and effective way. A safe way refers not only to physical safety, but also, and most importantly, to the safety of the sports results. Even if we always have to apply all the precautions in each case, we know that an athlete's body is usually stronger than the average person's, so it can endure more. But an athlete's optimal performance, built laboriously throughout the year, is very fleeting and can be easily destroyed by a wrong step. The consequences will not be harmful to athletes' health, but to practitioners' finances, when sports federations or athletes with multiple contracts sue and seek compensation. Even without a lawsuit, there will always be remorse that you have wasted a year or four years of work on someone who has sacrificed everything to succeed at the Olympics. Therefore, we have to follow the art of therapy, be familiar with and comply with all aquatic therapy and specifically WATSU indications, contraindications and precautions, know the physiology of training and recovery principles and comply with training goals set in the training plan.

Contraindications for water immersion

Aside from the general contraindications for water immersion which are covered in Chapter 2, there are some situations in sports where we must be cautious and sometimes skip WATSU sessions entirely. In winter sports, for example, if the training camp is held during a period of bad weather with low temperatures and strong wind, and access to the pool requires going outside back and forth, there is a risk of catching a cold. Hard training reduces the immune system's potential in general, and the risk of infection increases, so it's best to skip a session. In another case, if a marathon runner has just finished the race and is completely exhausted, has soreness in every part of the body, and is unable to walk normally, they are not a good candidate for a WATSU session. In this case, it would be better to take care of hydration, proper food intake to restore energy, sleep, and maybe a manual massage first. And after a few days, when muscle soreness is more or less gone and the energy level is well established, we may bring the marathon runners into the water. We occasionally have a person who cannot swim or is afraid of water for a variety of reasons. In such a case, we can begin by using other forms of aquatics to acquaint the person with water and reduce their fear before lying down in the water for WATSU. We can also apply classical hydrotherapy to introduce the healing benefits of water and easily convince people to receive a WATSU session.

Although the contraindications and precautions for water immersion are discussed in other chapters of this book, I would like to list them here for ease of recall (Schoedinger 2008):

- Cardiac instability
- All acute diseases with fever
- Acute pain
- Acute soft tissue injury, broken bones
- Active cancer
- Bowel incontinence
- Infectious diseases that may be spread by air, water or touch
- Significant open wounds
- Severe epilepsy
- Multiple sclerosis (warm and hot water)
- Sensitivity to pool chemistry
- Absence of cough reflex
- Significantly limited lung vital capacity (below 1000ml)
- Severe peripheral arterial disease
- Deep vein thrombosis
- Severe urinary tract infection
- Kidney disease with lack of compensation of fluid loss
- Severe ear infection, perforated eardrums
- Uncontrolled diabetes
- Recent cerebral hemorrhage
- Severe thermoregulatory control diseases
- Tracheostomy, gastrostomies, colostomies, ileostomies, catheters
- Autonomic dysreflexia
- Severe motion sickness
- Aggression, auto-aggression.

Contraindications for relaxation

Relaxation is the main benefit of WATSU sessions and is one of the most important tools used for therapy and for recovery in sport. However, in some cases, it may be a contraindication or require special precautions. For example, in acute ligament instability caused by trauma, or general hyper mobility of the body, when we relax the myofascial system, we make the situation worse. This may be the case with many gymnasts, but also we can find single cases in most disciplines. Applying WATSU in sports medicine, we need to remember there is another important contraindication connected with muscle relaxation. In most disciplines, athletes require a certain muscular tone for optimal performance. Sometimes they do specific, wake-up strength training on the day of the competition to achieve this optimal tone. Applying WATSU too early before the competition may destroy this tone and optimal performance ability. For this reason, we do not apply WATSU three to seven days before the competition, sometimes even more.

Contraindications for movement and bodywork in water

We have to deal with injuries all the time in sports. Some say it is a part of the game that we need to accept. Rehabilitation from an injury is a critical and delicate process. It requires time, which is limited, because athletes, coaches and sponsors want to come back to activities as soon as possible. Rehabilitation, on the other hand, necessitates precision and leaves no room for error. If any element of the soft tissue parts of the locomotor system is damaged, regardless of the level of this damage, there is a natural healing process in place, which engages an inflammation process to repair and rebuild damaged places, and this has its own timing, which can be shortened by intense rehabilitation. However, if we begin an activity by applying heavy loads, we risk damaging the tissue again, sometimes more severely, even resulting in a complete break. The secondary injury is much more difficult to heal and usually takes longer to recover from. For these reasons, the activities and exercises used during the rehabilitation process are critical—they must be done in a pain-free range of motion, with a low intensity at first, and with proper progression. The brilliant idea is to begin rehabilitative training in water with reduced gravity and then progress to land-based training. Because WATSU is basically a passive activity that leads to deep relaxation, it is possible to lose control over the body and go beyond the safe range of motion limits and to affect injured places.

For this reason, applying WATSU during rehabilitation time is a challenging task and requires precision and a focus on keeping it safe. When we apply stretching or bodywork in order to lengthen something, because, for example, we want to change our body mechanics and create a longer step and improve the result of running, we need to remember that even if we succeed in lengthening some structures and the step will be one or two centimeters longer, it does not mean we will improve the result automatically. The myofascial system, which forms a network around the whole body and is also an active part of the whole locomotor system, is adapting to the changes caused by the demands from the outside. According to the biotensegrity concept, the change created in one place does not affect only this place, but the whole system (Scarr 2014; Zagorski 2021). Lengthening or shortening in the calf will affect the hamstring work, which will affect the erector spinae muscle group, which will affect the neck muscles and the positioning of the head. The structures at the back of the body will affect the structures in the front and others. By elongating one part, we create a change in the system of tensions traveling through the whole network, and influence the conditions in the whole system. Sometimes the results are the opposite of what we expected; we may lengthen the steps slightly, but the running results are worse. For this reason, using bodywork in WATSU in order to change the biomechanical properties of the body should be well planned and done in consultation with the coach and body mechanics specialists who understand biotensegrity principles.

Key success factors in sports

In old Olympian times, when fairness in competition and fighting spirit were the most highlighted values, sport was simple and beautiful and we can say it was pure. Athletes were amateurs who did sports mostly as a hobby, and the highest prize was the glory of winning. Even in these difficult times, athletes recognize the importance of training to improve performance while also looking for other ways to improve performance. They applied oil to the skin before a fight, used massage to recover, and were looking for ways to improve the equipment, understanding the complexities of sports training and paying attention to the details that can already be seen in ancient sports. And when money and the media entered sport, they caused profound changes in sport itself and the approach to sport and the training process, including using doping to achieve additional advantages. Doping is a highly unethical issue that is not worth devoting time to here. However, it would be interesting to see how modern sport has become more complex and how many details can now play a significant role in sports success.

There are many similar cases, but I would like to focus on one case I was personally involved in: the 2016 Olympics in Rio de Janeiro, men's 200m sprint final (Zagorski 2018). Three athletes, ranging from third to fifth, were on the verge of finishing in the top five. Two-thousandths of a second decided the bronze medal. This amount of time is difficult to comprehend, but it determines whether you have a medal or not, whether you go down in Olympic history or not, whether you achieve your life's goals or whether you must wait and work hard for four more years, with no guarantee of success at the end. Athletes in fourth and fifth place were both close to and far away from sports heaven. And it was not only the athletes, but also the trainers and all the people involved in this preparation, as well as the families and friends of the athletes. I was lucky to work with the athlete who took bronze in the 2016 Olympics and we were in heaven for a couple of weeks. I was hired three years earlier in very difficult times when the athlete in question had had a series of injuries. The goal was clear—a medal at the Olympics—but the way to it was hard, including one serious injury three months before the main competition. This is a one-of-a-kind and personal story, but it adds to the picture of sports success preparation. I was privileged to assist other athletes to win 18 medals in international competitions over my 16 years of work in top-level sport, and I gathered a certain amount of experience that I would like to share with my readers. It could be another separate book, but I will try to be short and keep it specific to WATSU.

Physical preparation

The human body has an amazing ability to adapt to various environmental conditions and demands. For example, if we work in an office, we mostly sit, we sit in the car on the way to and from work, and rest at home after a long day, usually sitting or lying down, and it is difficult to find time for physical activities for many months. And then we go on vacations to nice places where we want to hike a lot. Even if the hike is short and easy, we find it very tiring for our bodies when we first start hiking. It is the effect of adaptation to an inactive life. Our bodies are adapted to sitting because there is no demand for physical effort, only for sitting. But if we keep going hiking, we may find it much easier at the end of a vacation, because the body gets used to the effort again. We do not need to go on a vacation to check it out. We can find out how it works when the elevator is broken and we need to use the stairs. After a couple of days, when our muscles are not painful anymore, we can feel the difference. A similar situation occurs in the bodies of athletes when they begin to train or take a longer break from training due to injury or other reasons. The body of an athlete adapts to specific demands, which we can control by implementing proper training and recovery.

Training

The training process is a key tool in shaping the body's functional capacity to exert the greatest amount of effort in a predetermined order (Elphinston 2013). The physiological aspects of training as well as the precise planning of training will be the subject of the next part of the chapter. Here, I would like to focus on the influence of this factor on overall success in sport. It is a fundamental one, especially in the senior age category, the main one for each athlete. Young athletes frequently win by utilizing their natural proclivities for a specific discipline, which we can refer to as talent. It means that talented athletes do not have to put in as much effort as less talented athletes to win junior competitions. When it comes to senior sports, talent is still very important, but it is not enough to win. Regular, well-planned training has begun to play a major role in athletes' ability to compete effectively. The optimal performance of the human body is linked to age, which limits athletes' sports lives and has an impact on age categories in sport. The main age groups are juniors under the age of 19, seniors under the age of 35, and masters over the age of 35. Professional sports focus on senior categories, whereas recreational sports have no restrictions, only different age categories every ten years. For example, we have a 103-year-old sprinter participating in competitions. There is a general understanding that young athletes should be protected from depleting their potential too early. Young categories have different equipment, shorter competition times, or do not compete in certain disciplines, such as the marathon. It reflects proper talent management in sport, when junior training should be only preparation, starting from just playing sport and building foundations for main training in the senior category. Unfortunately, the benefits of winning medals in the junior category are high for clubs and federations, which allows for very hard training for young people, leaving them physically and sometimes mentally depleted at a young age. This can result in a lack of functional capacity and resources for hard training in the senior category, and many athletes stop their career too early with the label of "good junior." The main reasons are frequent or serious injuries and this is a very common training mistake. Specific disciplines also have a correlation between age and optimal performance. For example, in endurance sports, the body has the optimal ability for effective performance between the ages of 28 and 32, assuming that the career was well planned and proper training was applied from the start. In disciplines where speed is important, the optimal age for best performance is 18–26, and athletes can try to maintain good results later in life. Also, there are some disciplines, like gymnastics, where training starts very early, maybe at the age of four or five years, and finishes earlier, because of the flexibility of the body during the developmental age, which plays a key role in performance. In general, in most sports disciplines, there are models of talent management and guidelines for the application of training in each age category according to the human body's development process. It is an ethical decision of every coach what kind of training will be applied, as well as political decision at club or federation level. It demonstrates how effective training can be in influencing an individual athlete's or team's career and sporting results.

Recovery

In professional sports, the training loads are balanced on the edge of human body capacity and injury. The goal is to expand the body's limits, but it is very easy to cross the line and break something in the body, usually the weakest or most overloaded point. This shows that training has certain limits that cannot be extended without damaging the structure or function. Therefore, athletes and coaches need to look for other ways of influencing performance improvement. And first, although not obvious to many, is the recovery process. Recovery is the natural consequence of every effort (Suchanowski 2001; Kellmann et al. 2018). When we get tired, the body wants to rest, so we slow down our effort, which is already a partial recovery. When we are extremely tired, we stop running, climbing, or doing whatever we are doing, and the natural, complete recovery process begins. We have increased our breathing until the body receives enough oxygen to pay the debt, and our muscles are stiff as a result of the high volume of lactic acid and depletion of energy substrate until the situation is resolved by the circulatory system, which washes out unwanted substances and brings in enough oxygen and energy. We can move on, but our next performance will be less effective. The body needs more time to rest completely, to be ready for the next heavy-load effort. This extra time needed to restore the functional capacity of the body is given by sleep and additional time without effort. These are natural ways to aid the body's recovery, but due to the nature of sports training, there are few opportunities to take days off. As a result, athletes and coaches are looking for natural and artificial ways to speed up regeneration and prepare for the next effort. I will describe the general rules, tools and methodology of biological regeneration applied to sport later. At this point, I would like to acknowledge that recovery is among the top three factors creating successful performance in modern sport.

Psychological aspects

Just a few athletes have strong, natural mental skills that help them to be successful competitors. It can be considered as a form of talent that an athlete brings to the table. Some athletes develop these skills throughout their career without external help, just by learning and gathering experience. Some hire sport psychologists who apply customized mental preparation programs. We also see some athletes who are very good at less important competitions but often fail at the main championships. Or, top soccer players who fail to convert penalty kicks that determine whether a team wins or loses a championship game. It could be an example of a lack of mental training.

Mental preparation

In normal daily life, the human body only uses a small percentage of its movement potential. Psychological experiments and real-life examples show that humans can be in high mobilization situations. We can use examples where a normal-sized mother can lift a car with one hand to get her child out from under it. This shows that the brain can overcome natural body limits and produce more effective performance when there is a need for it. Another piece of evidence comes from a psychological experiment on a death row inmate who was promised the cancellation of his death sentence in exchange for participating in a psychological experiment. It was a type of mental training based on visualization of specific situations: on a specific day and hour, in a specific room, the prisoner would sit and wait for someone to come in from the back and place hot metal on their back. This visualization was repeated according to the methodology of mental training. Finally, the day arrived, and the prisoner was sitting in the conditions described in the visualization when another person entered and placed neutral-temperature metal on the prisoner's back. However, the body reacted as if it were a hot metal, causing skin burn. This shows that the brain can sacrifice a part of the body in order to save the whole. In other words, it shows the supremacy of the brain over the body, as well as the power of visualization, which is a part of mental training.

In sports, the key area of mental training is the management of stress and activation levels (Gee 2010). Stress is beneficial for increasing the body's activation level and improving functionality, including sports performance according to fight or flight response activation. However, if stress or motivation is too high, it may result in a decrease in performance. Athletes can be paralyzed with fear, internal or external expectations, responsibility for results, and so on, and may make small or big technical mistakes, or not use their full ability for speed, strength and endurance. It can be explained by going into a certain level of freeze mode. Psychologists can help athletes with customized mental training programs (Blecharz *et al.* 2014). They diagnose athletes' needs by identifying their strong and weak points as well as areas for improvement. They use a wide range of tools, specific diagnostic tests, relaxation, visualization and mobilization, depending on the needs of the situation and the specific athlete (Bühlmayer *et al.* 2017). The overall goal is to prepare optimal psychological readiness for peak performance during the year's most important competitions, in conjunction with physical preparation and training.

The feeling of the day and luck
Athletes usually refer to it as "the flow." It is a situation in which everything goes smoothly, easily and as planned. Athletes frequently claim that it is easier than they expected. This is the result of well-planned mental training with detailed visualization of the main competitions. Obviously, it has to be connected with preparing the optimal performance functionality exactly for the day/period of competition at the physical level. It is also connected with optimal diet, hydration, good sleep and enough rest from previous efforts. Additional objective factors can increase the flow feelings. It could be a good qualifying round result and an optimal lane in the final, a preferred neighboring competitor, the wind on the back, and so on. Also, subjective factors can play a role. It can be the preferred number, preferred time of the day and weather or even the preferred color of the uniform or preferred color of the floor.

Athletes occasionally do not have a good day and may not have perfect preparation before a competition, but luck plays a role. It is possible that the main competitor, who has been unbeatable throughout the season, will suffer an injury just before the championships. It can be a supporting wind on the back, which is allowable in the rules. It could be a competitor who shares the tactical goals and sets the pace that allows the athlete to gather more strength to finish. And how can we call the situation where in one or two thousandths of a second someone has or does not have a medal after four years of hard work anything other than good luck? As Professor Jan Blecharz, a sports psychologist who has assisted many top-level athletes in winning medals and achieving extraordinary athletic feats, says, "Good luck favors the prepared mind."

External factors

Talent

Aside from training, talent is a second key factor in sport performance. In sports, talent is defined as a set of genetically determined properties that allow a person to perform at the highest level and compete effectively in a specific sports discipline. For example, in short distance running, the most important qualities are power and speed, generating maximal muscle effectiveness in moving from point A to point B in the shortest time. We can assess the type of muscle fiber content that we have inherited from our parents and their parents to determine our speed abilities. Muscles contain slow twitch fibers (STF), sometimes called red fibers, as well as fast twitch fibers (FTF), sometimes called white fibers. There is also a fraction of super-fast twitch fibers (SFTF) inside white fibers. In general, the more FTF and SFTF white fibers a person has, the easier it is to run fast and the greater their ability to participate in speed sports. The more STF red fibers a person has, the easier endurance sports are to do. You can't change the muscle content or the proportion of STF to FTF, especially if you can't create new FTF and SFTF muscles. And for this reason, the gene set is very important in sprinting. With endurance training, there is an adaptation that converts FTF to STF, causing the person to lose their speed abilities, which cannot be reversed.

You can also define talent as the physical and psychological ability to perform training at a high level of intensity and volume for an extended period of time without injury or overtraining. Talent and training are strongly bound together. Talented athletes usually win easily, but only at the entry and medium levels. To be effective in high-level competition, you need to connect proper training with talent. If we use only training without talent for a specific discipline, we can have some success in entry and medium-level sports, but never in the top level of competitions.

Selection system

The selection system or talent management is also an important part of sporting success and is usually done at the national or regional level. The selection system is based on a pyramid model, with the base being school physical education and youth sport. At the higher level, there are athletes at an average level in the junior and senior categories and, on top, we can have international champions. The general rule is that the larger the base, the easier it is to find and train champions. It is linked to the resources that certain populations have. We will have different resources in China and different resources, for example, in Lithuania. Hundreds of thousands of young people in China play table tennis and aspire to be champions. Through many regional and national championships, coaches can screen and select a very strong national team which will train hard to win international competitions. Such resources enable coaches to apply very strong training which eliminates the weakest athletes and selects the strongest ones. Even if the injury eliminates one or two athletes from Team A, there are five other candidates from Team B at a very similar level, ready to compete. Small countries do not have a wide base, and talent management is more difficult. Once a person with extraordinary skills is found, a much more careful training process needs to be applied in order to guide this athlete to a champion's level.

Financial resources

This factor is becoming increasingly important in modern sports. At the recreational level, there are some disciplines that you do not need to invest in so much and some are quite expensive. If you want to practice jogging, you need only proper shoes and comfortable clothes, whereas recreational golf or sailing are more expensive sports. But when it comes to professional sports, there are only expensive or very expensive sports. Even such a simple activity as running requires hiring a coach, physiotherapists and other specialists. You need to pay for the training facilities, including expensive training camps, and take care of many details, like proper diet, supplementation, high-tech aids and the best equipment. All these things create a huge annual budget, which is usually covered by the national federation when an athlete is on the national team, or by sponsors. And, in general, athletes supported by strong financial resources achieve better results. They are less stressed because they do not have to worry about finding resources for sport and for everyday life, in addition to the comfort of optimal preparation for competitions.

Equipment

Depending on the discipline, we need very simple and cheap or very sophisticated and expensive equipment. Running requires only shoes and running clothes for performance, which is relatively inexpensive and appealing to many people when compared to sailing, where the cost of equipment severely limits the number of competitors. Sports equipment is a step ahead of the technology currently available for people. It has to be the lightest, the fastest and the most comfortable, based on the newest innovations. Producers have their own competitions, which will provide the best equipment for the athletes. Even if top-level athletes' equipment is similar or has the same technology, top athletes demand updates and innovations to gain a small, sometimes psychological advantage over their competitors. In the running shoe market in 2019, the Nike company released a very advanced model that provided an additional recoil effect, making running easier and more effective. Runners wearing this model achieved the best marathon results. The other companies stayed behind with their products, and related to them, athletes who were obliged to run in other brands of shoes had worse results in general. And even in this situation, when a Kenyan runner made his attempt to run under two hours in a marathon, he got from Nike a customized pair of the best model. After some protests, the athletics authorities decided to ban this model and set up rules about using advanced shoes in official competitions, to avoid equipment doping. This example shows how important equipment can be in modern sport, and how it can give physical and mental advantages. Other companies have quickly provided their own solutions based on recoil technology, in accordance with current regulations, and the running shoe market has remained balanced.

Weather
The weather is the same for all athletes during the same competition. And we can't predict it perfectly, even if we have a high level of accuracy in our forecast. What we know is what kind of weather conditions we have, typically in specific places, at a specific time of the year. And we can prepare for such conditions by adjusting our training. In general, speed and power disciplines prefer warm and hot conditions because muscles have optimal performance in such conditions, while endurance disciplines prefer cold or moderate temperatures, because hot conditions mean that athletes spend extra energy on the thermoregulatory process during effort. I had the opportunity to witness the 2004 female Olympic marathon, which took place on the historical route from Marathon to Athens, and I rode almost the whole route in a technical car. The weather was extreme, with high heat and humidity. The big favorite, the current world record holder, did not fare well in these conditions because she had not trained in such high temperatures. The Japanese runners did, because they decided to prepare specifically for these conditions.

Other factors
The above factors are the main contributors to successful sports performance, but this is not an exhaustive list. Many other factors can play a key role in success, depending on the situation: sleep quality, correct acclimatization to the climate and time zone, a specific diet and many other things.

Sleep quality

Sleep is essential for the physical and mental regeneration of the body. Sleeping must be both sufficient and of high quality for each individual: deep enough, undisturbed, in a well-ventilated room and at an optimal temperature. We need to consider the time and quality of the last meal for good sleep quality as well as an optimal break from electromagnetic noise and other disturbing factors before falling asleep.

Correct acclimatization

The main competitions are announced usually three to five years or more before they start. Athletes are aware of the typical conditions at the location and time of competitions and strive to prepare for them as best they can. Athletes who live in similar conditions have certain advantages, because they compete in their natural conditions. Others must gradually adapt to challenges. They organize training camps in similar conditions, observe the adaptation process, and try different solutions. If they need to travel through many time zones to the competition they need to learn how to adapt to the new time. Many top-level athletes' performances have been ruined by jet lag.

Specific diet

Diet in sport is a very important topic. We must provide adequate energy, vitamins and micro- and macro-elements, while also ensuring that the digestive system is not overburdened. Food should be of good quality, diverse and well balanced. During specific training periods, athletes have their own specific dietary demands. For example, during a period when we are working on increasing muscle force, the body requires an extra amount of protein. In extensive endurance training, we need to provide more carbohydrates. Or in a situation where we can see the demand for a specific substance based on a blood test, we would supplement it.

And as the name suggests, it has to be supplemental delivery of specific content, which cannot be provided within a standard or modified diet. From my observation, athletes and coaches overuse supplements, which is not good in general, basically because most of these substances cause an additional load on the digestive system, the liver, the kidneys and even the brain. Some have side effects and possible interactions with other substances.

In addition, there is a specific diet before the main competitions, which varies depending on the discipline.

Training physiology

The human body has been developed as one of the most effective in terms of living in different, often stressful conditions, due to its adaptability. Training and competing are highly stressful conditions for the body, and adaptation skills are fundamental in the theory and practice of training. Coaches employ specific mechanisms to improve general functional capacity as well as specific qualities and skills in order to achieve peak performance during major competitions. The main tool in training is the training load on the athlete's body in order to achieve specific changes and adapt to training loads. We can distinguish the intensity and the capacity of training or applied loads. Intensity is a load quality that answers the questions of how fast, how strong and how far the movement was performed. Capacity describes the quantity of applied loads, and explains how long at certain intensity the effort lasts or how many weights have been applied. These two categories play a key role in planning for the training and managing the balance of work and recovery.

Biological adaptation

The adaptation of the human body to different conditions can be described as a desire to achieve homeostasis in the entire system of the body through the harmonious functioning of its various systems (Suchanowski 2001). For example, body temperature is regulated mostly by the blood system in order to adapt to external conditions. If it is cold outside, the small capillary system distributing blood to most superficial areas contracts and does not allow for large circulation there, and heat is not lost. In heat, there is an opposite mechanism. The blood is distributed to the surface to help eliminate heat from outside with different mechanisms like sweating in order to not allow it to rise to the core temperature too much and to protect internal organs and especially the brain, which is the most sensitive. Thermoregulatory mechanisms are important in sport and are often trained.

Another aspect of adaptation is the pH balance. The optimal blood pH is 7.4 and, at extreme physical effort, it can drop to 6.8–6.9, caused by releasing lactic acid (LA) from the muscles, which is caused by oxygen debt due to a high intensity of effort. Lactic acid circulates with the blood and is neutralized in the liver, usually up to two hours after the end of an effort. The level of LA, besides influencing overall pH balance, has an important role in functioning muscles, and when it is too high, it causes muscle stiffness and pain. For the human body, it is protective action against depleting energy resources and overall body acidosis, but for athletes is a key factor describing effort intensity levels and limiting duration of effort with high intensity. Many professional athletes use the blood LA level as a tool for measurement of the intensity of effort as well as to determine the overall level of how the body is trained.

The human body operates in cycles, which determine certain rhythms, beginning with the life cycle from birth to death, with all of the internal development, moving through the year-round cycle with different seasons, and concluding with the day and night cycle. In the life cycle of sport, we use the developmental phase and the time just after it, when the body has optimal performance ability. The periodization of training is determined by the year-round cycle, with the training plan based on one- or four-year training cycles (Bompa 1994). The day and night cycles are critical for human functioning as well as athletic performance. We need to balance daily activities with training and optimal recovery in order to increase functional capacity. Women have an important menstrual cycle that lasts about a month, which has implications for training.

To summarize, the body has enormous adaptability potential, and understanding the different cycles and body rhythms is the key to effective sports performance.

Phenomenon of super-compensation

The body has its own memory and recognizes things, especially bad things. When we were kids and we touched a hot object, we felt the pain and immediately removed our hand from the object. The primary reflex was applied, but we have learned something—this object is painful and it is better not to touch it again. It is a type of adaptation to the external environment; if something is bad, you avoid it. But not everything can be avoided; we are subjected to a wide range of unpleasant experiences. And the body, as an intelligent system, has discovered a solution: you can't avoid a difficult situation, but you can prepare for it and have a less difficult experience the next time. For example, if you need to run 300 meters very fast to catch the bus, you feel exhausted when you reach it. However, in addition to fatigue from effort, you may experience the next day a muscle soreness as a result of sprinting. You know this will happen frequently because you like to sleep well, so you decide to do some running training a couple of days a week, and you can feel the difference when you need to sprint to catch the bus the next time. The point is, extra effort gives extra abilities and this is the basis of the super-compensation phenomenon. The body remembers something difficult and adapts the system to be ready for the next time it goes through the same thing. To achieve super-compensation in any area, there are two conditions that must be applied. The first requirement is that the stimuli be significant, and, in this case, the effort be intense enough. The second condition is that the body needs to have enough rest between the end of effort and beginning of next effort, so the functional ability can rise above the initial level. If nothing happens and there will be no next challenge, the functional capacity will drop down because of a lack of demand (Zaitsev & Sazanov 2007; Brezhnev et al. 2011). This is the other side of the coin of human adaptability potential—if we do not use it, we lose it. The practice situation in sports is more complicated because different physiological processes have different timings for reaching the super-compensation phases. Successful planning of training is based on understanding of this process and practical application in a dynamic training process, which often becomes an art.

Overtraining and strategies for overcoming the problem

When we have a series of super-compensations and our overall performance ability rises, we have achieved the optimal result of training. This ideal situation can be disrupted by a variety of factors, which can be divided into two categories: excessive training and insufficient rest. The next intensive effort should start exactly when there is a super-compensation phase. Too early and too late will not have the desired effects. Too late rarely occurs because a training schedule is very tight and there isn't much free time available. More often than not, we see a situation in which effort is begun too soon, when the body is not fully recovered and does not reach the super-compensation phase. If the situation repeats, the overall performance ability drops down instead of rising and we can reach an overtraining state. There are several definitions of overtraining, and I would like to present my own, which says that overtraining is a chronic lack of sufficient recovery in terms of quality and quantity. There are many individual differences in the symptoms of overtraining, which will cause some difficulties with the management of the issue. There are numerous aspects and symptoms of overtraining that I will attempt to present, as well as potential solutions to the problem.

Sympathetic overtraining

The name comes from the symptoms suggesting a connection with the sympathetic part of the autonomic nervous system (ANS) responsible for activation of the body in general. Athletes seem to be active, vital, very keen on competing, but the results drop down and do not reflect the actual training. Overtraining of this type is more common in younger athletes with less experience, and it is most common in speed and strength disciplines. The symptoms can be similar to Grave's disease. We can observe sleep disturbance, decreased appetite, hyperactivity from external stimuli, anxiety and irritability. There is also an increase in heart rate during rest and a slower restitution of HR after an effort. When this overtraining is detected at the time, the process can be unwound in two to four weeks. But when a situation lasts longer with no intervention, it may turn to chronic overtraining, which is much more difficult to deal with and more costly in time.

The main treatment for the sympathetic overtraining is the detection and fast application of change in the training program and the intense application of recovery procedures. The training needs to have less intensity and volume. It is also good to change the applied stimuli, engage different groups of muscles, or change the equipment. In terms of increasing recovery, we need to influence both natural recovery (sleep, diet) and external recovery (massage, physical therapy and hydrotherapy). WATSU could also be helpful.

Parasympathetic overtraining

Parasympathetic overtraining is connected with another part of the ANS, responsible for slowing down the body, recovery and digestion. Athletes are often sleepy, apathetic, and lacking in energy and a desire to live. They do train hard, but there is no progress in results, so they train even harder and their results continue to decline. This type of overtraining is more common in older athletes with more experience and involvement in endurance sports. The symptoms can be similar to Addison's disease. We can see a decrease in HR during rest (what could be mistaken for normal adaptation to endurance training), a decrease in performance capacity, faster fatigue, and a lack of motivation for competition. Depending on how long it lasts and how deeply the process affects the system, treatment of parasympathetic overtraining can last for three to six months. In some cases, it can take a year to recover, but in all cases, it significantly alters or completely destroys an athlete's season. Treatment of this type of overtraining is long, difficult and complex, because of the complexity of the process. Detection is a first step, together with the change of training. Depending on the season and how seriously the body is affected, it may be necessary to stop training completely for a period of time and switch to another sport at a recreational level. Not only is the body affected, but the mind is also tired, so we need to apply psychological tools in order to refresh the mind too. Similar tools can be used as in the first type of overtraining, and medications may be used in some cases. WATSU has a very useful role here and can be one of the most important tools in overcoming the problem.

Psychological "burnout" and depression in sport

Sometimes, lack of success or improvement in results for a long time, together with repeated injuries and/or overtraining, may result in mental "burnout." Athletes do not see the point in continuing to train, especially if they are old and do not make a good living from the sport. There is no motivation to risk further destruction of health capacity and, in this way, many careers have been finished early.

Athletes can become so engrossed in their sport that they lose sight of their passions outside it. They may not be able to connect training with university education and thus have a low chance of landing a good job. Sometimes the training regimen, which requires 300 days away from home, does not allow them to have satisfactory relationships. Life can be complicated, and when bad things happen at the same time, there is a high risk of depression. And depression is a very complicated issue in sport. First of all, it is difficult to be honest with yourself and admit that you, such a strong and famous athlete, have depression. Second, coming out to the public is more difficult, too. What will the public say? What will sponsors, TV, the national federation say? I know personally several top-level athletes who suffered from depression and trained for a long time. It took a long time for them to come out, and it also took a long time for them to receive treatment. WATSU has a lot of potential in this area as well.

The weakest chain concept of injury

As already described earlier in the adaptation process, the body is a super intelligent machine. It wants to adapt to external conditions and to protect its integrity in these conditions. If some effort is too hard, metabolic changes (oxygen debt, energy depletion, LA accumulation in muscles) force the person to lower the intensity or stop the effort completely. If the situation is repeated with enough time for full recovery and the next hard effort begins at the super-compensation level, we have increased athletic potential. And if the situation repeats and there is not enough recovery and no super-compensation for a longer time, we can have different types of overtraining. But when the rest break is drastically short and efforts are very hard, the body will apply a self-protective mechanism which will allow for the breaking of a small part in order to protect the integrity of the whole. If the knee is painful, you cannot run anymore, and the time for healing the knee is also the time for treating the whole body's fatigue. And, because the body has its own memory, if such a strategy works one time, there is a good chance that the situation will repeat itself the next time the body is tired, and it will not be necessary for the same knee. Because muscles are not separate from the body but are connected within the entire body's myofascial system, which holds all the bones together, protects the organs and provides force transmission throughout the entire body, we must consider muscles and other selected anatomical structures (ligaments, tendons) as a part of the whole chain in action (Scarr 2014). When the body "wants" to stop activity and rest for some time, it chooses the weakest point of the system and allows it to be broken. It can also be the most overloaded part. Sometimes it is both, and we have a place where a doctor or physiotherapist will diagnose an injury. In this light, the first treatment for any injury would be to avoid overtraining and to seek appropriate restitution.

A specific area of the locomotor system is not always the weakest point that can stop body activity. There is a common understanding that hard work and fatigue decrease the immune system's capacity. We can see that an athlete has reached peak performance in two or three competitions before succumbing to the flu or another infection, which can be viewed as another weak point in the system. Being in good shape is connected with hard training and fatigue, which lower the immune system. For this reason, many top-level athletes take a lot of precautions in order to protect themselves from infections during the main competition period.

Biological regeneration

Biological regeneration in sport can be defined as a set of rules governing the management of recovery after athletic performance using specific tools. Understanding of fatigue and recovery mechanisms allows us to plan training and recovery and to use the most effective methodology (Suchanowski 2001; Crowther *et al.* 2017). Starting with natural resources like sleep or diet, we can progress to a variety of artificial means to accelerate the return of various physiological processes in readiness for the next effort.

Rules of recovery

Before applying any recovery tool, it is good to become familiar with the general rules listed below.

1. *Rule of conscious use of recovery.* Describes the application of physical treatments according to knowledge of performance physiology and recovery mechanisms, the characteristics of the discipline, and the main principles of physical therapy.
2. *Rule of individual selection of recovery tools.* Discusses the individual application of recovery tools based on an athlete's age, gender, health condition and sport level.
3. *Rule of specific selection of recovery tools.* Describes the need for selection of the tools according to the training period with its specific needs, physiological effects of short-term training, and targeting the next period and the characteristics of the training load.
4. *Rule of progressive application.* Discusses differentiation of applied tools in order to prevent the habituation of tissues and the whole body and lesser effectiveness of applied tools.
5. *Rule of complex application.* Requires the use of a variety of tools and methods of recovery in order to eliminate the phenomenon of adaptation of the body to one tool or method.
6. *Rule of cyclical use of recovery tools.* Discusses the correlation between the strict time schedules and repetition of individual recovery procedures.
7. *Rule of systematic use of recovery tools.* Advises athletes to be disciplined in their use of recovery procedures in order to have a more effective rest and be more prepared for the next effort.

Tools of recovery

Coaches have a variety of tools at their disposal to achieve specific adaptation effects, and each of these tools causes fatigue in different ways. Physical therapists, massage therapists and other specialists in charge of athletes' recovery have a wide range of tools at their disposal that allow them to meet the majority of demands. We have new recovery tools to use and serve athletes because science and practice are constantly striving for improvement. Here are the most important and commonly used ones.

Natural recovery resources (sleep, diet, supplementation)

Sleep: This is a very effective recovery tool. It reflects the basic day and night cycle, and, by its nature, sleep is the time when the body rebuilds using substrates from food, as well as when healing and recovery take place. Sleep has to be long enough and of good quality. In sport, we should avoid external factors disturbing sleep in order to fully use its recovery potential. Sleep is also a very important factor in adapting to a new time zone when traveling east or west through multiple time zones.

Diet: This is our natural source of fuel. We must provide athletes with high-quality food in sufficient quantities to meet their daily demands, which vary by discipline and training period. Quality means we need to deliver all the necessary substances: carbohydrates, proteins, fats, micro- and macro-elements. Besides normal daily life functions, there is a specific demand for physical effort. For the digestive system to be healthy and be ready for performance, quality food must be natural and easy to eat. Hard-to-digest and highly processed foods are not recommended during the hard training and competition period, and also do not support speeding up the recovery. Different sports necessitate different daily caloric demands; for example, cyclists competing in a race require a different caloric intake from gymnasts. Some disciplines, such as boxing, necessitate maintaining a specific body weight, which can also be controlled through diet. The general recommendation is that food needs to be well balanced in sport.

Supplementation: Sometimes we are unable to provide all of the necessary substances through our food, or we provide too little of something and must obtain it elsewhere. It is usually about vitamins and micro- or macro-elements, and the lack of specific substances can be detected by specific symptoms or by a decrease in performance. The best way to monitor the actual level of all needed substances is through a regular blood test, which will show specifically what is missing. In such cases, we can modify the diet and/or use specific supplements. I recommend using natural products when possible and avoiding artificial medications, which mostly have side effects and overload the digestive system, the liver and the kidneys. It is strongly advised to use something artificial only when there are no natural alternatives. Unfortunately, in modern sport, we have the opposite situation, and supplementation is commonly overused.

Physical tools

There is a wide range of physical tools that support and speed up the recovery process. More and more things are on the way, and I'd like to focus on the most commonly used ones and briefly discuss their benefits.

Massage therapy: I have noticed that many experienced and qualified physiotherapists and osteopaths working in sport are not keen on using a massage as a recovery treatment because they see it as too simple a tool, and instead they use sophisticated techniques or equipment that do not tire their hands. In my opinion, we cannot skip massage in sports, because during massage, we touch the muscles and physically remove metabolites after exercise and move them to the lymph tracts and nodes. We also increase blood circulation, which speeds up the recovery of the muscles. During massage, there is interpersonal contact and an athlete has an opportunity to talk and share, so we also speed up their mental recovery (Best *et al.* 2008).

Physical therapy: This category contains a very wide spectrum of application of different physical agents to human tissues in order to improve the healing process. This does have more application in the rehabilitation of an injury rather than in improving recovery after exercise. Different electrotherapy treatments with various biological effects, a wide spectrum of laser treatments, therapy that utilizes ultrasound, magnetic fields, infrared rays, shock waves and others help us deal with inflammation and the tissue rebuilding process, improve the elasticity and mobility of the tissue after immobilization and scarring, or just support manual techniques.

Thermal therapy is a distinct category in which we use cold or hot temperatures. Here we can trigger the adaptation processes and influence recovery after training and competition. Cold therapy can include the use of water or ice at temperatures ranging from 10 to 0° C. It is often applied in sprints and speed training, or after very intense training or competitions. Even if some research shows opposite results, athletes value this kind of treatment. Cryotherapy is connected with the application of extreme cold in the local area or to the whole body in a cryotherapy chamber. The temperature is in the range of −100 to −160° C, and the person stays there for three to five minutes, which gives an analgesic effect for several hours as well as strong hormone secretion, which can help in recovery. The sauna is on the opposite end of the temperature spectrum, ranging from 80 to 110° C. Such conditions necessitate a strong cardiovascular response in order to maintain the body's thermal homeostasis and are used to harden the body in order to improve immunity. It is recommended to do short, repeated sauna entrances. There are other kinds of saunas, like hammams and infrared saunas, but they have fewer applications in sport.

Hydrotherapy: Hydrotherapy is another wide category of treatments, which includes WATSU. Water is a great place for recovery and gives a wide range of healing possibilities (Cameron 2013). We have many different kinds of baths: pearl brine, mud, acid-carbon and herbal, with a wide range of therapeutic effects. We can apply underwater massage with precise jet application. We can use so-called Scottish whips with high pressure and different temperatures of water. An interesting option for recovery of the upper or lower limbs and the lumbar spine area is whirlwind massage in specially designed tubs. A form of recovery would also be drinking water rich in minerals, and inhalation of specific substances with specific inhalation equipment or using a graduation tower.

As we can see, classical hydrotherapy gives huge treatment opportunities for athletes' recovery and rehabilitation. Modern aquakinetic therapies, such as myofascial release in water (MRW) (Zagorski 2014), WATSU and other forms of aquatic bodywork, are also available. Flotation tanks have recently gained popularity, also in sports. These have, obviously, the whole list of benefits of warm water immersion, and can give you the feeling of sensory deprivation, which is a key point in the marketing of this service. The unspoken truth about floating is that the person is abandoned in claustrophobic conditions, which may trigger unwanted unconscious issues, especially if the person has mental issues. It may be a problem if someone is experiencing depression, for example.

Kinesiotherapy: This can be thought of as an application-specific movement system, for example Fascial Fitness, or as the use of tailored passive or active movements to solve a specific problem (Schleip & Muller 2013). This category also contains stretching and stabilization exercises. In general, the main goal of kinesiotherapy is to apply compensatory movement in order to give the brain stimuli different from the usual ones and to strengthen weaker parts of the body that are less engaged in the main movement. Aside from injury prevention, it may also help in recovery.

Specific tools: There seems to be a new gadget for sports therapists arriving on the market almost every year. Some of these tools serve a specific purpose and perform specific operations, while others simply relieve the therapist's hands. A clavitherapy pin is an interesting addition to the needles used in Traditional Chinese Medicine (TCM). It looks like a big pin with sharp ends. The application of treatment, which is a combination of TCM and modern neurology and pathology, is spectacular, because it is often very painful and there is usually an immediate release of pain and/or dysfunction. Athletes love it, and therapists love to show off with it—a placebo effect is at work. A massage gun has been a popular gadget in recent years. It looks like a gun, creates pressure and vibrations and has become very popular in sport, mostly because it is very convenient for therapists, who use it to replace a more tiring hand massage. Athletes like this gadget because it is new, gives an interesting sensation, so it is certain to work, and, most importantly, other good athletes use it as well. However, as a massage therapist with 25+ years of experience, I have seen many different tools and have not found any better than my own hands.

Psychological tools (relaxation, mental training, social balance)

Aside from the body, which must be well cared for after hard, repeated training, the mind must also be nurtured. The central nervous system governs the activity of skeletal muscles and gets tired too, which can manifest in impulse conduction between nerves, which is measurable. The psyche should also be a subject of recovery, especially in sports where coordination plays an important role.

Relaxation: This is the ability to release the tension on a physical and psychological level. Awareness and control of this process on a physical level is very important in sport, where we need to control muscle tension in order to achieve optimal performance. Psychological relaxation, the typical WATSU feeling of letting go, is also important, but is often underestimated in sport. A sportsperson's life is full of stress. Competitions are stressful, qualifications for competitions are stressful, living away from home and family, sometimes alone, is stressful, other things put stress on top of it and, as a result, we have people living in permanent tension. WATSU can provide a powerful dose of relaxation, a brief experience that is diametrically opposed to an athlete's normal feelings. It is of great value.

Mental training: This can be helpful, but will not replace the benefits of manual massage or hydrotherapy. It is especially useful when recovering from an injury (Podlog & Dionigi 2010). We can strengthen athletes' self-esteem, visualize goals, and ensure the progress of rehabilitation with correctly applied mental training.

Social balance: This is an important aspect of mental hygiene. It is important to have good relationships with loved ones, with peers, with colleagues from work and teams. Any tension in any of these areas will reduce the body's ability to recover completely and quickly. Awareness of the situation and active work to create a social balance is important for aiding the recovery process in sport.

Periodization of training and recovery

Periodization of training, connected with the training recovery process, is a consequence of the year-round cycle in nature. Different seasons of the year have different demands and humans adapt to these conditions. For example, in winter, we eat more calorie-rich food to have the energy to keep the body warm. Athletes' seasons are different, because the goal is to prepare for peak performance for a certain period. It has to be done progressively, and it is not possible to keep peak performance for very long, so it has to drop down to rise up again and there is a cycle.

Classical or block periodization

So far, classical periodization has been the most widely used (Bompa 1994). It uses a one-year cycle, starting from adaptation to training, making a wide functional base which narrows to specific training preparing for competitions, the competition period with the highest intensity, and dropping down to almost zero training in the rest period. Another cycle is the four-year Olympic cycle, where the intensity of training progressively rises each year to achieve a maximum in the Olympic year, and the next year is an easy one, a kind of recovery after progression. However, modern commercial sport, which introduces more and more important competitions at different times of the year, does not allow for only one peak per year. Sometimes it is two, three or more peaks, and the athlete needs to be ready to compete at the highest level at all of these competitions. In addition, the entire year's program is divided into training blocks. Each block can also have specific training goals, which should prepare the athlete for the most important competitions (Issurin 2008, 2016; Mujika *et al.* 2018). A major injury with a longer break in training may necessitate block periodization. The whole training program is significantly disturbed and the coach needs to save the situation with specific blocks of training.

An athlete's year plan

Every year of an athlete's career is different. The body is changing, functional and performance abilities are changing, attitudes and mental capacity are changing. We must adapt our training to these changes in order to have optimal performance at competitions planned for a specific time of the year. A step-by-step approach is applied, starting from a low level and increasing to the maximum during main competitions, after which there is a rapid decrease in training, and a rest period before the next year cycle, which we can call a macrocycle. I will use the example of athletics to illustrate the whole year's planning, and in athletics, we usually have the main competitions in August. Each macrocycle contains a number of mezocycles and is usually a month long. Each mezocycle contains a number of microcycles and is usually a week long. Each microcycle is built up of single training units.

Preparatory period

This starts at the end of October or the beginning of November and is usually 16–20 weeks long, until February or March. The main goal of this period is to generalize the body's preparation for future high-intensity training, beginning with easy and low-intensity training. All motor skills are being trained and the capacity of training is greatest in this period. In some athletic disciplines, like sprinting, jumping and middle distance, there are indoor competitions in January and February. If there are important competitions, athletes prepare a small peak disposition for these competitions using a block periodization. In other cases, participation in indoor competitions is a normal part of training, and some athletes skip the indoor season entirely in order to focus solely on summer competitions. For recovery goals, it is important to be in line with the specific goals of each mezocycle and focus on injury prevention from overload and prevention of overtraining. We can use WATSU during this period because there aren't many restrictions.

Pre-competition period

This contains two or three mezocycles in March, April and May. From a training perspective, the main goal of this period is to transform large-capacity general work from the preparatory period into more specific and more intense work, leading to the main period of competitions. Recovery work focuses on accelerating restitution after more intense training and preventing injuries, particularly those associated with higher intensity training. WATSU has fewer applications at this time, so we must exercise caution, especially before the most intense training in this period.

Competition period

This begins at the end of May and lasts until the end of August, sometimes as late as the middle of September. The main goal is to use maximal intensity training, including competitions, to prepare an optimal disposition for a specific period of major competitions. It is a long time, so usually, after a series of competitions at the beginning, there is a specific mezocycle of direct preparation for the main competitions, including a couple of control competitions. Aside from improving resting processes, the recovery goals are to take good care of warming up before intense training and to do compensatory work to avoid injuries. WATSU is used with caution here, and it is not used often, according to actual needs.

Recovery period

This begins in September or early October with an active rest. Usually, athletes go for vacations with their families, do some business which they cannot do during training, and refresh their heads. An important part of this period is a specific recovery microcycle, 10–18 days long, which should be done in a balneotherapy center with access to good natural resources. No specific training can be used here, other than simple activities that focus on body areas and muscles, such as golf. The important thing is applying a series of balneotherapy treatments to the most engaged/used or injured body areas. We can also do a general body-check and apply major changes in myofascial structures with Rolfing techniques on land and MRW techniques in the water if there is such a need. The change in the myofascial network will not affect performance. The body will have time to adapt to the changes, and the new training for next season will incorporate the changes. WATSU is a valuable tool here that can be used on a daily basis.

Examples of the application of WATSU in different sports

WATSU has been successfully applied in several disciplines already and has helped many athletes, including medalists at the Olympic Games and the World Championships. One of the first was a discus thrower, a medalist at the Beijing 2008 and Rio de Janeiro 2016 Olympics. He valued WATSU a lot as a tool for relaxation and recovery. A young Olympic hammer thrower from Poland loved WATSU sessions and regularly used WATSU when she had access to warm water during training camps. Members of the Polish whitewater kayaking team and Polish alpine ski team used WATSU sessions in some of their training camps. Two members of the 4x100m French relay team at the European Championships in Barcelona in 2010 used WATSU on a regular basis. In addition, many less-known or recreational athletes are using WATSU and its benefits to improve their performance and recovery. They also use social media to share training and recovery tips, and are a great source for the promotion of WATSU. I hope that this chapter raises awareness of the possibilities of WATSU and that its application in sports medicine will be more common.

Summary

This short chapter can only highlight the benefits and possibilities of the application of WATSU in sport at any level. As WATSU practitioners, we can help a lot when we apply it correctly, according to the physiology of training and recovery and in line with training goals. We can also destroy a lot when applying WATSU incorrectly. The limited frame of this text does not allow me to share all knowledge about the topic, and the reader is invited to take special training for working with top-level athletes and teams to deepen their knowledge. This training will fully answer the questions: when, how, how much to apply WATSU in sport. WATSU practitioners will be well prepared to spread WATSU in the sports medicine field and work with the biggest names in sports with this knowledge. This can benefit general WATSU recognition—when a famous athlete speaks on social media or on TV about WATSU benefits, it is a much more valuable promotion than many articles or limited, specific social media marketing. My big hope is that this small contribution will bring people closer to Harold's vision of everyone holding each other in warm water.

References

Becker, B. (2010). Biophysiologic Aspects of Hydrotherapy. In B. Becker & A. Cole, *Comprehensive Aquatic Therapy* (third edition), pp.23–77. Pullman, WA: Washington State University Publishing.

Best, T.M., Hunter, R., Wilcox, A. & Haq, F. (2008). Effectiveness of sports massage for recovery of skeletal muscle from strenuous exercise. *Clinical Journal of Sport Medicine*, 18(5): 446–460. doi: 10.1097/JSM.0b013e31818837a1.

Blecharz, J., Luszczynska, A., Scholz, U., Schwarzer, R., Siekanska, M. & Cieslak, R. (2014). Predicting performance and performance satisfaction: Mindfulness and beliefs about the ability to deal with social barriers in sport. *Anxiety Stress Coping*, 27(3): 270–287. doi: 10.1080/10615806.2013.839989.

Bompa, T. (1994). The Annual Plan. In T. Bompa, *Theory and Methodology of Training*, pp.167–232. Dubuque, IA: Kendall/Hunt Publishing.

Brezhnev, I., Zaitsev, A. & Sazanov, S. (2011). To the analytical theory of the supercompensation phenomenon. *Biofizika*, 56(2): 342–348.

Bühlmayer, L., Birrer, D., Röthlin, P., Faude, O. & Donath, L. (2017). Effects of mindfulness practice on performance-relevant parameters and performance outcomes in sports: A meta-analytical review. *Sports Medicine*, 47(11): 2309–2321. doi: 10.1007/s40279-017-0752-9.

Cameron, M. (2013). Hydrotherapy. In M. Cameron, *Physical Agents in Rehabilitation: From Research to Practice* (fourth edition), pp.323–357. St Louis, MO: Elsevier.

Crowther, F., Sealey, R., Crowe, M. *et al.* (2017). Team sport athletes' perceptions and use of recovery strategies: A mixed-methods survey study. *BMC Sports Science, Medicine and Rehabilitation*, 9, 6.

Elphinston, J. (2013). Building Progressive Programs. In J. Elphinston, *Stability, Sport and Performance Movement: Practical Biomechanics and Systematic Training for Movement Efficacy and Injury Prevention*, pp.199–318. Chichester: Lotus Publishing and On Target Publications.

Gee, C.J. (2010). How does sport psychology actually improve athletic performance? A framework to facilitate athletes' and coaches' understanding. *Behavior Modification*, 34(5): 386–402. doi: 10.1177/0145445510383525.

Issurin, V. (2008). Block periodization versus traditional training theory: A review. *Journal of Sports Medicine and Physical Fitness*, 48(1): 65–75.

Issurin, V. (2016). Benefits and limitations of block periodized training approaches to athletes' preparation: A review. *Sports Medicine*, 46(3): 329–338.

Kellmann, M., Bertollo, M., Bosquet, L. *et al.* (2018). Recovery and performance in sport: Consensus statement. *International Journal of Sports Physiology and Performance*, 13(2): 240–245. doi: 10.1123/ijspp.2017-0759.

Kulik, A., Rosloniec, E., Koszela, A. & Zagorski, T. (2016). Effects of Aquatic Therapy (WATSU) in Patients with Chronic, Nonspecific Low Back Pain. In *9th Interdisciplinary World Congress on Low Back and Pelvis Girdle Pain*. Singapore. pp.385–386.

Mujika, I., Halson, S., Balague, G. & Farrow, D. (2018). An Integrated, Multifactorial Approach to Periodization for Optimal Performance in Individual and Team Sports. *International Journal of Sports Physiology, 1*, 13(5): 538–561.

Orzel-Zagorska, P. & Zagorski, T. (2010). Watsu Provider – nowa propozycja dla ośrodków SPA [Watsu Provider – a new proposal for SPA]. *Refleksoterapia 1*, 25–29.

Podlog, L. & Dionigi, R. (2010). Coach strategies for addressing psychosocial challenges during the return to sport from injury. *Journal of Sports Science*, 28(11): 1197–1208. doi: 10.1080/02640414.2010.487873.

Scarr, G. (2014). Biotensegrity: A Rational Approach to Biomechanics. In G. Scarr, *Biotensegrity: The Structural Basis of Life*, pp.99–108. Edinburgh: Handspring Publishing.

Schleip, R. & Muller, G. (2013). Training principles for fascial connective tissues: Scientific foundation and suggested practical applications. *Journal of Bodywork & Movement Therapies*, 17: 103–115.

Schoedinger, P. (2008). Adapting Watsu for People with Special Needs. In H. Dull, *Watsu: Freeing the Body in the Water*, pp.119–133. Middletown, CA: Watsu Publishing.

Suchanowski, A. (2001). Theoretical Basic of Recovery Course. In *Variability in the Dynamic Process of Recovery in Sports Training Efficiency Control*, pp.26–45. Gdansk: Akademia Wychowania Fizycznego.

Tufekcioglu, E. & Çotuk, B. (2009). Comparison of heart rate variability in different body positions on land and in water. Niğde University. *Journal of Physical Education and Sport Science*, 3(3), Online. doi: 10.1186/1746-1340-15-19.

Zagorski, T. (2008). Watsu—nowy wymiar rehabilitacji w wodzie [Watsu—a new dimension of rehabilitation in water.] *Rehabilitacja w praktyce*, 3: 44–45.

Zagorski, T. (2014). Work on Fascia in Water—Benefits, Possibilities and Limitations of Application. In M. Bilska, R. Golonko & J. Soltan, *Movement Activities in Disabled Children and Youth*, pp.124–136. Biala Podlska: Akademia Wychowania Fizycznego Józefa Piłsudskiego w Warszawie. Wydział Wychowania Fizycznego i Sportu w Białej Podlaskiej.

Zagorski, T. (2016). Watsu for Athletes: Olympians set the trend. *Embody. The Magazine of the Complementary Therapists Association*. Spring Edition, London.

Zagorski, T. (2018). Therapy and recovery of sprinter: Rio de Janeiro 2016 medalist. Lecture at "Human in health and disease—health promotion, treatment and rehabilitation" Conference in Tarnow.

Zagorski, T. (2021). The Functional Aspects of Fascia During Human Performance and Sports. In R. Schleip & R. Fascia, *The Tensional Network of the Human Body*, Chapter 7.29. Edinburgh: Elsevier.

Zagorski, T. & Kulik, A. (2014). Physical and Psychological Benefits of Watsu Therapy. In M. Bilska, R. Golonko & J. Soltan, *Movement Activities in Disabled Children and Youth*, pp.151–161. Biala Podlska: Akademia Wychowania Fizycznego Józefa Piłsudskiego w Warszawie. Wydział Wychowania Fizycznego i Sportu w Białej Podlaskiej.

Zaitsev, A. & Sazanov, S. (2007). On the prediction of the supercompensation phase by determining the parameters of the living functional system of the body. *Biofizika*, 52(4): 727–732.

Further reading

Brezhnev, I., Zaitsev, A. & Sazanov, S. (2011). To the analytical theory of the supercompensation phenomenon. *Biofizika*, 56(2): 342–348.

Crowther, F., Sealey, R., Crowe, M. *et al.* (2017). Team sport athletes' perceptions and use of recovery strategies: A mixed-methods survey study. *BMC Sports Science, Medicine and Rehabilitation*, 9(6). doi: 10.1186/s13102-017-0071-3.

Decoster, L., Cleland, J., Altieri, C. & Russell, P. (2005). The effects of hamstring stretching on range of motion: A systematic literature review. *Journal of Orthopaedic & Sports Physical Therapy*, 35(6): 377–387.

Issurin, V. (2008). Block periodization versus traditional training theory: A review. *Journal of Sports Medicine and Physical Fitness*, 48(1): 65–75.

Issurin, V. (2016). Benefits and limitations of block periodized training approaches to athletes' preparation: A review. *Sports Medicine*, 46(3): 329–338.

Kulik, A., Rosloniec, E., Koszela, A. & Zagorski, T. (2016). Effects of Aquatic Therapy (Watsu) in Patients with Chronic, Nonspecific Low Back Pain. In *9th Interdisciplinary World Congress on Low Back and Pelvic Girdle Pain*, pp.385–386. Singapore.

Mujika, I., Halson, S., Balague, G. & Farrow, D. (2018). An integrated, multifactorial approach to periodization for optimal performance in individual and team sports. *International Journal of Sports Physiology and Performance*, 13(5): 538–561.

Orzel-Zagorska, P. & Zagorski, T. (2010). Watsu Provider—nowa propozycja dla ośrodków SPA. *Refleksoterapia* 1: 25–29.

Zaitsev, A. & Sazanov, S. (2007). On the prediction of the supercompensation phase by determining the parameters of the living functional system of the body. *Biofizika*, 52(4): 727–732.

Chapter 9

New Horizons in WATSU®
and Life Coaching

A Trust-Building Therapy

DR. ERTAN TUFEKCIOGLU AND DR. IFTIKHAR NADEEM

Life coaching and the somatic experience: Integrating the benefits of WATSU with life coaching strategies

This chapter highlights the definitions, foundational values, benefits, and approaches shared by WATSU and life coaching interventions. For life coaching, we used references that are in line with the International Coaching Federation's (ICF) principles.

This chapter aims to provide life coaching and WATSU therapy relations on a scientifically sound basis. We will explore the intertwined nature of the two modalities. The distinctions and nuances will also be apparent to the reader. In other words, how resourcefulness accessed via profound relaxation in WATSU is transformed into learning, change, and growth in life coaching. Since WATSU is considered a promising tool for personal growth, this chapter also aims to develop theories for life coaching practice and establish increased credibility for WATSU as a discipline.

Coaching is partnering with clients in a thought-provoking and creative process to inspire them to maximize their personal and professional potential (Rogers 2016). A successful coaching relationship depends on seeing the client as a powerful, resourceful, and wonderfully gifted person. The role of a coach is to be present, maintain a high level of awareness, listen holistically, and manage the session in the direction of the client's agenda. The questions are the tools to find the right direction in the exploration process, allowing the client to uncover their inner resources (Passmore & Sinclair 2020).

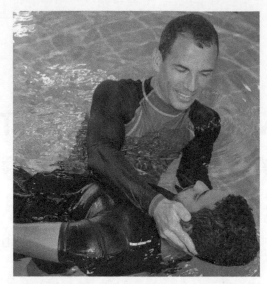

Figure 9.1: WATSU's quality of touch promotes clarity of mind

The ICF strives to collaborate with organizations and individuals that promote the highest standards of research to establish a discipline of coaching studies to support and further the profession. The ICF seeks to facilitate the exchange of information among researchers and practitioners studying coaching theory, methodologies, and outcomes (Dull 2008).

WATSU: A non-verbal communication for trust

Physical and physiological relaxation can enhance conditions, such as hypertonia, stiffness, pain, and sleep deprivation. Thus, daily movement functioning is improved. Likewise, emotional and mental relaxation can help improve cognitive and emotional functioning for higher learning, change, and personal growth.

Many interventions, including non-verbal somatic communication (WATSU aquatic bodywork), can significantly support life coaching. An aquatic environment may help establish safety and trust and encourage more productive verbal communication in coaching. In this regard, certain elements and values, including whole-person focus, promote WATSU as a promising intervention for better coaching results. WATSU works simultaneously on the physical and emotional levels. Adapting WATSU's established form to each person could create a space safe enough for the one in the therapist's arms to access every level of their being (Dull 2008). From the therapeutic point of view, it promotes deep relaxation, quieting the sympathetic and enhancing the parasympathetic nervous system activity, thus triggering self-healing in many ways.

In seeking better results, the combination of life coaching and WATSU, with a deep level of somatic and emotional experiences, can form a more empowering state/condition for the clients. Thus, the connection of the power of both interventions in professional hands can lead to deeper explorations of physical, intellectual, and emotional barriers and the removal of these energy blocks. These explorations can move the client to the most resourceful state, empowering the process of self-healing, change, learning, and having new perspectives. Trust established at an earlier stage and new ways of relating within the context of a safe physical interaction further support clients in their explorations.

First, both are concerned with the relationship based on trust, intimacy, confidentiality, respect, equality, and unconditional acceptance. Like mutual unconditional respect in a coaching conversation, a client is held in unconditional positive regard in WATSU. As the coaching client is supposed to be actively engaged in a coaching session, a tractable and floating WATSU client may indeed be in a very active state of improving interoceptive awareness. The interoceptive transmissions of how we organize our body from the inside out may enable our clients to better process and regulate their emotions.

WATSU's physical movements and techniques help the client to explore new perspectives beyond visible and physical boundaries. In coaching, questions are the tools of a coach to explore new perspectives and deal with issues beyond the intellectual level. Neuroscience research has shown that the main contribution to one's decisions comes from emotions. Every coaching conversation and WATSU session must flow in line with emotions to make the most individualized, client-centered, and beneficial sessions. The client-centric approach requires holistic listening, full presence, and intuition as quality prerequisites in both interventions.

Holistic listening helps notice the subtle changes in the emotions, resistance to the moves in WATSU and feelings triggered by the questions in life coaching.

The initial motivation to receive WATSU may be more problem-focused as stress-related physical and mental symptoms. In contrast, a coaching client seeks personal and professional development, change and learning, solution-focused coaching. An intimate WATSU approach in warm water before a coaching session can contribute to emotional awareness and meanings. At this point, WATSU may be considered a solution-focused preparatory intervention. Life coaches need to develop and maintain an open-minded, curious, flexible, and client-centered mindset in line with the competencies needed for WATSU professionals. Curiosity about the client's health and condition before a WATSU session leads to finding the best techniques and to modifying techniques. In short, practicing WATSU can help coaches improve an open and flexible mind with a constant focus on the totality of the client.

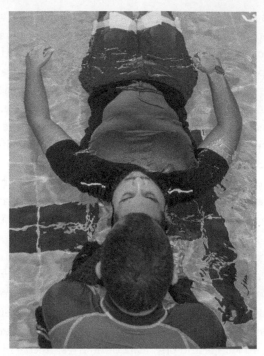

Figure 9.2: Somatic moments provide opportunities for a higher mind

Both interventions' enriched and mutually beneficial relationship practices can uncover the client's wisdom toward emotional, mental, and spiritual empowerment and self-healing in the physical dimension. The empowerment process helps clients enter resourcefulness which is a productive and creative process for self-exploration. However, all of the above qualities depend on the core competencies determined by the years of research and observation in both interventions. Table 9.1 shows the two interventions' common and similar core competencies through the International Coaching Federation and the Worldwide Aquatic Bodywork Association (WABA).

Table 9.1: Core competencies required by the ICF and WABA

ICF core competency	WABA professional
Demonstrates ethical practice. The ICF coach demonstrates coaching aligned with the ICF Code of Ethics and will remain consistent in the role of coach.	The WABA professional follows the WABA Code of Ethics in creating relationships that honor the responsibility and privilege of touch.
Embodies a coaching mindset—a mindset that is open, curious, flexible, and client-centered. It is a process that requires ongoing learning and development.	Is directed toward a sense of duty and responsibility, invited to grow through study, practice, and increasing self-awareness.

Establishes and maintains agreements. The coach partners with the client to identify or reconfirm what the client wants to accomplish in this session, including measures of success and importance.	Demonstrates a sincere commitment to providing the highest quality professional service, including a safe, healthy, and appropriate environment with unconditional acceptance.
Cultivates trust and safety. A coach acknowledges and respects the client's unique talents, insights, and work in the coaching process. They also show support, empathy, and concern for the clients.	Demonstrates compassion, support, and non-judgment. WABA professionals conduct their professional activities with integrity, honesty, respect, and compassion.
Maintains presence—in response to the whole person of the client—and partners with the client by supporting the client to choose what happens in the session by allowing for silence, pause, or reflection.	Committed to the quality of presence. Develops an ever-greater presence, unlearns whatever keeps them from being present. Strives continuously for progress especially for being present, being in free flow.
Listens actively—questions and observations are customized using what the coach has learned about the client and the client's situation. The coach inquires about the words the client uses and explores the emotions, energy shifts, non-verbal cues, or behaviors.	Listens intuitively. The WABA professional engages in holistic listening to acknowledge the client as a whole. Sees the client as a totality of mind, body, and emotions.
Evokes awareness—the coach asks questions about the client, such as their current way of thinking, feeling, their values, needs, wants, beliefs, and behavior. The coach shares observations, intuitions, comments, thoughts, and feelings, and invites the client's exploration through verbal or tonal invitation while allowing the client to do most of the talking.	Provides a safe environment for clients to experience and identify emotions released. Always aware of their state that is "doing" or "being" self. Ends each session by allowing clients to enjoy and be in their own space in silence. Helps clients realize that whatever "love" or "oneness" they feel during or after sessions is universal and not personal.
Facilitates client growth. The coach invites the client to explore progress toward what the client wants to accomplish, and designs post-session thinking, reflection, and action. The coach partners with the client to consider how to move forward, including resources, support, or potential barriers, and designs the best methods of accountability for themselves. They also celebrate the client's progress and learning and partner with them on how they want to complete the session.	Discusses these feelings when the client and WABA professionals agree on appropriateness if professional counseling is not required. Protects the confidentiality of such communications. Assists in obtaining further professional help for their physical, mental, and emotional well-being. Directs the client to other well-qualified professionals when the problem falls outside the practitioner's competency boundaries.

Mechanism of emotions

Emotional regulation is complex and never down to one biological or hormonal factor. However, a deeper understanding of neurobiological mechanisms of emotional processing is necessary, especially when using the intimacy of aquatic bodywork connection for coaching. This combined method can help clients master their emotions and increase mental clarity. Our sensations (internal and external inputs to the brain) play a critical role in establishing an emotional balance. The afferent input is intertwined through all the sensory systems (auditory, visual, gustatory, olfactory, tactile, vestibular, proprioceptive, and interoception). However, the contribution rate of these systems to emotional processing may vary from person to person.

A variety of sensory inputs is processed through the complex cooperation of multiple brain systems for emotional regulation. The prefrontal cortex (PFC) and anterior cingulate cortex (ACC) connect with other areas such as the amygdala, lateral hypothalamus, brain stem centers, hippocampal region, and orbitofrontal cortex—ventral striatum that have autonomic, memory, and reward-related functions (Dixon *et al.* 2017). The ACC plays a significant role in mediating the emotions' cognitive influences with connections to both the "emotional" limbic system and the "cognitive" prefrontal cortex. This complex structure for emotional regulation is the cortico-limbic system, dysfunction of which is manifested as specific psychopathologies and pain (Stevens *et al.* 2011).

One of the most significant inputs for emotional quality sensation is gentle touch as physical contact. In general, tactile inputs are the primary determiner of the emotional state from infancy to senescence. The transformation of physical contact or gentle stroke to pleasant and emotional touch forms the earliest connections and empowers individuals at the beginning of their lives. The infant-mother connection is one of the earliest primarily physical connections human beings make. Thus, gentle tactile strokes (input) can contribute to resilience and mitigate mood and anxiety symptoms (Breit *et al.* 2018).

This empowering sense of connection is bound to nerve receptors in the skin, C-tactile (CT) fibers, through which the afferent affiliative touch is transformed into feelings. C-tactile fibers appear to be tuned for interpersonal touch (i.e., "caress sensors"). They are found mainly in hairy skin, wrapped around hair follicles. CT neurons may also be present in the glabrous skin with different biochemical and structural characteristics (Nagi & Mahns 2013). Thus, the emotional neural circuits and brain's emotional modulation centers process these tactile stimuli, perceived as emotional quality touch. However, in neuropathic pain conditions, a light touch can elicit unpleasant sensations due to a loss of their normally pain-inhibiting role (Liljencrantz & Olausson 2014).

C-tactile afferents (CTs) have specific importance for socio-emotional responses and psychological well-being. CTs are tools to help convert soft and caring touch to the sense of affective touch. CTs increase social motivation and reduce physiological and behavioral reactivity to stressors (Walker *et al.* 2017). They improve positive feelings, reduce stress, and influence psychomotor function and cognitive performance (Schitter *et al.* 2020). Pleasing emotional experiences and a sense of hedonic environmental features for homeostasis and well-being may be correlating with oxytocin (Field 2019). However, research suggests that touch does not increase prosocial behavior without meaningful social and psychological connotations. Any touch-related effects on prosocial behavior likely depend on the situation's ecological validity (Rosenberger *et al.* 2018). In this regard, the WATSU environment forms a great ecological situation in which gentle affective touch can be easily transformed into feelings of well-being, resilience, connection, trust, and safety (Pawling *et al.* 2017). CTs are tuned to respond to tactile stimuli with the specific characteristics of a gentle caress delivered at typical skin temperature. This provides a peripheral mechanism for signaling pleasant skin-to-skin contact in humans, promoting interpersonal touch and affiliative behavior (Ackerley *et al.* 2014). Also, in such an environment with pleasant touch, eye contact, and empathy, oxytocin levels may show a significant rise (Ito *et al.* 2019).

Interestingly, CTs demonstrate "fatigue" with repeated stroking stimuli (Macefield 2009), which suggests a time limit for specific manipulation, movement, or tactile input to the client. In addition, CTs have been shown to reduce pain, depending on the context of the stimulus (Shaikh *et al.* 2015), but this tactile stimulation may not be perceived to be identical across participants and result positively (Gatti *et al.* 2018). The individual's past experiences and avoidance of painful emotions might considerably affect positive feelings and they may benefit from the company, tactile stimulation, and solitude (Schitter *et al.* 2020). The inability to regulate emotions and the effort to suppress painful emotions promote undesirable changes in behavior (Stevens *et al.* 2011).

Modalities offering various somatic experiences, including manipulations, mobilizations, stretches, and gentle strokes through holistic quality, are vital for a feeling of connection and empowering emotions. In addition to enriched tactile inputs in the intimate WATSU approach, tailored activation of the vestibular and proprioceptive (kinesthetic) system in a warm pool can further contribute to the feelings of warmth, safety, and relatedness. Thus, altering afferent input makes WATSU a unique and powerful somatic experience. A client can clarify the interrelationship between emotional, physical, and cognitive functioning necessary for intuitive understanding in a session. Clients can achieve this mindfulness and focus on the physical self by eliminating external and internal stressors (thoughts, pent-up emotions) in WATSU. Clients can become better prepared to explore deeper issues in the life coaching process that are chronically ignored.

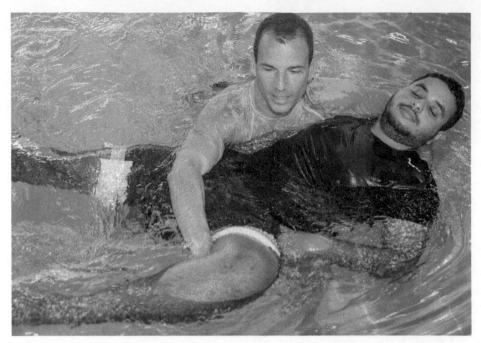

Figure 9.3: The support of mindfulness, consciousness and the feeling of wholeness

Mindfulness is the base for transforming into resourcefulness, where hidden and triggering emotions come up to the conscious level. In neuroscience, this can be explained as the brain's mode shift from the activity of specific brain areas to a more general brain activity called the Default Mode Network (DMN). The DMN is considered a backbone of cortical integration (Alves *et al.* 2019) and is negatively correlated with other networks in the brain, such as attention networks (Broyd *et al.* 2009).

DMN activation possibly contributes to avoiding psychosomatic diseases (Buckner 2013). The DMN is activated when individuals are focused on their internal mental-state processes, such as self-referential processing, interoception, autobiographical memory retrieval, or imagining the future. The DMN is deactivated during cognitive task performance (Ekhtiari *et al.* 2016).

The DMN increases our capacity to overview body, emotions, others, and cognition, resulting in increased mindfulness and self-awareness. This state is where one can begin to notice the energy blocks created over a long period. A meditative state can increase awareness, a cognitive ability that involves controlling the DMN and task-specific attention requiring brain networks (Ramírez-Barrantes *et al.* 2019).

Higher self-awareness is the starting point to developing higher emotional control, resilience, and psychosocial functioning (Martinez-Pons 1997) that is the base for successful coaching.

Biological base for transformation and self-awareness

Affective touch can help release negative emotions and enhance positive emotions concerning the safety and warmth of the environment. CTs' emotional quality touch sensation activates the emotion-related brain areas and increases oxygen levels, especially in the PFC and ACC guiding decision-making. Movements in the isolated pool with reduced gravitational forces on the joints and muscles (i.e., less noise for the body), help clients become internally focused. Exploration of personal values via increased emotional process is supported by gentle stroke sensation from CTs. These altered afferent inputs are interpreted as supporting touch, higher emotional quality, and safety.

When the client's mind is silent and free of responsibilities due to whole-body support, they benefit more from inner guidance and listening. Feelings of safety and physical support can help identify stressful thoughts and emotions that need to be released. Thus, WATSU, as non-verbal communication, can form the first step leading to deeper self-exploration. It can provide a period to rediscover the emotional blockages, realization, and dispatching of stressful thoughts in warm water. Realizing the current feelings and thoughts is likely to induce relief from the emotional and physical tension. In WATSU, the altered inputs via vestibular, kinesthetic, and tactile sensory systems can shift the brain from the task-oriented high activity in specific brain regions to the DMN. The DMN forms the base for mindfulness and self-awareness, enabling people to explore new perspectives through uncovering unidentified emotions. This enhanced awareness enables WATSU clients to open up more in seeking full self-expression. Because these positive senses bring the best out of clients and their willingness to share their most profound issues to be resolved, this is the desired state for high-quality life coaching sessions. The emotional, physical release or catharsis in WATSU is transformed into full self-expression in the coaching room. This state can be used as an excellent opportunity for coaching to pre-shake up the preconceptions for self-awareness and understanding others.

WATSU for awareness-based life coaching

"The quieter you become, the more you are able to hear." (Rumi)

We live in an age of ultra-information and relentless demand for tasks requiring high cognitive energy. In addition to high cognitive demand, the strains of modern life cause pent-up frustrations and emotional disturbance and diminish our empathy toward others and ourselves. Constant external focus underpins superficial thinking with quick decisions and reacting rather than responding. We feel forced to develop habits for the sake of saving time and money, causing a loss of our awareness, social interactions, deeper connections, and productivity. We live our lives with the continuous stress of due dates. In addition, fast-food style dietary habits prevent us from having natural and refreshing breaks, leading to various disorders, including digestion or other vicarious health issues. A psychological or emotional sense of being "drained" is, therefore, manifested as unproductivity.

In contrast, entering a safe and silent zone without the noise of our daily tasks provides the pause, silence, presence, and strong connection human beings need. Thus, one can see life from a new perception. This new perspective is strengthened by the connection between the client and the practitioners in both interventions to initiate the change and enrich one's life. The depth of experiences and exploration of deeper resources in both interventions provides spontaneous adaptation for more transformational results. The deeper the connection with self and others, the more awareness there is and the longer-lasting changes we can make. WATSU and life coaching integration help clients dig deeper for the most profound exploration.

Coaching and WATSU using visible, audible, and physical techniques are only for getting to its heart. Thus, WATSU- and coaching-induced DMN activation can significantly contribute to exploring emotions and social understanding. It is known that the DMN is an indispensable part of the social understanding of others (Wanqing *et al*. 2014). Thus, a deep resting and relaxing state of WATSU provides the potential for improved resilience and emotional intelligence.

WATSU's contribution to emotional intelligence and life coaching

Although there is a dire need to focus on one's self and explore the most profound values, beliefs, and emotions, the day-to-day tasks force us to always live in a fast phase. The constant need for mental work and for the quick refreshment of mental energy is relentless. One cannot entirely refresh mental energy without shifting between physical, emotional, and spiritual dimensions. In this regard, an allotted time of stillness and an isolated environment away from stressors can be enriching. Decoding the emotions and their meanings is critical for being able to change from the inside out. Mastering our emotions and their meanings helps us define priorities, set more attainable goals, identify the triggers, and defer immediate results for long-term success. Thus, self-awareness and self-management as building blocks of emotional intelligence (EI) have great potential to strengthen individuals against socio-emotional conflicts.

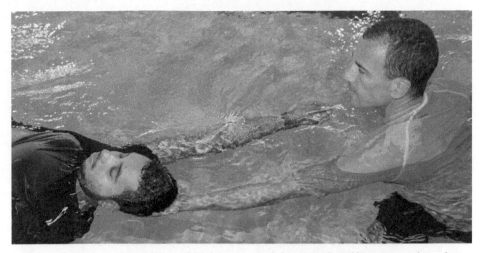

Figure 9.4: Coaching the need for learning and change induced by a strengthened client-practitioner connection provides high-quality outcomes

In life coaching, exploration of emotional driving forces or blocks is the main target. Because neuropsychology has shown that decisions are emotionally led, not rationally, this further describes the central role of EI in one's life in seeking change, growth, and success.

EI consists of elements of life self-awareness and self-management. EI implies that one can insert a pause between action and reaction, allowing time to process emotional and intellectual inputs. The moments of no reaction to a stimulus underpin our attention to recognizing moods and emotions (Martinez-Pons 1997). Inserting a pause before an act can be done in different forms and environments, such as deep breathing practices, immersion, or traveling. Thus, the more time and focus to monitor one's emotional states, the better the response one can form in any situation. As different forms of intervention to help people, WATSU and life coaching share the power of focusing on emotions in the sessions. Both interventions value the moments of stillness in different forms, leading to emotional awareness. WATSU's safe physical guidance supports positive feelings. Especially in the "distant stillness" technique, minimum physical contact and movement promote connection and oneness with others. In the highest feeling of connection, WATSU therapists devote themselves entirely to being present and listening holistically. This provided space for emotional processing can increase resilience.

From here on, the client takes the lead invisibly, making the client feel/sense a high quality of emotional connection and physical support from the therapist's gentle and light touch. The emotional strain can be replaced with the most potent emotional forces for regulation and self-healing in these moments of connection. Feelings of gratitude, safety, trust, relaxation, self-awareness, and being understood are triggered in this connection. These positive emotions and their awareness empower the cognition that moves the clients into a higher meaning-making process. Validation and acceptance are also promoted in coaching and WATSU, enhancing EI and leading the client into resourcefulness.

EI helps identify and understand the other's feelings, needs, and viewpoints. In addition to that, EI contributes to impulsivity control and mitigates careless decisions, stereotyping, and judging (Martinez-Pons 1997). It increases comfort with change and ease. This outward competency is based on the inward-looking quality of identifying emotions and their roots. This inward-looking quality eases the process of how to act to resolve the situation with the best possible outcome.

Positive emotions do not always imply positive thoughts. Consequently, the notion that positive thinking produces positive outcomes may not always be accurate. The meaning of awareness goes beyond positive thinking and emotional state, which then avoids fooling our mind into perceiving that we have already attained our goal, slackening the readiness to pursue it. In general, achieving goals necessitates a balanced approach, with an ability to perceive the positive aspects of the events or earnings and the unpleasant side of them.

Heart rate variability: Monitoring autonomic and emotional influences

Balanced autonomic nervous system activity is the key to well-being. The ANS coordinates multiple dimensions of our being acting together to ensure an overall balance and proper reaction to the environment. The ANS also synchronizes the coordination of bodily systems and socio-emotional functioning.

Measuring the adaptation of ANS activity helps determine the healing effects of interventions. It has been known for decades that ANS activity and emotions are reflected in our heart rhythm patterns. The rhythmic pattern in the body is generated primarily by the heart due to its responsivity to afferent inputs and ANS modulation. The heart rhythm transmits neurological, hormonal, pressure, and electromagnetic patterns processed by the brain. These cardiac afferent signals evaluated at the cortical level play a role to regulate emotional and autonomic activity (McCraty 2019).

The ANS is quantified by measuring the RR intervals (the time between successive heartbeats). The continuous interplay between sympathetic and parasympathetic influences the heart rate from beat to beat. Many physical and psychological factors that affect the ANS influence the variation in RR intervals. Therefore, analyzing heart rate variability (HRV) enhances our understanding of ANS balance (Kaikkonen 2015). This constant variation in milliseconds between heartbeats, HRV, indicates the heart's ability to respond to different situations. Thus, HRV biofeedback can help determine emotional and behavioral regulation at ANS level (Kim *et al*. 2015).

HRV analysis provides insight into autonomic flexibility, stress-coping levels, self-control abilities, willpower, attention, and cognitive functioning. For example, the experience of anger, frustration, or anxiety reduces HRV (McCraty & Shaffer 2015). In addition, low HRV has been associated with panic symptoms, depression, poor attentional control, emotional dysregulation, and inflexibility of behavior (Kim *et al*. 2015). This socio-emotional response is critical to understand the specific and overall effect of interventions (Field & Diego 2008; Tufekcioglu *et al*. 2010). Therefore, HRV can give us insight into ANS dynamics, susceptible to emotional states and attitude changes.

The activation of the corticolimbic system correlating with increased HRV promotes emotional memory processing and enhances conciseness and socio-emotional functioning (Meier *et al*. 2020). Future studies can help establish a stronger link between WATSU and the activation of the corticolimbic system. It is known that sustained positive emotions, such as appreciation, love, and compassion, are associated with higher HRV patterns (McCraty 2019). Higher HRV implies altered cardiac afferent inputs to the brain (i.e., activation of the corticolimbic system, promoted regulation of emotions, and shrunk amygdala in size) (Fredrickson *et al*. 2008), which can form a biological base for central integration of afferent inputs and self-awareness. This is a condition for the best coaching experiences for explorations and learning.

WATSU's HRV-increasing effect has been shown (Tufekcioglu *et al*. 2010). WATSU-like interventions provide the experience of a new afferent input pattern deviating from the established memory (McCraty 2019) that can activate the corticolimbic system and stimulate feelings. Moreover, gentle stroking carrying emotional quality tactile input via CTs in WATSU can significantly contribute to the higher HRV (by activation of the vagal nerve). Thermo- and mechano-sensitive skin receptors enable us to feel the thermo-neutral water that further promotes the sensation of affective quality touch. Further, breathing becomes more conscious, deeper, and slower. Conscious breathing is known to enhance HRV and emotional control. The higher the HRV, the better autonomic flexibility and socio-emotional processing (Guan *et al*. 2014). This processing has been witnessed in many WATSU sessions as crying or laughing. These emotional expressions are likely to form healing cathartic releases.

Non-invasive HRV recordings are now more accessible and practical with the numerous user-friendly apps for digital devices. HRV biofeedback can be used to enhance cardiovascular coherence, self-awareness, and regulation (Kim *et al*. 2015). Although the signal recording methods vary, the cost-efficient method for individuals is the non-medical heart rate sensors connected to a smartphone with an HRV app or an Oura ring. It is critical to know that each person's HRV is unique. Therefore, a comparison of HRV to one's averages can better show the efficacy of the interventions.

In conclusion, monitoring overall well-being via HRV biofeedback can reflect the effectiveness of WATSU and life coaching on an emotional and physiological level as verbal or non-verbal interventions. Of equal importance, healthcare professionals can adjust therapeutic work doses using HRV biofeedback.

Exploration through movements in WATSU and questions in life coaching

Calming the mind through emotionally penetrating movements in WATSU before coaching may have a great potential for deeper explorations, and thus long-lasting change and transformation. The practice of intuitive listening and whole-person focus while suspending, floating, pushing, and pulling the client into therapeutic positions enables the therapist to notice subtle changes. Coaches could question the underlying issues of these observed changes in a WATSU pool for validation of the emotions and deeper exploration. This type of somatic coaching is a part of life coaching in general. Moreover, the clients can easily sense intuitive listening, presence, and full engagement. Being listened to holistically in the nurturing arms of the WATSU therapist may enable clients to explore deeper emotional values, resulting in higher awareness levels. Full engagement of the therapist illuminates the client's way toward further self-exploration.

The movements in WATSU and questions in life coaching support exploration to a higher level in a combined way. Thus, the use of WATSU movements in combination with coaching questions is likely to be a powerful tool for quality presence, awareness, and self-regulation.

Presence and resourcefulness

"Consciousness is the birthplace of change." (Anonymous)

WATSU is one of the most valuable practices to establish a *being* self rather than a *doing* self. Being with a client and quality presence can be manifested as the ultimate connection. This strong connection can lead to the most powerful emotions such as gratitude, appreciation, feeling understood, and thus healing. Having no concern about the next moves in WATSU or following questions in coaching is critical to being present and allowing the client to be fully open. The point is shifting from using specific techniques to "being in the flow and the moment." Flowing at the moment is best described as "free flow" in WATSU.

This kind of harmony between the coach and the client can be called being in the flow. This state is sought in coaching for more openness and authentic presence to contribute to the client's resourcefulness. Being in the present moment helps the coach and the client ensure that their emotions are not coming into the process in an unhelpful way. This pure presence enables the client to focus on the feelings and sensations, leading to higher openness and deeper understanding.

For deeper explorations, it is critical to move from "doing" self and physical movements to "being" self. The moments of stillness in which inward-looking and self-listening are promoted can move the person from a "mind the problems" to a "mind the present moment, body, and existence" state. The Water Breath Dance (WBD) technique is considered a mindfulness practice for reconnection with self. The self-observation in WBD provides an opportunity to detach one's self from intrusive negative thoughts. The ability to stop negative thoughts and feelings getting in the way is required in both professions to enhance exquisite concentration on the now. This moment! This pool! This me! (i.e., presence, acceptance, and awareness). Reconnection in WBD makes it easier to enter the flowing moments with physical movements.

A similar practice is needed in life coaching sessions when the feeling of pointlessness and extended questions are taken over. The anxiety of thinking about the next question triggers subjective listening to take control over intuitive listening. In this situation, life coaches need to bring peace, get rid of the stress of asking good questions one after another. Otherwise, the state of worry can diminish the connection and the desired results in both professions. If coaches are trapped in asking long questions, they need to take deep breaths, take a pause, and gather thoughts to feel the presence. If WATSU practitioners are trapped by the concern about the next move and unsure how to continue in the session, they need moments of stillness to regain the connection and match their breathing with the client. These kinds of pauses or moments for reconnection are critical to reinforce and nourish the body's ability to rest within a "being" state rather than a "doing" state.

Fluidic early access to resourcefulness

People in a high state of emotional arousal, passing through negative feelings of rage, anxiety, and fear, are not coachable. This unbalanced emotional state is the reflection of amygdala activation over the prefrontal cortex. In this state, the cortisol and adrenalin stress hormones switch the brain's learning region off. The most energy (i.e., blood and oxygen) is moved to the amygdala to respond as quickly as possible, known as the fight or flight response of the ANS. In general, this is when anger blinds the mind, and the truth disappears. ANS imbalance created must be resolved for maximum coaching achievements.

Creative potential is related to the capacity to relax (Meier *et al.* 2020). A state of anger, stress, and anxiety does not produce a refined mind. However, in rare moments when there is not any perception of threat or demand on us, and when our bodies and passions are comfortable and quiescent, we have the privilege of being able to access the higher mind, called the neocortex in neuroscience. The neocortex, the seat of imagination, empathy, and impartial judgement, when activated, unlatches our hold on our egos. Thus, we ascend to a more universal and less biased perspective, casting off a little of the customary anxious self-justification and brutal pride.

WATSU helps us ascend to the deepest self. Achieving the awareness of the deepest self in WATSU can propel life coaching clients to the highest awareness. In such states, the mind moves beyond its particular self-interests and cravings. This common quality makes two interventions go hand in hand and form protection from invasion of fear for the past and worries for the future. Empowering WATSU helps clients get the most out of their resourcefulness. Once clients enter their resourcefulness with WATSU, they can easily recognize firmly held personal values, after which coaching helps link these values to the clients' goals more efficiently. Therefore, calming the ANS with WATSU (Tufekcioglu *et al.* 2010) acts as preparatory work for coaching by providing a base for better learning and exploration in the coaching session. Research has shown that positive emotions, induced through loving-kindness meditation, build consequential personal resources (Fredrickson *et al.* 2008).

In this regard, a regular life coaching process can benefit significantly from pre-accessing the resourcefulness state. With the client already in this state, a coach finds it easier to facilitate learning, expand thinking, and add new perspectives to their agenda.

Support and trust in WATSU and life coaching

The support in the WATSU pool and the coaching room is a critical element for the success of therapists and coaches alike. In WATSU, the support requires intimate and close physical contact while floating, rocking, and gliding the clients. Other support elements are warm water properties, including buoyancy, density, viscosity, and water resistance.

WATSU's physical support ends with the session. On the other hand, support in coaching is sustained for years, depending on the relationship between coach and client. In this regard, physical and emotional support in the pool can be augmented and extended to years with the life coach's emotional and social support in daily life.

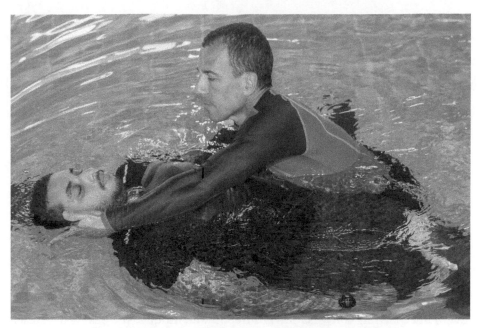

Figure 9.5: The physical support at WATSU therapy can be
extended by the coach's support in daily life

Conducting the proper physical and emotional challenge is critical in WATSU and life coaching. The clients should be challenged in an individualized manner, considering their physical, mental, and emotional limitations. In contrast to what many people believe, the challenge is an indispensable element of professional support and essential for maintaining trust in both modalities. Challenging may give sufficient input for self-healing in WATSU and change in life coaching.

Although a client in WATSU does not seem to be challenged, some moves and stretches are applied with a reasonable challenge to improve range of motion, mobilize the joints, and decompress the spinal column. Gentle physical input/manipulation is adjusted according to the client's limits and resistance to movements. In case of stiffness or any limiting factor, the movement is adapted or replaced to improve the condition. This is another form of support achieved by somatic interaction.

On the other hand, life coaching requires a good level of challenge to balance support. A good challenge helps the coach to shake up the client's preconceptions and accelerates the process of change. The balance in coaching support and challenge intends to eliminate the client's fear of transformation and growth. The success in the desired transformation depends on the coach's skill, wisdom, empathy, and the willingness of the client to be open. Similarly, the impact of personal characteristics and skills can significantly contribute to the success of a WATSU session.

The main contribution of WATSU to the coaching process is to improve these required competencies needed in the coaching room. Receiving or giving WATSU provides benefits for the success of a coaching relationship. WATSU's non-verbal communication, non-judgmental listening, and unconditional acceptance increase awareness and potentially contribute to exploration and learning in the coaching room. Therefore, working in the pool is likely to improve the competencies for working in the coaching room to address life issues presented by a coaching client, such as clarity of goals, anxiety, procrastination, stress at the workplace, and limiting beliefs.

Finally, support and challenge are the tools to empower the connection, safety, and trust in both interventions. WATSU-induced resilience and resourcefulness can prepare clients for enormous challenges in a coaching session.

Life coaching models and WATSU principles

Every life coaching conversation is different and unique. The best way to ask a powerful question is to be deeply connected to the client and the conversation; to be present, to listen with all of the senses.

In universal eclectic coaching, the person-centered approach posits that change is naturally triggered by fundamental conditions such as warmth, genuineness, and unconditional positive regard (Passmore *et al.* 2020). As healing in WATSU necessitates all of these competencies, WATSU has the potential to form an excellent base for change and growth to start.

The Gestalt approach is another coaching model to help clients live more in the present moment and reconnect with their whole selves. The goal is to find out how meaning takes shape in human perspective in the here and now. In other words, the best coaching is co-created in the moment and is led by the client's needs (Passmore *et al.* 2020). The best WATSU sessions are co-created in the moment, based on the needs of the client, too.

The Gestalt approach emphasizes full presence, and the focus should be on the individual as a totality of mind, body, emotions, and spirit (Passmore *et al.* 2020). Equally, the experience of the integration of all disparate parts helps the clients discover and experience the wholeness, energy, pattern, and shape of their existence in a typical WATSU session. Life coaches using the Gestalt approach can benefit from the experience of fullness in WATSU to empower the client. The Gestalt approach intends to bring these parts together by self-reconnection to become totally what they already are. It seems that a combination of both interventions can provide an original impetus for further settlement and a journey to become a better self.

In the same way, the whole body is concerned about leading to better self-awareness in the somatic coaching approach. Somatic coaching aims to deepen understanding of self and enable clients to explore faulty thinking and hidden emotion at a deeper level, which is a key to change in coaching, whereas deepening understanding of self and emotions is the key to healing in WATSU.

On the other hand, the humanistic coaching approach posits that the individual's subjective experience is the most crucial element of self-actualization. For this subjective experience, the liquid elements of WATSU provide an excellent condition. One can achieve and experience a state of flow leading to the sensation of deep concentration, enjoyment, and fulfillment in a warm WATSU pool. In this state, conscious and unconscious motivation are easily aligned with personal values. The alignment in WATSU's therapeutic environment can significantly prepare the client for a higher emotional, cognitive, and even physical performance. Specifically, the state achieved leads to space and time to think free of concerns. Intuitive and holistic listening and unconditional acceptance in the coaching room further support this improved thinking pattern. Consequently, WATSU's fundamental principles, values, and physical environment can help the client hear a message meaning "you matter."

The OSKAR model in coaching mainly focuses on solutions rather than problems (Passmore et al. 2020). It requires a listening skill to find a hint of a solution and use it as the element to reflect on, directing the conversation forward. With this in mind, modification of the techniques and adapting the session for more benefits can deepen the client's experience in WATSU. For instance, many clients report that the movements and range of motion realization occurred beyond their imagination. In the same way, WATSU clients can re-explore their physical limits and the many more ways of feeling emotions beyond the self-limiting beliefs. For example, release from the pain and physical restrictions helps shift the attention from physical boundaries to their higher spiritual and emotional freedom. After that, the client leaves their limiting belief for the desired result with this freed mind.

Focus on the solution within the physical interaction may include identifying the unexpressed emotions and eliminating the ugly return of the emotions later. However, interaction in WATSU is always open to transference and counter-transference of feelings as another source of information about the client and the opportunity to practice self-management. Despite this, unnoticed counter-transference of feelings can get in the way of the work in both professions.

The integrated model in coaching focuses on behaviors, conscious-unconscious cognition, emotions, body, and system (Passmore et al. 2020). Nevertheless, working with the body, even without the intimacy of in-water WATSU therapy, can be uncomfortable for some coaches and clients. If the mind and body integration is not kept in mind, some may consider aquatic bodywork therapy beyond the boundaries of coaching. On the contrary, understanding our bodies and using them to enhance our performance is vital for coaches to help clients be their best selves.

The bodily sensations are most of the time the reflection of psychological needs. At the same time, the physical sensations can be the signals of the current emotions or deeper and longer-term issues. Similarly, somatic coaching or mindfulness body scan promotes the connection of mind and body, leading to a better understanding of the physical messages. Of equal importance, promoted bodily sensations in WATSU can provide an excellent tool for somatic coaching seeking the blind spot.

In conclusion, the competencies of therapists and WATSU values are aligned with many elements of coaching. Using the WATSU method for coaching can bring clarity in synthesizing our mass of learning, multiple models, ideas about change, and different tools and techniques. In this regard, dual background and professional certifications are necessary for establishing trust and enhanced outcomes.

Although many reports indicate that WATSU, a holistic experience, supports the coherence and forms a feeling of a unified whole, future studies will be highly valuable to confirm the efficacy and effectiveness of WATSU in coaching interventions.

Lastly, WATSU can be a valuable tool to help life coaches adapt and flex to meet the different needs of individual clients, inviting the use of a diverse range of approaches.

Free flow

WATSU requires and reinforces us to just be within the moments that flow towards the strongest emotions of trust, understanding, and connection. Trust is likely to flourish in the sense of warmth, which underpins the success of the WATSU experience and coaching process. The ability of the practitioner to create a strong connection in the climate of warmth, holistic listening, and acceptance invigorates the feelings of being understood and validated.

These feelings are the best safeguard from entering the negative feeling zone of uneasiness, aloneness, and irritation. The feeling of being understood is a prerequisite for benefiting from other emotional resources. It helps clarify one's mind for existence, appreciation, let off, and love, and eliminates self-alienation (Seltzer 2017). Moreover, feeling truly "gotten" is to feel deeply, rewardingly validated, which helps us to perceive life from a more positive perspective.

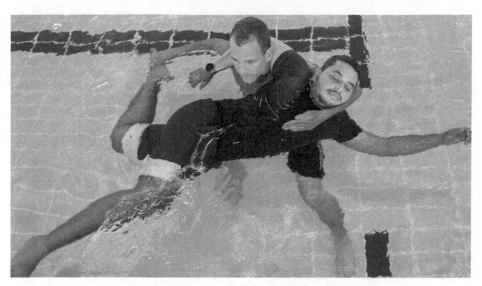

Figure 9.6: WATSU is a journey toward the feeling of being understood

The depth of feeling understood explains why *free flow* in a WATSU session empowers the connection. In the peak moments of *free flow*, movements are decided in coherence with the clients non-verbally. This is where the WATSU session is completely transformed into an active interaction. The transition from one movement to another is spontaneous, flowing, and seamless. Being in the flow is the time of energy peak but always under control and full of explorations. *Free flow* can be in fast or slow forms without following a pre-planned sequence. Surprises and rewards emanate and strengthen the connection. *Free flow* provides moments for the uplifted feelings of being understood and acceptance of being imperfectly self. *Free flow* clarifies self-perception and helps internalize self-acceptance resulting in eased self-expression. In coaching, eased self-expression is desired by coaches where they can initiate change and growth significantly.

Both professions are deeper than applying a technical sequence of movements and asking questions in a structured order. Their shared values (Table 9.2) and using the power of now form a more solid and more profound experience for the clients to have the correct direction of flow in their life.

In consideration of common elements, shared tools, and similar benefits, coaches and clients can start using WATSU to prepare themselves for learning, exploration, and change. Soon, WATSU may have a role beyond relaxing aquatic therapy.

Table 9.2: Common quality attributes and benefits of coaching and WATSU

Attributes			Benefits		
Mutual respect	Intuitive listening	Unconditional acceptance	Self-management	Holistic experience	Feeling understood
Openness	Surrendering	Confidentiality	Mindfulness	Self-expression	Relaxation
Support	Stillness	Genuineness	Empowerment	Transformation	Self-healing
Safety	Silence	Empathy	Self-exploration	Change	Stress relief
Wholeness	Harmony	Warmth	Self-acceptance	Self-awareness	Trust

Presence, Connection, Free flow, Relatedness

Summary

In conclusion, we hope this chapter illuminates a new horizon toward integrating the therapeutic benefits of WATSU with life coaching not only to innovate and enhance the processes but ultimately to improve the quality of life of the clients we have the privilege and great responsibility to work with.

References

Ackerley, R., Wasling, H.B., Liljencrantz, J., Olausson, H., Johnson, R.D. & Wessberg, J. (2014). Human C-tactile afferents are tuned to the temperature of a skin-stroking caress. *Journal of Neuroscience*, 34(8): 2879–2883. https://doi.org/10.1523/JNEUROSCI.2847-13.2014.

Alves, P.N. *et al.* (2019). An improved neuroanatomical model of the default-mode network reconciles previous neuroimaging and neuropathological findings. *Communications Biology*, 2: 370.

Breit, S., Kupferberg, A., Rogler, G. & Hasler, G. (2018). Vagus nerve as modulator of the brain-gut axis in psychiatric and inflammatory disorders. *Frontiers in Psychiatry*, 9: 44. doi:10.3389/fpsyt.2018.00044.

Broyd, S.J., Demanuele, C., Debener, S., Helps, S.K., James, C.J. & Sonuga-Barke, E.J.S. (2009). Default-mode brain dysfunction in mental disorders: A systematic review. *Neuroscience & Biobehavioral Reviews*, 33(3): 279–296.

Buckner, R.L. (2013). The brain's default network: Origins and implications for the study of psychosis. *Dialogues in Clinical Neuroscience*, 15(3): 351–358. doi:10.31887/DCNS.2013.15.3/rbuckner.

Dixon, M.L., Thiruchselvam, R., Todd, R. & Christoff, K. (2017). Emotion and the prefrontal cortex: An integrative review. *Psychological Bulletin*, 143(10). doi:10.1037/bul0000096.

Dull, H. (2008). *WATSU: Basic and Explorer Paths*. Middletown, CA: WATSU Publishing.

Ekhtiari, H., Nasseri, P., Yavari, F., Mokri, A. & Monterosso, J. (2016). Neuroscience of drug craving for addiction medicine: From circuits to therapies. *Progress in Brain Research*, 223: 115–141.

Field, T. (2019). Social touch, CT touch and massage therapy: A narrative review. *Developmental Review*, 51: 123–145.

Field, T. & Diego, M. (2008). Vagal activity, early growth and emotional development. *Infant Behavior Development*, 31(3): 361–373. doi:10.1016/j.infbeh.2007.12.008.

Fredrickson, B.L., Cohn, M.A., Coffey, K.A., Pek, J. & Finkel, S.M. (2008). Open hearts build lives: Positive emotions, induced through loving-kindness meditation, build consequential personal resources. *Journal of Personality and Social Psychology*, 95(5): 1045–1062.

Gatti, E. *et al.* (2018). Emotional ratings and skin conductance response to visual, auditory and haptic stimuli. *Scientific Data*, 5: 180120.

Guan, O.L., Collet, J.P., Yuskiv, N., Skippen, P., Brant, R. & Kissoon, N. (2014). The effect of massage therapy on autonomic activity in critically ill children. *Evidence-Based Complementary and Alternative Medicine*, 656750. doi:10.1155/2014/656750.

Ito, E., Shima, R. & Yoshioka, T. (2019). Hypothesis and perspective: A novel role of oxytocin: Oxytocin-induced well-being in humans. *Biophysics and Physicobiology*, 16: 132–139.

Kaikkonen, P. (2015). Post-exercise heart rate variability: A new approach to evaluation of exercise-induced physiological training load. *Studies in Sport, Physical Education and Health*, 224: 94.

Kim, S., Rath, J.F., McCraty, R., Zemon, V., Cavallo, M.M. & Foley, F.W. (2015). Heart rate variability biofeedback, self-regulation, and severe brain injury. *Biofeedback*, 43(1): 6–14. doi: 10.5298/1081-5937-43.1.10.

Liljencrantz, J. & Olausson, H. (2014). Tactile-C fibers and their contributions to pleasant sensations and to tactile allodynia. *Frontiers in Behavioral Neuroscience*, 8: 37. doi:10.3389/fnbeh.2014.00037.

Macefield, V.G. (2009). Tactile C Fibers. In M.D. Binder, N. Hirokawa & U. Windhorst (eds), *Encyclopedia of Neuroscience*. Berlin, Heidelberg: Springer. https://doi.org/10.1007/978-3-540-29678-2_5865.

Martinez-Pons, M. (1997). The relation of emotional intelligence with selected areas of personal functioning. *Imagination Cognition Personality*, 17: 3–13.

McCraty, R. (2019). Heart-Brain Neurodynamics: The Making of Emotions. In S.B. Schafer, *Media Models to Foster Collective Human Coherence in the PSYCHecology*, pp.191–219. doi:10.4018/978-1-5225-9065-1.ch010.

McCraty, R. & Shaffer, F. (2015). Heart rate variability: New perspectives on physiological mechanisms, assessment of self-regulatory capacity, and health risk. *Global Advances in Health and Medicine*, 4(1): 46–61.

Meier, M. *et al.* (2020). The opposite of stress: The relationship between vagal tone, creativity, and divergent thinking. *Experimental Psychology*, 67(2): 150–159. https://doi.org/10.1027/1618-3169/a000483.

Nagi, S.S. & Mahns, D.A. (2013). Mechanical allodynia in human glabrous skin mediated by low-threshold cutaneous mechanoreceptors with unmyelinated fibres. *Experimental Brain Research*, 231(2): 139–151.

Passmore, J. & Sinclair, T. (2020). *Becoming a Coach: The Essential ICF Guide*. Cham: Springer Nature Switzerland. https://doi.org/10.1007/978-3-030-53161-4.

Pawling, R., Cannon, P.R., McGlone, F.P. & Walker, S.C. (2017). C-tactile afferent stimulating touch carries a positive affective value. *PLOS ONE*, 12(3): e0173457. https://doi.org/10.1371/journal.pone.0173457.

Ramírez-Barrantes, R. *et al.* (2019). Default Mode Network, meditation, and age-associated brain changes: What can we learn from the impact of mental training on well-being as a psychotherapeutic approach? *Neural Plasticity*, 7067592. doi:10.1155/2019/7067592.

Rogers, J. (2016). *Coaching Skills: The Definitive Guide to Being a Coach* (fourth edition). Maidenhead: Open University Press.

Rosenberger, L.A. *et al.* (2018). Slow touch targeting CT-fibres does not increase prosocial behaviour in economic laboratory tasks. *Scientific Reports*, 8: 7700. https://doi.org/10.1038/s41598-018-25601-7.

Schitter, A.M., Fleckenstein, J., Frei, P., Taeymans, J., Kurpiers, N. & Radlinger, L. (2020). Applications, indications, and effects of passive hydrotherapy WATSU (WaterShiatsu): A systematic review and meta-analysis. *PLOS ONE*, 15(3). doi:10.1371/journal.pone.0229705.

Seltzer, L.F. (2017). Feeling understood—even more important than feeling loved? *Psychology Today*. Available at: www.psychologytoday.com/intl/blog/evolution-the-self/201706/feeling-understood-even-more-important-feeling-loved.

Shaikh, S., Nagi, S.S., Francis, M. & Mahns, D.A. (2015). Psychophysical investigations into the role of low-threshold C fibres in non-painful affective processing and pain modulation. *PLOS ONE*, 10(9): e0138299. doi:10.1371/journal.pone.0138299.

Stevens, F.L. *et al.* (2011). Anterior cingulate cortex: Unique role in cognition and emotion. *Journal of Neuropsychiatry and Clinical Neurosciences*, 23: 2: 121–125.

Tufekcioglu, E., Perlitz, V., Müller, G. & Cotuk, B. (2010). Heart rate variability during naive relaxation on land and receiving WATSU in water. Deutscher Kongress für Psychosomatik und Psychotherapie, Berlin, 2010.

Walker, S.C., Trotter, P.D., Swaney, W.T., Marshall, A. & McGlone, F.P. (2017). C-tactile afferents: Cutaneous mediators of oxytocin release during affiliative tactile interactions? *Neuropeptides*, 64: 27–38. doi:10.1016/j.npep.2017.01.001.

Wanqing, L., Xiaoqin, M. & Chao, L. (2014). The default mode network and social understanding of others: What do brain connectivity studies tell us? *Frontiers in Human Neuroscience*, 8: 74. doi:10.3389/fnhum.2014.00074.

Chapter 10

A Water Journey Through Pregnancy and Parenthood

JURGITA SVEDIENE

I want to invite you on a water journey through the world of pregnancy and parenthood, where I have found my vocation and constant interest that encourages me to explore this special period of becoming a human. To me as a midwife, pregnancy is an authentic, physical and transforming process. It's truly a bodily experience and it offers us ways to connect with the world, how to be in the world and how to understand it (Matulaitė 2012). Parenting opens up previously unfamiliar capabilities and unfolds the complexity and richness of life.

As aquatic bodyworkers, we work with alignment and physical structure in the water where there is no gravity. In WATSU, you cradle, fall with the breath, rise, float, rock, stretch, arch and fold. WATSU awakens and highlights significant things, widens the boundaries of perception. It's the world where you remember human touch, and the touch of water lingers longer than words.

WATSU and fertility

The act of creation of human life begins from movements. Inside the woman's body, the egg starts its journey to the warmth and darkness of the uterus. The sperm enters the body and travels to the place of the unknown. At the moment of conception, the new form starts to grow and the new human life begins. This continual process is full of stimulus and growth. At every moment, cells divide and differentiate, creating organs and systems. Within the amniotic sac, the fetus is moved and starts to move by itself, developing its nervous and vestibular systems. In nine months, the balance between "doing" and "being" in the womb prepares the future human to grow and be ready for birth.

The inability to conceive naturally can cause feelings of shame and guilt;

low self-esteem may affect intimate relationships. These feelings bring huge emotional and mental turbulence and can change safe living habits into harmful ones: alcohol consumption, malnutrition, insomnia. This may lead to various degrees of depression, anxiety and distress (Rooney & Domar 2018). Often couples hear advice from friends and relatives: "Just relax... Quit your stressful job... Take a vacation... Accept your hidden self..." These words become insensitive and lack an empathic tone when couples are struggling to conceive. Infertility is a silent life struggle. Just as there is no single answer to why some couples can conceive easily and others cannot, so there is no simple causal relationship between stress and pregnancy. One of the most compelling mind/body questions comes up: *does infertility cause stress or does stress cause infertility?*

The connection between these two is complex and subtle. The answer about the relationship between distress and infertility may not have a clear cause and effect direction (Rooney & Domar 2018). The more research that is done, the clearer it becomes that different methods of infertility treatment are needed to overcome this complexity.

When spontaneous pregnancy does not happen for a long time, couples may utilize assisted reproductive technologies and may use different non-invasive methods to get pregnant: the cognitive behavioral treatment approach, awareness practices, relaxation training, hatha yoga, progressive muscle relaxation, imagery, meditation, art therapy, singing, changes in diet and lifestyle. The cognitive psychology activities and mindfulness-based psychological interventions in everyday life could be effective in the treatment of the emotional aspects of infertility, may increase self-compassion and may lead to higher conception rates. All these methods are helpful and several studies confirm that such treatments show significant decreases in anxiety, depression and fatigue, increased vigour, and may increase pregnancy rates (Domar, Seibel & Benson 2004; Li *et al.* 2016; Patel, Sharma & Kumar 2020; Rooney & Domar 2018).

Observations

I want to share observations that are gratifying and pave the way for wider research.

I gave sessions to women who applied WATSU as part of their natural treatment of infertility, as a tool to:

- break the vicious circle of a belief that "I will never have children," "My husband will leave me"
- be embodied
- trust the life flow

- acknowledge the fears of being pregnant and being a mother in the future, the fears of death.

These women had individual WATSU sessions once in two weeks and participated in WATSU Circles for expectant mothers once a week in the hope that this practice would awaken the forces in them that would help them to conceive. Some women said they wanted to feel the world of abundance, love and empathy, and to listen to what pregnant mothers spoke about and felt.

All women got pregnant without using medical assistance. WATSU floats us into a meditative state, a space of silence in which irritating thoughts calm down and the body relaxes. Calming down provides clarity on how to proceed and reduces self-pity and dissatisfaction.

Although there are no comprehensive studies that accurately capture the knowledge that stress affects pregnancy, an analysis of the connection between them suggests that self-esteem, self-knowledge, the ability to feel safe in the world and relaxation may affect conception.

These findings show that WATSU, together with other methods of treatment, could be a gentle and relaxing remedy for healing. It can be added to any complementary treatment for infertility. We need more studies and confirmation of the impact of these observed effects.

Pregnancy time

In happy pregnancies, mothers say that the baby is a gift, a mystery, a possibility to become a better person. Though pregnancy and parenting involve huge hormone surges and biological and psychological adaptations, they bring excitement and wonder in creating a close relationship with the new personality. During pregnancy, a woman becomes more emotional and intuitive, sometimes vulnerable. Mood changes, sensitivity to smells and sounds, switching desires, anxiety, sensuality and joy that changes to tears in a moment fill her being. Sometimes she is angry for advice and constant teaching, sometimes she is frustrated that nobody advises her on how to be. *Doesn't that resemble adolescence when states of being change so fast that you don't have time to comprehend and understand them?*

Several studies show that a woman's brain and body undergo dramatic changes to support her transition to motherhood during the perinatal period (Kim 2016; Kim & Strathearn 2016). Distinct neural plasticity characterizes the female brain during this period. The changes may reflect a process known as "synaptic pruning," a brain phenomenon that eliminates certain connections between brain cells to encourage the facilitation of new connections (Hoekzema *et al.* 2017).

These changes seem necessary and adaptive: since the survival of the young is dependent on the mother's efforts, her brain seems to have evolved in ways that promote mother-infant bonding and sensitive caregiving (Barba-Müller *et al.* 2019). And if in adolescence our brains have to develop for us to become functional and skilled adults, then during pregnancy our brains prepare us to become attentive, understanding and good mothers, and to manage the challenges of motherhood.

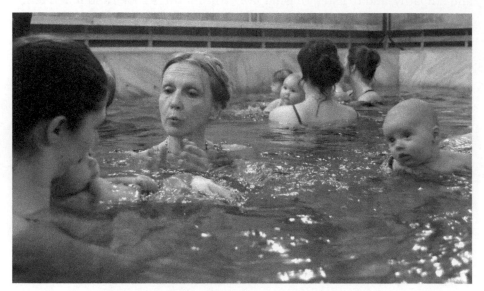

Figure 10.1: Gathering to learn Baby WATSU in a circle
(Photographer: P. Malukas. The national photo project "Lithuania and We")

Dynamic transformations are important for maternal care, maternal memory of one's own infant, bonding, absence of hostility towards the newborn, lactation. There are many things we "learn" as mothers that we aren't even aware of. These natural brain changes benefit women throughout motherhood, but they may also be advantageous later in life, when women need to take care of their grandchildren or assume other caretaking roles (Pawluski, Lambert & Kinsley 2016).

The changes in the morphology of a mother's brain can last for at least two years postpartum. One more piece of evidence is emerging that these changes might not be specific only for mothers. Fathers, adoptive parents, grandparents, nurses might experience shifts in brain function to make them more effective guardians once they begin caring for a child (Rutherford *et al.* 2015).

The maternal brain receives a rich spectrum of tactile cues from the unborn infant, new and subtle signals from the body, and new visual and auditory information about parenthood from books, childbirth educating classes and friends, which in turn activate the brain regions that are involved in learning how to be a parent. And later on, high levels of interaction with the infant may structurally augment these brain areas (Lonstein, Lévy & Fleming 2015).

Some research provides evidence that stressful experiences, whether from the past or present environment, are associated with altered responses to infant cues in brain circuits that support maternal motivation, emotion regulation and empathy (Kim 2021). If stress can be one of the trigger effects then we are looking for ways to reduce, change or eliminate those effects.

WATSU from early pregnancy to one year after birth is a tool for reducing the stress level as it activates the parasympathetic nervous system and brings relaxation and complacence.

The first clinical study investigating the effects of WATSU during pregnancy shows notable benefits of WATSU with regards to stress, pain, mood and mental-health-related quality of life (Schitter *et al.* 2015). It shows that WATSU can be useful not only at the third trimester of pregnancy but in the earlier stages, too.

The unborn baby as the teacher

We all attended our first ecological "school" in the womb. The human brain registers touch, and sensory integration begins in the womb when the fetal brain senses the movements of the mother's body (Ayers 2005).

The baby felt his first WATSU in a warm, silent space where he could explore his hands and legs and experience different rhythms of various movements when the mother walks, exercises or dances. Even when the mother is asleep, the heartbeat, breathing and the work of the internal organs introduce the baby to various rhythms. The baby learns many things: how to eat and sleep, how to suckle and swallow, how to turn, bend, straighten and kick from the uterine wall, how to respond to different impulses from the outside of the world.

The woman feels how the baby touches her from within—the kicks, hiccups, overturning. It's mysterious and interesting, and invites the mother not only to feel the impact but also to respond. The mother gets to know the child, learns to recognize his/her non-verbal language through these small movements. It's a moment when she begins to distinguish where she is and where the baby is. The boundaries of the mother and child connection start to expand.

Day by day, the woman learns to understand this new world without words and this time will help her to take care of the newborn baby later. She is learning to be with her unborn baby by accepting her newly formed body in response to her unexpected needs (Matulaitė 2012), singing and talking to him/her, asking to behave more gently: "Please, don't kick my ribs and liver." She is opening her intuition as a tool for the cognition of the world. And then comes the question: "Who am I? Who does this body belong to—to me or my baby?"

In WATSU, the similarity of body and water temperatures, the state of silence and weightlessness creates a sense of lightness and an altered perception of gravity and time. During WATSU, the baby sometimes becomes more active and curious, sometimes calms down. Boundaries expand and create a new way to communicate in a peaceful state.

WATSU in pregnancy: Preparing to listen

In childbirth classes, when mothers-to-be spend their time in a cozy atmosphere while doing something together, deepening knowledge about birth and mothering or contributing their experience, expectant fathers have their personal—men's—time. Here they can share their expectations, hopes and worries, meet with new fathers and learn from them.

WATSU and other water modalities are part of my childbirth educating program and help to develop a calm, curious state of mind, to reduce fear, to accept and value the changes.

The Uno WATSU session is individual, Duo WATSU is for pairs and couples and WATSU Circle explores the topic of parenthood in a group setting. The warm water provides a vessel for compassionate listening and conversations between exercises. I have found that these WATSU Circles soften the fears and anxieties.

WATSU Circle for expectant mothers

Until the moment a mother recognizes her body as wise and begins to trust it, there is a period when she wants to control various prenatal conditions. The body begins to change and the woman has to accept these changes and not worry non-stop.

Once or twice a week, expectant mothers meet in the water for relaxation and movement explorations. Here mothers find support, grace and affirmation instead of standard advice and guidance. They open their courage, allow their intuition and awareness to guide their touch. Mothers take turns in several roles: to work individually, to be a holder, to be held. These are small lessons to perfect self-awareness and drop into embodied experience. The Sisterhood of Motherhood is a special bond shared by women. This bond helps to overcome the ambivalence and to prepare for birth by socializing and voicing fears and joys in a safe group setting. A WATSU Circle is a non-threatening, therapeutic and compassionate way of being with the person and transferring this experience to the moment when expectant mothers will hug and cradle their babies themselves.

Sharing within WATSU Circle

WATSU in women group gave me a very deep relaxation that I had not experienced for a long time. Given the difficult start to my pregnancy and the otherwise intense pace of life, I am very happy and it's a great value to me… I felt that after all the "spins" in the water, some compressed energy was released, and after a longer respiratory hold (which I sincerely did not know that I could do), I started to have more self-confidence, I think it affected the successful birth. What excitement, a communion of women, chatters and sincere sharing for all.

WATSU Circle was full of peace and relaxation and was recharging for the whole week. Very interesting sensations when it seems that you are lying alone in the water and you are carried by a current somewhere and are diving and agitating, and forget that maybe at that time there are five people around you…you are alone in your own universe that protects you. I really enjoyed the exercises "stars" as well as accepting them and passing through the touches of the massage to the other mom, and the tenderness of calm relaxation.

WATSU's activities were one of my best pregnancy desserts… It's much more than just a swim in the pool—for me it was going to myself, to my baby, diving into the past and something I can't understand yet… I felt that the water can hug, can gently surround the body; I have experienced that water is infinitely soft and gentle; that my skin can feel the smallest tickles of water… This is my first time having this physical experience. On the physical plane, I always knew that babies live in water. But it was the knowledge of the mind, that knowledge was not in the heart. During WATSU's gatherings, when I was rocked like a baby by another mom, I saw that little creature in the womb calmly waving at his mom. I saw his completely relaxed face, bent arms and legs. It seemed to me that I was experiencing what the baby is experiencing in the womb—a quiet gentle swing in infinite peace…

In WATSU Circle for the expectant parents, they become aware of what it is to be present, how to hold the space for each other and feel supported. They learn how to touch the partner peacefully without judgment. They may experience a state of safety and weightlessness similar to that which a baby may experience in the womb, being together as one…

Couples WATSU

During Couples WATSU, the father perceives how silence and relaxation affect the body and appreciates the quality and subtlety of the other person's touch. He can become more attentive to his partner, can sense and bond with his unborn baby deeply. Non-verbal and non-sexual communication expands knowledge and enriches feelings, and helps to understand the importance of welcoming a partner with unconditional respect and the newborn with unconditional love. This can become an impetus in forming a new attitude toward the partner as they both are feeling overwhelmed and unprepared for the changes that parenthood brings.

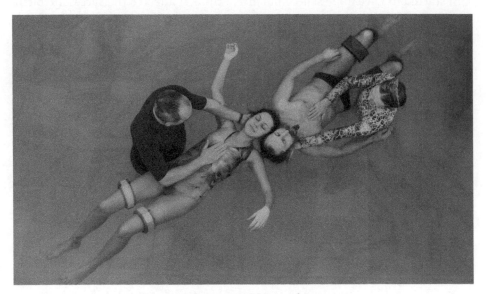

Figure 10.2: Duo.WATSU couples session
(Photographer D. Ivaskaite)

Fathers share their thoughts

As new waves, still new people, it's all very interesting and vivid. I went out full, and the scale of that fullness ranged from confusion to euphoria. It takes a lot of motivation to search. I rediscovered the fun and joy of being and exploring.

Very new experience and good relaxation. If the baby feels in his mother like this, it is safe to be. I think I will go to the pool with the baby in the future.

Welcoming the woman to WATSU

WATSU could be honored as a prenatal bodywork. A pregnant mother can also appreciate the nurturing, relaxing or tonifying session to open herself to the inspiration and complexity of motherhood.

When she comes to WATSU, she is greeted with all the sensitivity of the current situation. As practitioners, we must create a harmonious relationship; she needs to know that we are here not to correct or heal her but to hold the space for her experience. It's a safe place for her and she is accepted as she is. Her expectations for the session, her fear of water, should be addressed. A clear conversation is an appropriate prelude to a session.

A woman's verbal expressions in the first and second trimesters of pregnancy are different from the expressions in the third trimester. You often hear in early pregnancy: "I can't concentrate, my brain is numb; I am crying too much; I am sleepy and have no energy; I do not like my reactions, they do not come from me, maybe from the baby? I don't want to be intimate, I feel so scared." And in late pregnancy you can hear: "I feel scared that nobody will listen to my wishes during the birth; I trust my body; I wish to be more connected with myself and my baby; I need to learn how to relax and how to breathe; I want to be more grounded."

When it comes to the experience of a pregnant woman, there is no one objective truth and it is impossible to know another person's experience or feelings. Giving WATSU, we see some objective changes—decreased muscle tone and pain, increased range of motion, relaxation, deep exhales, the difference in the color of the face. This is information we can describe, structure and analyze. However, part of the experience and its reflection is only alive in the moment it is experienced. Later, it seems to evaporate or change. This shows that the experience belongs to a person, it's hidden from our eyes, and what is invisible to us now turns into words or actions later.

One of the important criteria in how pregnancy will run psychologically is the pregnant woman's earlier relationship with her own mother. This relationship can be powerful and respectful or can be challenging.

Sometimes, WATSU brings a sense of unity with mother, sometimes the body remembers the feeling of separation. With whatever experience a woman gets from WATSU, she can start a dialogue with her mother before her baby is born.

The bodily experience through WATSU client insight

In the session, I let the practitioner take care of me. I surrender to the care of another person. This is how I learn to trust the outside world, but also my instinct and intelligence. It will help me in raising my baby. I feel how respectfully the practitioner holds me. In the same way, gently and respectfully, I will hold my baby in my arms and float, introduce him/her to the water anew; in the same way, I will float my husband for him to experience the magic of our pregnancy. Through water I experience the baby as a separate but close being, as a personality with whom we share one air, one home. I experience myself as a baby and accept with all my cells the message that water is safe and that being in the water is safe. I go back to myself and find my source of strength there. The baby trusts me, my decisions. And I don't have to doubt the understanding that unfolds through building a relationship with a baby in the water.

What additional support can we as practitioners provide after the WATSU session?

- Drink after the session and increase the amount of water you drink for the rest of the day.
- Be careful while walking out of the water as the body feels heavier.
- Get more fresh air.
- Remember that silence and minimal talk helps to prolong the effect of relaxation and serenity.
- Do what your body wants to do—sleep, rest, spend a day alone or go for a walk, finish the work, dance, be kind and sensitive to yourself.

Physiological benefits of WATSU during pregnancy

- Increases blood and lymph circulation, brings more nutrition to all parts of a woman's body, including the placenta, and aids in the removal of waste products (Knaster 1996). This can lead to having more energy.
- Improves breathing by addressing postural deviation for increased mobility of breathing muscles, rib cage release.
- Stimulates peristaltic action of the gastrointestinal tract and eases constipation and flatulence.
- Reduces blood pressure and heart rate, musculoskeletal pain, strain and swelling.
- Releases holding patterns of the mandibular, which sometimes are caused by anxiety and stress.
- Contributes to the kinesthetic awareness needed to fully participate/ dive into the birth experience and process.

Emotional and somatic benefits of WATSU during pregnancy

- Enables the mother to experience that the body is wise and changes as necessary for a successful pregnancy and birth.
- Improves patience, stimulates creativity.
- Opens the possibilities to learn how to relax in preparation for the birth (Knaster 1996).
- Fosters appropriate touch and nurturing, supports the experience through various transitions.
- Allows endorphin release into the bloodstream, leading to a deep state of unity and oneness.
- Brings joy and a pleasurable experience.

WATSU precautions in pregnancy

Before we even recommend WATSU or other aquatic modalities to our prenatal clients, we must consider their current health history and the evolving nature of their pregnancy. As with any symptom that may be contraindicated for water therapies, if your client has a history of recurrent miscarriage, ruptured membranes, early labor, a weak cervix, multiple pregnancies or heart and lung disease, she may want to take advice from her midwife or physician. The lists below are areas to consider before beginning treatment.

Prenatal precautions

- Uncontrolled blood pressure (be careful of water temperature).
- Placenta previa (if not bleeding).
- Twins, triplets.
- Hypersensitivity (to light, sea sickness, chlorine).
- Contractions (first stage of labor).
- Multiple sclerosis (may not tolerate warm water).
- Small open wounds.
- Unstable angina, diabetic.
- Severe aquaphobia.

WATSU contraindications in pregnancy

- Fever over 37.5 C, and contagious diseases.
- Severe lower abdominal pain (the sign of retained placenta).
- Vaginal bleeding.
- Broken water sac.

- Uncontrolled epilepsy.
- Cardiac failure.
- Severe urinary tract infection, bowel incontinence.
- Open bleeding wounds.

WATSU considerations for the practitioner—tricks of the trade

- Awareness and precise supporting of the head and pelvis.
- Constant elongation of the spine.
- Respectful support and touch; ask if it is appropriate to touch the belly.
- Purposeful moves and tools for adaptation.
- Compassion.

Temperature

- The temperature of the water could be 33–35 C. In the first/second trimester, the mother-to-be may prefer warm water (34–35 C); in later pregnancy, they often feel better in 32–34 C water. Anything higher than 37–38 C may cause fetal distress (Odent 1997).

Position

- From 36–40 weeks, the baby's position refers to the relationship of its presenting body part to the pelvis. In headfirst presentations (cephalic), the back of the head (occiput) is the reference. As you float in the water, a woman's body sinks more on the side where the baby's back is facing. It is suggested to either put floats of different sizes or to place them on the different leg areas to elongate and extend the body horizontally.
- Half noodle under the knees and a head pillow can be used temporarily if you cannot reach the feet or help keep the hips and trunk slightly folded.

Motion sickness/vestibular concerns

The pregnant mother may have a sensitivity to motion sickness and the low tolerance of vestibular stimulation may cause vertigo, facial sweating and dizziness. It may be useful during the session to:

- travel head-first (direct the water toward her head)
- be slow, avoid spacious rotations and circling, be very slow in changing positions (from supine to upright position (various saddles))

- use only linear movements
- suggest opening the eyes
- give WATSU in an upright/sitting position, when the ears are out of water; gentle ear massage relieves uncomfortable senses
- suggest the mother eats a bit and drinks water an hour before the session. Heartburn and reflux can come with hormonal changes, and in late pregnancy, it can be caused by pressure on the stomach and intestines from the growing baby. It is a good idea to change the position from horizontal flow into a seated position.
- avoid extension of the lumbar area, especially if you see *diastasis recti*.[1] Lumbar pain can be linked to pregnancy hormones, compression of the lumbar-sacral nerve roots, increased pressure in the abdomen, incorrect posture, softening of the ligaments around the back and some other causes.
- use gentle traction and precise support of the head to release psoas muscles and sacroiliac joints while decompressing the neuro-skeletal system.

Fear of water

Aquaphobia or fear of water can vary from fear of splashes on the face to severe panic looking at a big pool or the sea. There is no "one size fits all" treatment, but if the goal is to become more comfortable around water, there are many ways to overcome it.

As we know, the changes in the maternal brain during pregnancy are tremendous, and this should be because the mother must learn what they are not even aware of. An example of this could be when the expectant mother comes to WATSU with the idea that she wants to overcome a fear of water *now*, before birth. She wants to accept water, start to trust it and "tame" it. Over time, through the series of WATSU in groups or individually, through small successes, her confidence increases. And then the mother can present the water world to the newborn without fear, with the ability to swim and them both to be in the water environment in the future.

Babies in a breech position

Babies in a breech position occurs in 3–4 percent of pregnancies. The delivery can be without difficulties, but sometimes it can bring complications to both mother and child (Hannah *et al.* 2000).

When the baby is still in breech position at 37 weeks, the mother has several options for birth:

---

1   *Diastasis recti* is the partial or complete separation of the rectus abdominis of the stomach muscles, which meet at the midline of the stomach. It is very common during and following pregnancy.

- Undergo a natural cephalic version.
- Undergo an external version with precise medical care.
- Give birth in breech with knowledgeable care.
- Undergo a cesarean-section (C-section).

A successful natural and external cephalic version depends on uterine tension, the amount of amniotic fluid and the size of the baby's head. External cephalic version attempts to move the baby to a better position can be successful if there is enough amniotic fluid for turning, low uterine tension and clear parameters of fetal position and placental location (Kok *et al.* 2008). Then the natural version to a head-down position can happen even at 39 weeks of gestation if the baby is not big.

The first clinical study of WATSU in pregnancy shows that it yields therapeutic benefits for pregnant women and that the lowered tone of the uterus may encourage attempts at cephalic versions when the baby is in a breech position. This warrants further research (Schitter *et al.* 2015).

My private practice one-year observations about mothers and their babies in a breech presentation

Observations/considerations: Seven expectant mothers with babies in a breech position, pregnancy time 35–39 weeks. One baby was in a footling position, one in an incomplete breech position, five others in a frank or complete breech. The average age of the mothers was 33–37 years, three of them were primiparous, the others, multiparous. All mothers were healthy, conscious and wanted to give birth naturally. They attended the medical examination, took pregnancy movement classes, visited childbirth education classes and did mindfulness exercises.

Once a week they had WATSU sessions for 45 minutes. To our surprise, all the babies effortlessly changed their position to "head down" without any other intervention. We can assume that this change was influenced by various factors both on land and in water. The empirical data suggests that the lowered tone of the uterus, enough amniotic fluid, relaxed emotions and conscious connection with the baby encouraged babies to turn head-down naturally before the due date. The spontaneous cephalic version happened and mothers gave birth vaginally.

These "home-made" observations are not interpreted scientifically, but this may be a good idea for future in-depth research.

Birth as the rite of passage

The day is approaching when a woman says goodbye to her pregnancy.

What kind of childbirth do I want for myself and my child? Do I entrust childbirth to others, or will I take full control and indulge in the flow of childbirth? Am I powerless or discreet? Is it a woman's time, or is there room for a man in it?

The mind chatter becomes stilled. You feel boundless as water. What part of our being is affected by WATSU if a mother-to-be can clearly define what her needs are or what kind of birth she wants for her child?

It becomes clear that what is important to her, her baby and her family is not the people who are constantly advising and offering them the ways they like best. It is not uncommon for a woman to feel that she wants to immerse in water during labor or birth. She is struck by the clarity with which this thought is embodied in the body after WATSU. And then she starts searching for information, classes and people to find support and fulfill what she decided.

Going through labor and giving birth in water as a practice started to increase in the 1970s, mostly in midwifery-led units, and is now accepted across many countries. Midwives' insights and stories of women's experiences of using water during birth should hopefully encourage further studies as it is important to understand more about the benefits of water immersion for women and newborns, along with any risks (Cluett, Burns & Cuthbert 2018).

Commonly we describe labor in three stages. The first stage is when the cervix opens to 10cm dilated. The second stage is when the baby moves down through the birth canal and is born. The third stage is when the placenta is delivered.

In water births the available data has produced two core categories: "Getting *to* the water," which revealed the impact of preparing for and anticipating the water, and "Getting *into* the water," which provided a sanctuary and a release from pain (Maude & Foureur 2007).

Women use water to gain a greater sense of freedom and privacy; they feel cradled, soothed, protected and relaxed during contractions.

They use water to lower their fear of pain and childbirth by itself and to have a greater sense of control and comfort (Maude *et al.* 2007). It is easier to cope with pain, not necessarily to remove or diminish it.

Laboring in water, women make more rhythmical movements in the tub than in bed. A greater range of positions facilitate labor progress and help women to concentrate and avoid unnecessary interventions (Stark, Rudell & Haus 2008). Water affects pain relief and may reduce the use of regional analgesia (Cluett *et al.* 2018; Shaw-Battista 2017).

Hydrotherapy during labor affects neuroendocrine responses that modify psychophysiological processes and reduces maternal anxiety and fetal malpresentation; the buoyancy in water lowers a woman's pain perception, helps to cope with pain, increases maternal satisfaction with movement and results in cervical dilation progress equivalent to standard labor (Benfield *et al.* 2010; Shaw-Battista 2017).

Water can be used in any form: shower, bath tub, birthing pool. A warm shower (35–37 C) on the lower back or the whole body for 10–20 minutes helps with relaxation. Women feel cared for and comforted, and have a more positive overall experience (Lee *et al.* 2013).

When there is no possibility of being in water, then the sound of running water or music with the murmur of waters can be calming and bring comfort.

Land birth

As we know, the birth experience shows us the unique connection between active and passive, between personal and beyond the personal.

WATSU brings the celebration of connection with oneself and with the baby, sometimes with the invisible life force which helps during the labor. Mothers giving birth on land share that remembering the feelings of WATSU—weightlessness, freedom of movement, floating—helped them to immerse in the birth process and trust it. They remembered how to breathe rhythmically and deeply, how to relax the jaw and throat, how to divert attention from the pain to the outside and be connected with their baby.

> During the last contractions when they were only one minute apart, I remembered the feeling of WATSU floating, when all the cells were relaxed and I relaxed my eyes, jaw and throat, my hands dropped into the imaginative WATSU waters, and it helped me not to scream and shout...

Water birth

Women are seeking settings for a birth that respects their choice. For some women, it is important to find a unit that honors their ability to have a natural birth without interventions. A water birth can increase the chances of attaining this goal.

The option of water birth for women at low risk of complications is available in hospitals, birth centers, midwifery units and at home. A growing body of evidence reveals the safety and efficacy of labor and birth in water. A Cochrane review and many other studies found no data to support safety concerns over water birth (Cluett *et al.* 2018).

It is essential to examine whether immersion in water during the first and/ or second stage of labor has the potential to maximize a woman's ability to accept the labor pain, work with it, and have a normal birth without increasing the risk of any harmful event. Adverse situations could be perineal tearing, hemorrhage and increased risk of infection to women and newborns. Several reviews of the literature provided no evidence that laboring in water increases these risks (Cluett *et al.* 2018; Dahlen *et al.* 2013).

Results suggest that water birth is associated with a high level of maternal satisfaction with pain relief and the experience of childbirth, with fewer perineal traumas and experiences of postpartum hemorrhage (Dahlen *et al.* 2013; Nutter *et al.* 2014). One study about hospital-based underwater deliveries states that water birth had a lower risk of neonatal intensive care unit or special care nursery admission (Sidebottom *et al.* 2020). Many studies highlight that water birth does not cause harm or additional risk to neonates (Bovbjerg, Cheyney & Everson 2016; Dahlen *et al.* 2013; Taylor *et al.* 2016).

In between contractions, water wraps the mother gently, gives her a rest from physical pain and tensions and brings her to a peaceful state of mind. WATSU is a beautiful way to prepare for birth, to invite surrender to your life and to honor the mother's journey.

Miscarriage, stillbirth or death of a baby

When you lose a baby, days become as long as a century; it raises many strong feelings: anger, guilt, despair, confusion, loss, emptiness. Again and again, the woman questions: "What is the meaning of this experience? What could be done differently?" She wants to share her experiences, but those around her are not always ready to listen in a way she wants to be heard. Then she decides to stifle her feelings and goes through the emptiness alone. She is shy, ashamed, questioning her femininity... At the same time, there are unexpected feelings about the future. There are often fears about how to get back to work, whether to get pregnant, whether the loss will happen again.

How does the parent cope after the death of a child? Together with colleagues from the family center Gimtis we invite women to meetings where they can share the feelings of loss, their discoveries about self, the ways they go through grief—anything that they wish to share. Experience has shown that the conversations are effective; they not only help a woman to express her deepest insights, but also enable those around her.

WATSU can be used by those who work with and support grieving families. It can be tremendously beneficial not only for the mother but for family members—husband/partner, parents, grandparents. They can "dilute" in WATSU waters, accept the experience and find a meaning that helps them to live. WATSU is an unconditional acceptance of a person, it is a guarantee that you will not be "lost or left alone." It is an opportunity for a person to get to know their various reactions and accept their new reality.

Observations

Often, death experience freezes the body and the resulting physical tension prevents the emotional tension from being released. The emotional and physical release doesn't come easily—sometimes it takes months or a year to reveal these feelings.

I noticed that in different stages of mourning process (denial, isolation, anger, bargaining, depression, reconciliation) I come across different body language. Here I will share only a few observations.

When the person is in the place of denial or anger, the muscle spasticity increases, the range of motion decreases, the breath becomes superficial and short. You can hardly notice the exhale. The body is motionless, sometimes stiff. Be cautious. Many essential WATSU moves (accordion, rotations, roles, legs over) may not be suitable. The practitioner should question whether their experience and hands-on practice meet the needs of the client. Sometimes it's better to stay and just be with the person with less movement. Less is better.

When the person is in the state of bargaining, the tiny involuntary vibrations at different intervals start to come but do not relax the body. You can sense that these vibrations are infusing life and energy. When the person is in the state of forgiveness/acceptance you may hear a deep exhale or voice, notice the fluidity of the body, see the tears.

These are just personal observations that I treat with respect and I do not draw far-fetched conclusions.

Postpartum WATSU

Mothers who come to WATSU regularly in pregnancy and visit at least once after giving birth notice that WATSU during pregnancy and WATSU after the birth are different. The right time for postpartum WATSU is when you stop bleeding when the wound heals in the perineum area when the cesarean scar has healed. Before the session, it is helpful to talk about the birth experience and to disclose the true attitude towards it—maybe a mother has soul scars?

There are a few reasons why moms come back to experience WATSU again as a part of a journey to become a mother:

- She wants to close one stage (pregnancy) and prepare to accept the next stage (motherhood).
- She wishes to understand the relationship with the body after childbirth: "Where do 'I' begin and where do 'I' end?"
- She wants to learn how to strengthen personal boundaries and be clearer in communication with others and their advice.
- Following an increase in sleepless nights and wakefulness, she wants to rest, get more energy and joy, relax and sleep well.

This new connectivity, a new attitude to her body, which she sees as wise after

giving birth, and a new approach to her freedom bring the new aspect of acceptance—the transition to motherhood is a truly rewarding experience.

The touch from the outside world

If we agree with the idea that birth is the extraordinary moment where functional and complex changes happen to prepare a newborn to live outside the
womb then we can agree that birth is the bridge between gestation in the womb
and gestation outside the womb (Montagu 1986). And then we can accept
the idea that the newborn is continuing his gestation in the outer world near
his mom's breast, hearing the familiar heartbeat, through his parents' voices,
facial expressions and eye connection. Every tactile experience the newborn
gets brings a lot of information as the skin is an active source of sensations, an
organ of communication and the cognition of the world. Replete with sensory
receptors, the skin is our outward connection to the central nervous system
within (Knaster 1996).

Through the mother's body, the baby makes his first contact with the
outer world and starts to "digest" first experiences of warmth and comfort;
through the father's hands the baby is immersed in a fountain of security and
playfulness.

The first year is special for all human beings—we bring the baby to the land
of rhythms, sounds, colors. The baby is welcomed, new parents are greeted as
the family and adults. A baby begins his long-life journey of metamorphosis to
become a human and this journey has its specific basics. This time should be
slow, gentle and peaceful. The baby feels safe when life is predictable when he
knows we sleep, now we are awake, now we eat or play or bathe. It is beneficial
to the health of the child when one or other actions are performed at the same
time of the day.

If we delve into the basic principle of WATSU—to be, not to do—then
through using WATSU with the baby, we learn the basics: to observe, to respond,
to be truly present because babies are 100 percent present and authentic in
their response.

WATSU and babies

Before WATSU became an integral part of rehabilitation, one study showed that
placing premature babies in gently oscillating waterbeds improved their behavioral development and reduced breathing and heart rate problems (Korner *et al.*
1975). Another study revealed that if a premature infant (27–34 weeks) is either
touched, rocked or cuddled daily in the first weeks, he has fewer non-breathing
(apneic) periods and enjoys increased weight gain (Montagu 1986).

Observations

After giving WATSU (twice a week) to several premature baby girls (32–33 weeks) it was observed that the general level of sensitivity raises and facilitates smooth adaptation to the world. Such soft postpartum cutaneous stimulation fills in early lost stimuli. Rocking or swaying moves in WATSU stimulate the vestibule apparatus and the skin.

Later, the bathtub could be the place for the father to participate and initiate the bond between him and the newborn. Though the parent's touch is therapeutic, it's important to be attentive and not overstimulate the fragile infant.

WATSU for newborns

WATSU for a baby is different from water exercises, therapeutic moves, joyful plays, diving or training to swim. These styles and methods are valuable and useful for sensory integration and getting to know the world's diversity. They may be a part of you and your child's life later. The first months are an extended gestational period when the outer world is experienced through the senses of gravity, movement and touch, through sight, smell and taste.

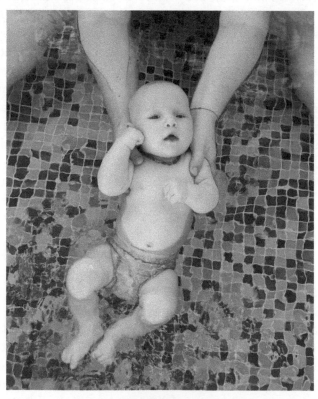

Figure 10.3: Baby Patrik in a soft seaweed
(Photographer B. Burneike)

We should remember to always protect the senses, not overstimulate the baby. WATSU is a peaceful stimulus for the baby to integrate into the world. Let the first bath or "return home" come at the right time when your child is awake, full and open to a new experience. Parents will learn to deduce from the baby's facial expressions and movements when the time is right for these experiences. During the first months when mothers are recovering, WATSU bathing time can be the father's privilege.

My body remembers WATSU as very deep peace... The feeling of peace returns to me every time I bathe my daughter... As soon as I start putting her into the water, I see how her body relaxes... As soon as her body comes into contact with the water, the miracle of peace shows up: she relaxes and falls asleep. I, surrounded by a veil of peace, float my daughter in the water, her arms and legs slowly swing from side to side like seaweed, being completely merged with the water... Now she is not sleeping in the bath but relaxing very deeply... These are the miraculous moments of the evening, when I travel back to WATSU in my mind because during the sessions I experienced the softness and calmness of the water. I repeat this experience every evening.

Observations

- When the baby is restless, sleeps poorly, when his stomach hurts, he is tired or irritable, when he gains little weight, WATSU helps and tends to make the baby calm and happy.
- When you put a baby into the tub (lower him/her) he may grasp the air with his arms and legs. This is one of the first total-body motor patterns (Ayres 2005).
- When water touches the cheeks, a baby starts moving his head.
- When you put the baby on the stomach, he makes alternate crowing motions or "drops" his extremities in deep relaxation.
- Sometimes we see the chaotic movements, then stillness or quiet minutes of integration; later these moves will evolve and be well organized.
- Soft rocking calms the baby.
- The baby is not alone in the bathtub—one of the parents holds him in the warm water, and takes time. Parents learn to be aware, alert and relaxed at the same time.
- The touch sensation of the water—its temperature, viscosity, waves— are the source of emotional satisfaction for the baby.

WATSU for infants

WATSU for babies is always about being, not about doing. It is quality time, one-on-one bonding. Young parents mostly are convinced that they need "to teach babies" to sleep, eat, walk, swim. In reality, we need to set an example in various kinds of activities, and we should create an open space for babies to be, play, learn or rest, to help, if they need support, and not to hurry them to get to the result, for example to start loving water and feeling safe in it. Parents want to see some results quickly as the fulfillment of their effort.

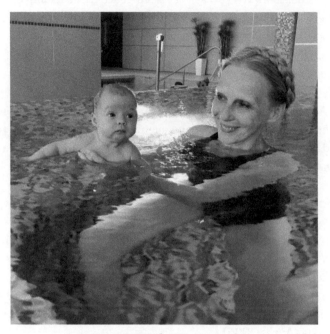

Figure 10.4: Baby Morta wonders
(Photographer I. Jankaviciene)

What we should pay attention to:

- Babies are honest in their response. Body language is created for communication, and through the baby's gestures, parents can decode emotions. Parents should change the move or position, to calm the flow if it disturbs the baby.
- Babies do not close their eyes during WATSU so the connection is constant.
- At about four months, babies do not like to float on their back, as they are learning to flip from the tummy to the back on the ground. They bend more in the water, raising their heads and shoulders to look around. It's time for a creative approach—follow the moves that

the baby initiates and give WATSU in a more vertical position, hold the baby closer, skin-to-skin.

- A baby is a rhythmic creature. During WATSU, we should understand what rhythm is appropriate to the baby—slow or fast, spiral or linear.
- If after many days spent in the water the baby does not feel comfortable and cries, the WATSU practitioner can suggest mother-baby or father-baby WATSU when the baby is lying on the parent's chest. Floats, noodles, pillows can be used for support.

With peacefulness and patience, we enable the baby to grow into a toddler and child who, because he feels safe and because life is predictable, is a pleasure to be with, both for himself and others.

Final thoughts

While writing this chapter, I remained personal because the topic of WATSU in pregnancy and parenthood resonates emotionally. By providing examples and insights, I pursued a clear goal of presenting WATSU's applicability and mean-ingfulness. I have used WATSU in thousands of hours of work with pregnant mothers, babies and children with special needs. We are not only interested in quantitative changes, which would certainly contribute to the improvement of perinatal care and the extended attitudes of midwives, nurses and doctors. WATSU is a phenomenon and each session could be a qualitative study that would reveal factors in a person's internal dynamics that would be useful in the healthcare system. WATSU interconnects us all and what rises is a deep feeling of belonging.

References

Ayres, J.A. (2005). *Sensory Integration and the Child: 25th Anniversary Edition*. Torrence, CA: Western Psychological Services.

Barba-Müller, E., Craddock, S., Carmona, S. & Hoekzema, E. (2019). Brain plasticity in pregnancy and the postpartum period: Links to maternal caregiving and mental health. *Archives of Women's Mental Health*, 22(2): 289–299. Accessed on 13/03/21 at https://doi.org/10.1007/s00737-018-0889-z.

Benfield, R.D., Hortobágyi, T., Tanner, C.J., Swanson, M., Heitkemper, M.M. & Newton, E.R. (2010). The effects of hydrotherapy on anxiety, pain, neuroendocrine responses, and con-traction dynamics during labor. *Biological Research for Nursing*, 12(1): 28–36. Accessed on 13/03/21 at https://doi.org/10.1177/1099800410361535.

Bovbjerg, M.L., Cheyney, M. & Everson, C. (2016). Maternal and newborn outcomes following waterbirth: The Midwives Alliance of North America Statistics Project, 2004 to 2009 Cohort. *Journal of Midwifery & Women's Health*, 61(1): 11–20. Accessed on 13/03/21 at https://doi.org/10.1111/jmwh.12394.

Cluett, E.R., Burns, E. & Cuthbert, A. (2018). Immersion in water during labour and birth. *Cochrane Database of Systematic Reviews*, 5(5): CD000111. Accessed on 12/03/21 at https://doi.org/10.1002/14651858.CD000111.pub4.

Dahlen, H.G., Dowling, H., Tracy, M., Schmied, V. & Tracy, S. (2013). Maternal and perinatal outcomes amongst low risk women giving birth in water compared to six birth positions on land. A descriptive cross sectional study in a birth centre over 12 years. *Midwifery*, 29(7): 759–764. Accessed on 13/03/21 at https://doi.org/10.1016/j.midw.2012.07.002.

Domar, A.D., Seibel, M.M. & Benson, H. (1990). The mind/body program for infertility: A new behavioral treatment approach for women with infertility. *Fertility and Sterility*, 53(2): 246–249. Accessed on 13/03/21 at https://doi.org/10.1016/s0015-0282(16)53275-0.

Hannah, M.E., Hannah, W.J., Hewson, S.A., Hodnett, E.D., Saigal, S. & Willan, A.R. (2000). Planned caesarean section versus planned vaginal birth for breech presentation at term: A randomised multicentre trial. Term Breech Trial Collaborative Group. *Lancet* (London, England), 356(9239): 1375–1383. Accessed on 13/03/21 at https://doi.org/10.1016/s0140-6736(00)02840-3.

Hoekzema, E., Barba-Müller, E., Pozzobon, C. *et al.* (2017). Pregnancy leads to long-lasting changes in human brain structure. *Nature Neuroscience*, 20(2): 287–296. Accessed on 13/03/21 at https://doi.org/10.1038/nn.4458.

Kim, P. (2016). Human maternal brain plasticity: Adaptation to parenting. *New Directions for Child and Adolescent Development*, 2016 (153): 47–58. Accessed on 13/03/21 at https://doi.org/10.1002/cad.20168.

Kim, P. (2021). How stress can influence brain adaptations to motherhood. *Frontiers in Neuroendocrinology*, 60: 100875. Accessed on 13/03/21 at https://doi.org/10.1016/j.yfrne.2020.100875.

Kim, S. & Strathearn, L. (2016). Oxytocin and maternal brain plasticity. *New Directions for Child and Adolescent Development*, 2016 (153): 59–72. Accessed on 13/03/21 at https://doi.org/10.1002/cad.20170.

Knaster, M. (1996). *Discovering the Body's Wisdom: A Comprehensive Guide to More than Fifty Mind-Body Practices That Can Relieve Pain, Reduce Stress, and Foster Health, Spiritual Growth, and Inner Peace.* New York, NY: Bantam Books.

Kok, M., Cnossen, J., Gravendeel, L., van der Post, J., Opmeer, B. & Mol, B.W. (2008). Clinical factors to predict the outcome of external cephalic version: A metaanalysis. *American Journal of Obstetrics and Gynecology*, 199(6): 630.e1–e5. Accessed on 13/03/21 at https://doi.org/10.1016/j.ajog.2008.03.008.

Korner, A.F., Kraemer, H.C., Haffner, M.E. & Cosper, L.M. (1975). Effects of waterbed flotation on premature infants: A pilot study. *Pediatrics*, 56(3): 361–367. Accessed on 12/03/21 at https://pubmed.ncbi.nlm.nih.gov/1080560.

Lee, S.L., Liu, C.Y., Lu, Y.Y. & Gau, M.L. (2013). Efficacy of warm showers on labor pain and birth experiences during the first labor stage. *Journal of Obstetric, Gynecologic, and Neonatal Nursing: JOGNN*, 42(1): 19–28. Accessed on 13/03/21 at https://doi.org/10.1111/j.1552-6909.2012.01424.x.

Li, J., Long, L., Liu, Y., He, W. & Li, M. (2016). Effects of a mindfulness-based intervention on fertility quality of life and pregnancy rates among women subjected to first in vitro fertilization treatment. *Behaviour Research and Therapy*, 77: 96–104. Accessed on 13/03/21 at https://doi.org/10.1016/j.brat.2015.12.010.

Lonstein, J.S., Lévy, F. & Fleming, A.S. (2015). Common and divergent psychobiological mechanisms underlying maternal behaviors in non-human and human mammals. *Hormones and Behavior*, 73: 156–185. Accessed on 13/03/21 at https://doi.org/10.1016/j.yhbeh.2015.06.011.

Matulaitė, A. (2012). "I've got you under my skin": The embodied relationship with the baby within. *Studies in the Maternal*, 4(1): 1–22. Accessed on 12/03/21 at http://doi.org/10.16995/sim.50.

Maude, R.M. & Foureur, M.J. (2007). It's beyond water: Stories of women's experience of using water for labour and birth. *Women and Birth: Journal of the Australian College of Midwives*, 20(1): 17–24. Accessed on 13/03/21 at https://doi.org/10.1016/j.wombi.2006.10.005.

Montagu, A. (1986). *Touching: The Human Significance of the Skin* (third edition). New York, NY: Perennial Library.

Nutter, E., Meyer, S., Shaw-Battista, J. & Marowitz, A. (2014). Waterbirth: An integrative analysis of peer-reviewed literature. *Journal of Midwifery & Women's Health*, 59(3): 286–319. Accessed on 13/03/21 at https://doi.org/10.1111/jmwh.12194.

Odent, M. (1997). Can water immersion stop labor? *Journal of Nurse-Midwifery*, 42(5): 414–416.

Patel, A., Sharma, P. & Kumar, P. (2020). Application of mindfulness-based psychological interventions in infertility. *Journal of Human Reproductive Sciences*, 13(1): 3–21. Accessed on 13/03/21 at https://doi.org/10.4103/jhrs.JHRS_51_19.

Pawluski, J.L., Lambert, K.G. & Kinsley, C.H. (2016). Neuroplasticity in the maternal hippocampus: Relation to cognition and effects of repeated stress. *Hormones and Behavior*, 77: 86–97. Accessed on 13/03/21 at https://doi.org/10.1016/j.yhbeh.2015.06.004.

Rooney, K.L. & Domar, A.D. (2018). The relationship between stress and infertility. *Dialogues in Clinical Neuroscience*, 20(1): 41–47. Accessed on 13/03/21 at https://doi.org/10.31887/DCNS.2018.20.1/klrooney.

Rutherford, H.J., Wallace, N.S., Laurent, H.K. & Mayes, L.C. (2015). Emotion regulation in parenthood. *Developmental Review*, 36: 1–14. Accessed on 13/03/21 at https://doi.org/10.1016/j.dr.2014.12.008.

Schitter, A.M., Nedeljkovic, M., Baur, H., Fleckenstein, J. & Raio, L. (2015). Effects of passive hydrotherapy WATSU (WaterShiatsu) in the third trimester of pregnancy: Results of a controlled pilot study. *Evidence-Based Complementary and Alternative Medicine*, eCAM, 2015: 437650. Accessed on 13/03/21 at https://doi.org/10.1155/2015/437650.

Shaw-Battista, J. (2017). Systematic review of hydrotherapy research: Does a warm bath in labor promote normal physiologic childbirth? *The Journal of Perinatal & Neonatal Nursing*, 31(4): 303–316. Accessed on 13/03/21 at https://doi.org/10.1097/JPN.0000000000000260.

Sidebottom, A.C., Vacquier, M., Simon, K. *et al.* (2020). Maternal and neonatal outcomes in hospital-based deliveries with water immersion. *Obstetrics and Gynecology*, 136(4): 707–715. Accessed on 13/03/21 at https://doi.org/10.1097/AOG.0000000000003956.

Stark, M.A., Rudell, B. & Haus, G. (2008). Observing position and movements in hydrotherapy: A pilot study. *Journal of Obstetric, Gynecologic, and Neonatal Nursing: JOGNN*, 37(1): 116–122. Accessed on 13/03/21 at https://doi.org/10.1111/j.1552-6909.2007.00212.x.

Taylor, H., Kleine, I., Bewley, S., Loucaides, E. & Sutcliffe, A. (2016). Neonatal outcomes of waterbirth: A systematic review and meta-analysis. *Archives of Disease in Childhood. Fetal and Neonatal Edition*, 101(4): F357–F365. Accessed on 13/03/21 at https://doi.org/10.1136/archdischild-2015-309600.

Further reading

Batten, M., Stevenson, E., Zimmermann, D. & Isaacs, C. (2017). Implementation of a hydrotherapy protocol to improve postpartum pain management. *Journal of Midwifery & Women's Health*, 62(2): 210–214. Accessed on 13/03/21 at https://doi.org/10.1111/jmwh.12580.

Dull, H. (2008). *Watsu: Freeing the Body in the Water.* Middletown, CA: Watsu Publishing.

Harper, B. (2014). Birth, bath, and beyond: The science and safety of water immersion during labor and birth. *The Journal of Perinatal Education*, 23(3): 124–134. Accessed on 13/03/21 at https://doi.org/10.1891/1058-1243.23.3.124.

Simpson, K.R. (2013). Underwater birth. *Journal of Obstetric, Gynecologic, and Neonatal Nursing: JOGNN*, 42(5): 588–594. Accessed on 13/03/21 at https://doi.org/10.1111/1552-6909.12235.

von Mohr, M., Mayes, L. & Rutherford, H. (2017). The transition to motherhood: Psychoanalysis and neuroscience perspectives. *Psychoanalytic Study of the Child*, 70(1): 154–173. Accessed on 13/03/21 at https://doi.org/10.1080/00797308.2016.1277905.

Chapter 11

The Poetry of WaterDance

Going Underwater and Being Reborn

ARJANA C. BRUNSCHWILER

WATA is the abbreviation of the German "**WA**sser**TA**nzen" (WaterDance). Water-Dance is a form of sub-aquatic therapy in which the receiver (wearing a nose clip) is gradually guided underwater in a three-dimensional therapeutic landscape.

Introduction

WaterDance (WATA) is essentially a technique to bring about a state of profound aquatic relaxation. It is a therapy that uses the healing properties of warm water along with the calming effects of suspended and fluid breathing. The individual who receives the session is first brought to the water's surface and alternately moved, mobilized, stretched and massaged. Psychic tensions, blockages of emotional and psychological origins, may soften or even disappear entirely.

Using a nose clip, the nose is blocked and the client is progressively brought underwater in a three-dimensional, gravity-less state. The touch of the water, the work on the breathing and the fluidity of the dancing movements have calming effects. The body relaxes. The mind relaxes. The emotions calm down. The energy field expands. As the treatment progresses, the breath is naturally held for longer and longer periods of time, depending on the particular capacity of the individual. A liberation of the movements in the water follows naturally, creating a form of sub-aquatic dance. A time-space distortion may transpire from whence springs a modified state of consciousness, a feeling of profound relaxation. Sensations of pleasure and deep joy frequently result. Thus, Water-Dance brings together a natural playfulness along with fluidity and harmony.

WaterDance shares influences with the moves of Aikido (the Japanese martial art), the grace and agility of classical ballet and the undulating liberty of dolphins. Sometimes, WaterDance provokes a regression to the fetal state, our link with the energy of the mother, the vastness of the sea with its expansive effects, to the very source of life that hides within.

The underwater and surface sequences depend greatly on the individual respiratory capacity and rhythm.

WaterDance (WATA) was created by me and Aman P. Schröter in 1987. We are both of Swiss origin.

The history of WaterDance (told by Aman Schröter)

This has been freely adapted from the book *WasserTanzen: Aquatische Körperarbeit Aurum* (Schröter & Brunschwiler 1990).

What I have not already learned and practiced: swimming, massages, body psychotherapy, contact improvisation, tantra, breathwork. All of these techniques revolve around the body: a source of constant fascination for me, and most of all this wonderfully crazy experience of a shift of space and time: infinite vastness, timelessness and weightlessness. Then, when playing in water, diving or swimming with dolphins, another door opened for which the connection between breath and water was the key.

In 1980, during a training in Gentle Dance with John Graham, we entered the warm water of a spa and moved each other, one actively, the other passively: gently holding, rocking, pulling the head through the water. Little seemed to be done, but much was triggered. Some people cried, others laughed, a woman even crawled on all fours as she had regressed to a toddler.

Fascinated by this, I played and practiced with friends in water until one of them once brought a nose clip. It clicked for me—now it was possible to put a person underwater. Gently I guided his face underwater and played with all kinds of movements and rhythms. The longer he was underwater, the more relaxed his face became. At first, he was still worried about his breath, but he soon surrendered more and more to the game and with time he forgot breathing completely—it happened by itself.

In 1987, I met Arjana Brunschwiler in a 35° C warm pool, which was kind of a "refreshment" since our meeting was quite intense and passionate. But water helped us get in tune with one another, and it created an atmosphere of trust and devotion. In the love play between yin and yang, passive and active, we invented new variations of releasing and moving. We started to write down certain movements and sequences, we experimented in public pools and danced in front of an audience who must have found such performances very unusual. Nevertheless, our dance created a meditative space around us that others seemed to be fascinated by.

Soon we started to teach our creation to interested people. We found this work to be a wonderful combination of aesthetics, play and therapy. And so the name WasserTanzen (WATA) was born. Christian Larsen, MD and expert of spiral dynamics, was one of the first to come into contact with WaterDance. He described this new therapy as connecting the primordial water element with dance movements. He said that the therapeutic effect of WATA is based on the existential meaning that the combination of water and movement has always had for human beings.

At the time, I was still running a practice in body-oriented psychotherapy and soon I began to invite my patients into water. Here I discovered the phenomenon of the diving reflex, which is triggered by wetting the face with water. All metabolic processes are slowed down, so that people can stay longer underwater. In the best case, the breath is forgotten, and when the face reappears, the cooler air contact causes the reflective inhalation.

The moment a client was brought underwater proved to be of crucial importance. For people who associated unpleasant memories with water, it was necessary to work much longer on the surface. This is when Arjana and I discovered WaterShiatsu (WATSU) and the work of Harold Dull. Shortly after this, Arjana was trained by Harold Dull and became one of the first Swiss WATSU teachers.

In autumn 1993, together with Helen Schulz and Shanti Petschel, we founded the Institute for Aquatic Bodywork (IAKA) in both Switzerland and Germany. The IAKA offers a holistic training concept including bodywork in water and land, deep breathwork, meditation, communication skills, anatomy and emotional process work. In this sense, the IAKA also has the task of reviewing and developing existing training guidelines and keeping the aquatic bodyworkers up to date through supervision and training groups. Its members are also in contact with the Worldwide Aquatic Bodywork Association (WABA) based in Harbin Hot Springs, California.

The history of WaterDance (told by Arjana Brunschwiler)

This has been freely adapted from the book *WasserTanzen: Aquatische Körperarbeit Aurum* (Schröter & Brunschwiler 1990).

Meeting Aman Schröter in summer 1987 created a big change in my life. I was only 26 when he introduced me to the art of tantra in his own gentle way. We are both distinct body people, fascinated by our moving bodies and their numerous possibilities. Although we were different in age and temperament, the idea for WaterDance sprouted between us and grew up to become our "child." Today we watch our common "child" like proud parents as it grows bigger and stronger, and slowly develops independently in the world.

It was not a big step to bring our joy of movement and dance into water. In the early days of WaterDance, we spent almost every weekend in public thermal baths where we danced and played together for hours. I was the ideal WaterDance model; I let myself be moved with enthusiasm and ease and never shied away from going underwater. On the contrary, the longer the better! As I am flexible, new forms and figures could be invented easily and came up almost by themselves.

At that time, I had already gained some experience with meditation. I was familiar with the hustle and bustle of the human mind and knew how much practice it took to get into one's own stillness and center. With great astonishment, I soon realized how quickly and effortlessly I entered a deep state of silent meditation when being moved harmoniously underwater. There was a feeling of expansion and opening, and the contact of the water with my skin was no longer perceptible. Water and body seemed to merge into an energetic unity. From deep meditations, I already knew I could enter a space where suddenly everything became very quiet and peaceful. The difference with WaterDance, however, was the regularity with which I was able to experience this phenomenon.

In the beginning, I could never get enough of these sensations and always wanted to go back in the water. However, later on, I encountered another, new characteristic, which I had not noticed at the beginning. After very long stays in warm water I started to feel as if I was dissolving. My physical body became softer and more flexible, while my energetic and emotional body felt wider and boundless. My whole being seemed to become permeable. I very much enjoyed staying in this particular state. However, awakening from it was always a hard and painful experience.

By looking and observing carefully, I learned over time to distinguish between three basic states of being: *holding on and controlling, giving up on and losing oneself, devotion and surrender*. Being of the Capricorn zodiac sign not only gave me the pleasant qualities of a strong grounding and sense of reality, but also the less welcome trait of holding on. However, underwater I could effortlessly and completely transform the state of being that I was familiar with: from holding on to completely letting go. This new state touched a deeply hidden longing in me. My womanhood awakened, my yin part asked for more of this. But then, after an intensive weekend in the water, it sometimes became very difficult for me to regain a foothold in everyday life. I remained in a dreamy state of suspension and it felt as if I had left a part of me in the water and in the arms of Aman. It felt as if I was losing myself.

This quiet painful oscillation between "being in control" and "self-abandonment" finally presented me with a new goal and task. I began to consciously search and integrate the golden mean between the needs of my "inner woman" (the yin part) and the needs of my "inner man" (the yang part). Some years have passed since the birth of WaterDance and today I feel much closer to my "inner holy wedding." I have understood that true devotion is an act of humility and surrender to the divine spark within me. Today, when I step into this ecstatic space while dancing in water, I remain in my own inner being and I return strengthened and free to my everyday life, able to tackle my tasks with ease and joy.

Parallel to my personal learning path with WaterDance, Aman and I started to teach WaterDance in small groups. We noticed that other people were also confronted with the same issues of dissolution of boundaries and/or difficulties with letting go of control. We observed that "yang people," who had their life well under control, first of all realized underwater that it was not so easy to let go of arms, legs, head and especially the breathing, while "yin people" had to be careful not to get lost in a nebulous state of delimitation.

Today, supporting students in approaching these topics with awareness and self-responsibility is an integral part of every WaterDance training. WaterDance teaches us to draw healthy boundaries in order to be able to expand them safely. Once this difference is understood, we can discover in water how devotion eventually leads to freedom.

WaterDance in comparison to WATSU

In WATSU, the nose and face are always above the water surface, while in WaterDance, the receiver wears a soft nose clip and is fully immersed underwater at intervals.

One of the specificities of WATSU is its nurturing body-to-body contact: the receiver is cradled throughout the whole session, which is why WATSU is also sometimes called "bonding therapy," referring to the first bonding we had with our mother. This first connection with our mother is a survival-based human need, or more explicitly, bonding is the biologically anchored basic need for emotional openness, together with physical closeness to others. Through the limits of the core family and the stress of everyday life today, children in Western culture often experience a deficit with regards to physical and emotional attention. In that sense, WATSU can help practice new physical and emotional closeness in a trustful and supportive environment.

WATSU's intention to be with someone in the water was not bound by a need or goal to transport the receiver back to these beginning attachment periods, nor was this a goal of WaterDance. However, the dynamic holding of WATSU coupled with the independent dance-like underwater suspension of WaterDance anecdotally can bring memories of developmental formation and attachments to the surface for the receiver. Traditionally, combining these two modalities within a session can create deeper states of self-introspection and improved body and emotional awareness within the "yin-like" holding of WATSU and the "yang-like" fully submersed world of WaterDance.

This same intimate and close touch is present in WaterDance, although the main experience is more one of dance and freedom. In WaterDance, the receiver is regularly released into the depths of water, with little physical contact with the giver. In that sense, WaterDance is a moving and dancing art, which proposes the exploration and stimulation of our natural fluidity and non-resistance in the physical body. It is an aquatic body- and dance-work, using breath, apnea, movement, and the continuous and whole embrace of warm water.

Together, WATSU and WATA form a wonderful couple, which complements each other perfectly well: the cradling of WATSU and the letting go into freedom underwater of WATA. I think of WATSU as the mother and WATA as the father of all aquatic bodywork, the two pioneering forms, and all the other aquatic modalities as their children and grandchildren.

WaterDance as a dance/meditation/spiritual practice

We have been asked so many times why we call our method WaterDance. Many people seem to think that this term is not professional for a therapeutic method. Or maybe the word "dance" makes them think of synchronized swimming. But the name we gave our creation right at the beginning has remained with it to this day—and I still think that this name suits it perfectly well.

WaterDance as a dance

Dance has always accompanied man as a form of expression. Dance seems essential to our survival as human beings. Many vital issues were expressed or dealt with in this way: life transitions, war and hunting, Shamans use dance for healing the sick and for communication with the spirit world; dance is practiced as religious magic by priests, and agricultural dance forms mime planting and harvesting food. Any dance tradition or technique represents movement patterns that those people have found useful for connecting them to something they perceive as having value. And, whether tribe or tradition, pleasure or skill, community or divinity, dance as movement is inherently relational. In all these primeval forms of expression, dance is an art, which always leaves imprints on the physical, emotional and spiritual being that we are. Dance is therefore a *healing dialogue between the body and the soul.*

WaterDance now brings new impetus to the long history of dance. Surely this is not about tribe or tradition, nor religion or art as such. But since time immemorial, man has strived to overcome gravity in dance to escape the heaviness of earth-bound existence for the duration of the dance. That is where water comes into play: water as the element that lets us experience weightlessness and effortlessness in the body, lightness and playfulness in the heart, limitlessness and boundlessness in the soul. People are able to express pleasure in experiencing their body and the surrounding liquid environment in new and special ways. As gravity is suspended in three-dimensional water, WaterDance offers a time- and space-less environment in which the healing process can happen in a whole new context.

The fact that we are virtually weightless in water helps us to let go of physical and emotional tensions, as well as holding patterns. Many WaterDance sequences are based on wave- and snake-like spiraling movements, which stimulate the flexibility and energy flow in the spine, and thus in the energy centers (*chakras*). WaterDance receivers describe sensations of expansion and presence beyond the limit of their skin. Some would call it a rising of the *kundalini* energy or *srana*, the life force, which keeps the subtle bodies activated. Some perceive vivid colors, like shades of blue, violet, green, red and yellow. Others describe deep states of meditation in a silent breathless place with no thoughts, only light.

WaterDance as a meditation

From scientific studies, we know that when a person is immersed in meditation, the *brainwaves* of this person slow down from beta frequencies to alpha and theta frequencies.[1] At the same time, these frequencies become very coherent. This signature affects the autonomic nervous system and the different areas of the brain begin to communicate and synchronize with each other. A new

---

1   There are four categories of brainwaves, ranging from the most activity to the least activity. Here is an overview of the different brain frequency patterns (by Joe Dispenza, 2014):

- High-frequency beta waves: Measurable in emergency situations and stress, show incoherence, the focus constantly jumps from one thing to another, chaotic brainwaves.
- Middle-frequency beta waves: Increased attention and concentration.
- Low-frequency beta waves: Everyday state in which we absorb and process external stimuli and information, analytical thinking.
- Alpha waves: Imagination, creativity. Thinking is less analytical, more in images, and the holistic inner world is more in the foreground, external impressions are perceived only from the side lines.
- Theta waves: The body falls into "light sleep" (deep relaxation) and regenerates; the gateway between consciousness and subconsciousness is open and new information can be absorbed directly into the subconscious. This frequency range is ideal for reprogramming the subconscious and pre-programming body and mind for a new future.
- Delta waves: Deep sleep, in which the body deeply recovers and regenerates.

order is created in the brain, which affects the whole physical and emotional body. By slowing down the brain waves to alpha and theta frequencies, our awareness opens the door to the subconscious and we learn *to be conscious in the subconscious*, we step aside as an observer, which allows new solutions and possibilities to emerge.

This seems a coherent explanation why so many WaterDance receivers share that the worries and burdens they brought to water suddenly appear in a completely new light after a session, so that solutions and new approaches appear as if by magic.

WaterDance as a spiritual experience

In water, we are also back in the *origin of life*. The memory of ocean water and the amniotic fluid in one's mother's womb comes to life again.

For most people, being completely immersed underwater (with body and head) and at the same time being danced or held in stillness by a skillful Water-Dancer seems to trigger a deep longing and reaching out for the divine. In this state, WaterDance receivers long to re-experience that ultimate peace and clarity, acceptance and ecstasy. It is a yearning for something unspeakably and unchangingly beautiful, good and holy. It is not easy to say with precision what that longing is. But it seems that people urge to be absorbed into the vastness of the ocean, into the void, into the unified field, freed from the rules of the three-dimensional reality. The Sufis refer to it as "the sweetness that was before honey or bee," recognizing a time when our soul was together with God, the space and time between lifetimes, that brief taste of wholeness. In this state, people feel an incredibly strong love and a feeling of wholeness. This is how I understand my favorite quote from the Persian poet and Sufi master Rumi: "You are not a drop in the ocean. You are the entire ocean in a drop."

WaterDance as a heart opener

After such an experience, WaterDance receivers are naturally more mindful, more conscious and more loving. The heart is touched; it opens up and reaches out. The part in us that thinks that we are too vulnerable to open our heart and creates the boundaries of separation between the others and us is naturally located in our mind, in our thoughts. However, when brain waves modify and bring us to a relaxed and coherent state, the heart feels safe and flows into a coherent beat-rhythm. It then radiates an enormously powerful magnetic field.[2]

---

2   Measurements by the HeartMath Institute in California have shown that the heart's magnetic field, which is the strongest rhythmic field produced by the human body, not only envelops every cell of the body, but also extends out in all directions into the space around us. Its magnetic field is 500–5000 times stronger than that of our brain—depending on how open and loving the heart is.

Conversely, the heart also supports and strengthens the coherence in the brain and so heart and brain support each other in this process. Together, they send a clear, powerful electromagnetic signature into the field. The body comes into a more balanced state, the immune system and self-healing powers are strengthening and people have immediately more energy available and feel better in a holistic way. As mentioned previously in Chapter 1, we continue to reiterate the scientific facts that heart coherence and the connection permeates not only with WATSU but also with WaterDance. As Pema Chödrön (2001), an American Tibetan Buddhist ordained nun, said: "When you begin to touch your heart or let your heart be touched, you begin to discover that it's bottomless."

The first immersions

Being led by someone underwater is a kind of initiation. As WaterDance practitioners, we guide the receiver across a threshold into another world, into another element, even into another dimension. Not only does the receiver leave us their body, but they also entrust us with their breathing (their very first basic need), which is unique in the therapy field. This is why we should never underestimate the physiological and psychological impact a WaterDance session can have.

Building trust and confidence

A session always starts with a dialogue and trust-building between practitioner and client. Indeed, the person may or may not have some reservations or even fears about going underwater. In any case, we want to create a safe space and an environment of love and protection and confidence for them to express their experiences with water and/or the issues they bring into the session. As certified practitioners, we are expected to have acquired skills to provide our clients with a supportive and caring guidance through whatever might come up before, during or after a session. It is our responsibility to ensure the comfort and safety of the receiver by allowing as much time as needed to initiate the unique experience of being danced underwater. Our primary goal in these first WaterDance experiences is to foster a sense of trust with our clients and begin to understand and acknowledge their therapeutic intentions and aspirations for venturing into this unique form of aquatic bodywork.

Sometimes, "water games" can create a joyful and playful atmosphere, which can help reduce negative associations with water. This might be a gateway to explore the underwater world in a playful way and allow receivers to take responsibility for going underwater on their own before they learn to trust someone else to do it for them. We must also give them time to adjust to the nose clip once it is put on. Specific breathing exercises can help them get used to breathing through the mouth. Contrary to free diving, in WaterDance, we release air bubbles in order to relieve the lungs and chest from pressure, and ultimately to let go.

Once the person is in our arms, we may do movements at the surface to stretch the body and invite deep breathing as a preparation. When the client is ready, the client puts on the nose clip and their underwater journey can begin.

The very first immersions are done in slow motion. If the movements are too fast or there are too many, this is distracting in a moment when a rich inner experience is taking all the receiver's attention. We carefully observe the face and the way the inhalation comes back when the head reaches the surface. We should not miss any signs of discomfort. If all is well, the WaterDance session can unfold in its own and unique way.

Signaling

At this stage of WaterDance, we usually signal our intention to take receivers underwater by giving two (or three) signals at the end of an exhalation. By giving enough time between signaling and taking them underwater, we enable them to fully inhale in a relaxed way. We never take them by surprise, or rush them. With more experienced receivers, we might leave the signal out and just tune into their breathing rhythm.

This *initial synchronizing* with the breath is *crucial* for building *trust* between the receiver and the giver! We follow the breath as closely as possible as we want to be absolutely sure of where the receiver is in his breath cycle, taking no chance that we are off.

The breath

It seems obvious that we cannot talk or write about WaterDance without also speaking about breathing.

Research has found that breathing exercises can enhance parasympathetic (inhibit neural responses) tone, increase the vagal tone of the vagus nerve, decrease sympathetic (excitatory) nervous activity, improve respiratory and cardiovascular function, decrease the effects of stress, and improve physical and mental health (Velkumary & Madanmohan 2004).

In WaterDance, we can use this knowledge and regularly incorporate proper slow breathing exercises with our students and future clients.

Everyday experiences of breathing for most untrained individuals are much more inconsistent than one would assume. We often first teach individuals to observe their own breath to ultimately familiarize themselves with the sensations of breathing. Thus, one meaningful aspect in learning breathing techniques is the awareness of the difference in smooth, even breathing and erratic breathing. Modifications in respiratory patterns come naturally to some people after one lesson, but it may take months to replace bad habits and ultimately change the way one breathes (Sovik 2000). The general rule, often noted in studies, and particularly observed by Gallego, Nsegbe and Durand (2001), is that if a voluntary act is repeated, learning occurs, and the neurophysiological and cognitive processes underpinning its control may change.

To breathe or not to breathe: Breath retention and the diving reflex

By practicing *pranayama* and regulating the flow of *prana*, the mind calms down. When this happens, we can allow the energy we normally spend engaging with and processing the world to turn inward.

This is what yoga teaches with *pranayama*. What does this Sanskrit word mean? Although *prana* is related to the *breath*, it is not the breath. *Prana* is the life or universal energy, which pulses through the body along a network of subtle body channels, the *nadis*. *Yama* means control. In this respect, *pranayama* can be translated as breath control, which means in practice "regulating and channeling one's breath and energy."

WaterDance testimonial

I had always had a profound fear of drowning or suffocating that seemed to come from another lifetime experience, although possibly it may have originated from something that happened as a baby in this life, as I was sexually violated by the nurse "caretaker" who I was left with aged around nine months when my parents went on vacation for two weeks. To go underwater for me was terrifying! Fear shifts you right out of the moment and the body closes up in panic. I could stay for two to three minutes on land without breathing... having built up this practice starting as a child and evolving an internal body-breath-awareness in my meditation as a healing process I discovered from a car accident. Going underwater brought back the old panic, so I used images for my mind to shift from panic to bliss and my knowledge of deep relaxation to make that breakthrough. Once free...I felt I could stay underwater without breathing, having re-discovered my organic origins and become one with the water itself! Those sessions were long ago and with the most sensitive, skilled and highly experienced instructors and practitioners. Obviously, the experience of WaterDance will be unique and different for each person and is dependent on the skill, presence and sensitivity of the practitioner. For this reason, it is not possible to assess the healing potential other than a broad recommendation.

For me it was physically and emotionally transformative. I recovered a state of total freedom and fluidity as well as an ancient internal remembering that led to a truly spiritual experience. This I believe is the essence of healing on any and all levels. (Angela Farmer, world renowned yoga practitioner and instructor, Lesvos, Greece)

The *pranayamas* are classified into the following four stages:

- *Puraka* (Inhalation)
- *Antara Kumbhaka* (Inhale-retention, a voluntarily controlled suspension of breath after an inhalation)
- *Rechaka* (Exhalation)
- *Bahya Kumbhaka* (Exhale-retention, a voluntarily controlled suspension of breath after an exhalation).

When the WaterDance receiver is in complete relaxation and in a surrendered state of being, these moments of breath retentions provide a bridge between the individual self and the universal soul, which means that the person is stepping into a deep state of meditation. Recent research is also beginning to reveal how controlled breathing can powerfully affect every system in our body (the cardiovascular, nervous, endocrine, lymphatic, immune, digestive and, of course, the respiratory system). However, this does not occur if the receiver is under stress, caught by fear, or in a control mode. In that case, the mind stays occupied and restless, and the emotional state of the person is activated.

Usually, a person can hold their breath for 25–75 seconds. However, with practice, yoginis and yogis manage to hold their breath much longer, which leads them to "ecstatic states under conscious control." Yogic breathing techniques can also have profound physiological effects, such as rejuvenation or healing. No other body function has as many diverse effects as breathing does. It is the interface between body, soul and spirit.

But what about not breathing?

Kumbhaka (conscious breath retention in yoga) is about mastering the breathing center (medula oblongata), located between the spinal cord and the midbrain. It is connected to everything in the body: from the brain to the vagus nerve (which as part of the parasympathetic nervous system ensures digestion, rest and relaxation), the sensory organs, the psyche, as well as the muscles. All these body parts can therefore be influenced via the breath.

Moreover, breath retention leads out of linear time into no-thought areas, with the awareness that "something in me continues to breathe," which is often accompanied by light phenomena.

The diving reflex

Surprisingly, in WaterDance, we come more spontaneously and more easily to prolonged breath holds (*Kumbhaka*) than in *pranayama*. An important role is played here by the diving reflex which is activated as soon as certain sensitive nerve endings around the mouth and nose get in touch with water—heart rate and metabolism decrease to supply the vital organs with oxygen. The trigeminal nerve, which is composed of three major branches (the ophthalmic nerve, the maxillary nerve and the mandibular nerve), is the nerve responsible for sensation in the face and motor functions such as biting and chewing; it is the most complex of the cranial nerves. In this context, sensation refers to the conscious perception of touch-position and pain-temperature information, rather than the special senses (smell, sight, taste, hearing and balance) processed by different cranial nerves and sent to the cerebral cortex through different pathways.

Interestingly, about three months before birth, the first breathing movements appear in the fetus. This practice of a function that is vital only later on serves to train the diving reflex, which automatically closes the airways of the nose, throat, bronchial tubes and lungs when a person is brought underwater, causing a respiratory stop. In babies, the diving reflex can be activated as well, at least until the age of four months. In adults, the small bronchial branches of the lungs are still drawn together when the reflex goes underwater, reminiscent of the diving reflex. At the same time, the heartbeat frequency is reduced by half, the blood withdraws into the trunk and head, the entire metabolism is reduced and oxygen consumption is lowered.

In principle, the diving reflex is not subject to voluntary control. However, with extensive relaxation with a complete letting go of the will to breathe, as well as a profound trust and devotion to the water element, it seems possible to influence the diving reflex and extend the time spent underwater far beyond common human limits.

During a WaterDance session, people occasionally say that they "breathed on" underwater. Time becomes a relative term in this space; it seems to flow from the common idea of Chronos toward Kairos, a subjectively determined, psychic time.

Although WaterDance quickly allows for longer stays underwater, it is essential to work first on the emotions, injuries and traumas that can resurface with water therapy, before breath retention is considerably prolonged and ecstatic states are reached.

Vagal tone

The longest nerve in the body, the vagus nerve is highly stimulated with breath-holding and deep breathing, which in turn improves vagal tone and decreases sympathetic nervous responses. Vagal tone is extremely important as it is a part of our "gut instincts" that transmit ascending and descending messages between the gut and the brain. These sophisticated transmissions determine how we respond to emotional and physiological symptoms of depression, anxiety and PTSD, as well as influencing our gastrointestinal, inflammatory and the immune response systems in the body. With emerging science on the benefits of vagal nerve stimulation, WaterDance could be a new and natural way to stimulate this key tenth cranial nerve. By doing so, we can improve the gut and brain axis that is essential to having balanced responses and basic instincts for everyday life.

The eight categories of movement in WaterDance

In WaterDance, the movement categories seem to match basic patterns, not only of the body but also of the water itself. All WaterDance moves can be gathered into eight basic forms: snakes (or waves), aikidos, rolls, embraces, releases, somersaults, parachutes and inversions.

Snakes

The snakes are the most frequent and most powerful forms of movement as they create waves to undulate the body. From foot to head, or from knees to head, a wave travels through the body, affecting all joints, one after the other, and releasing energy blockages on its way up. With snakes, the entire body can be moved, including the head and neck.

The snakes are used in foot or knee snakes.

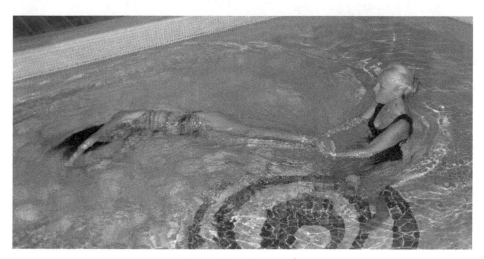

Figure 11.1: Foot snake

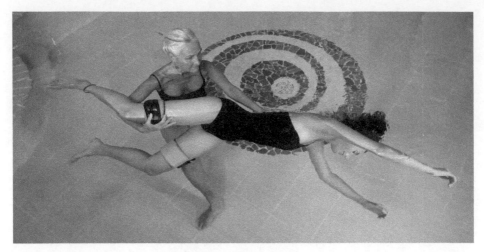

Figure 11.2: Knee snake

Aikidos

Aikidos are movements in which arms or legs are used as levers to bend or stretch the body around the main joints. The joint on which the pivot point is located is opened, freed from tension and provided with an extended range of motion.

The aikidos are used in arm, leg and knee aikidos.

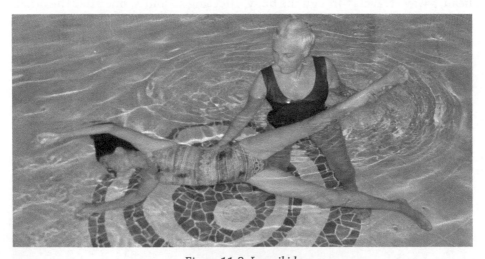

Figure 11.3: Leg aikido

Rolls

Rolls are movements around the longitudinal axis of the body. For taking down or surfacing the partner face up, rolls are ideal and used often.

The rolls are used in thigh rolls or full body rolls.

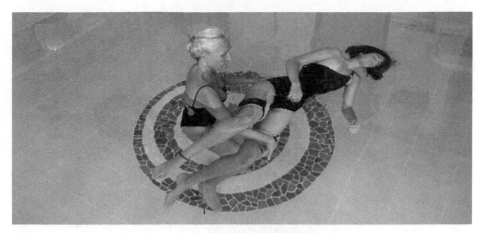

Figure 11.4: Full body roll

Embraces

Embraces are positions or moves in which the body is wrapped up and folded together. These close positions are the counterpoint to the open and free movements of WaterDance. They offer security and closeness, as well as strong stretching effects.

Embraces are used in accordions, coffee mills and embryos, or in double side foot snakes.

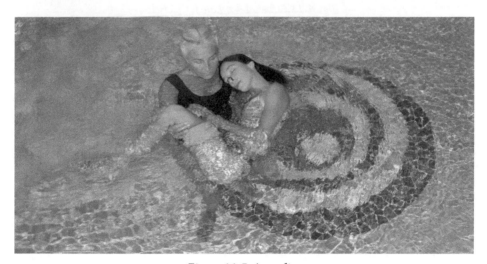

Figure 11.5: Accordion

Releases

Releases are the counter-movements to embraces. They are open moves in which the WaterDancer practitioner lets go of all body parts of the receiver and lets the person float freely in water. Some releases are done with an impulse, sending the receiver through water on their own in order for them to experience complete freedom and weightlessness. Releases are an important part of WaterDance, as they attract the receiver's attention to water as a supporting element.

Releases can be used as a transition between moves or as an exit after the deep down position.

Somersaults

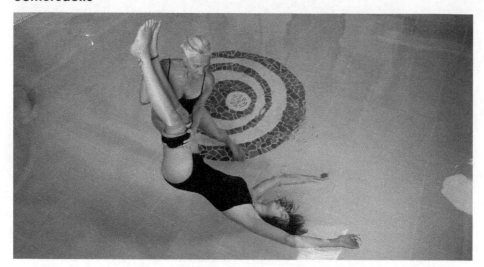

Figure 11.6: Two-leg aikido half-circle

Somersaults are slow turning figures rotating around the *hara*, the center of gravity of the body. The receiver is either held in an inverted and bent into a fetal position (head down), or turned around the longitudinal axis of the body in an open position. The receiver loses their "above and below" landmarks; spatial perception is dissolved.

Somersaults are applied in embryo positions or in two-leg aikido half-circle.

Parachutes

Parachutes are turning moves that wave the body out and away from the Water-Dancer practitioner. Executed with speed, they often generate enthusiastic reactions from receivers, who enjoy the fascinating sound of water rushing by, as well as the feeling of weightlessness, flying and soaring.

Parachutes are applied in the carousel and the half-side foot snake.

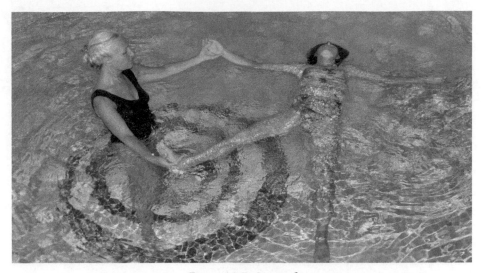

Figure 11.7: Carousel

Inversions

In WaterDance, an inversion is a position in which the receiver's body is gently swayed or held motionless with the head below the pelvis. This unfamiliar position sometimes brings about surprises, as the receiver may remember times in their mother's womb and react to these with emotions. Inversions should be initiated slowly so that the receiver can get used to them and learn to cope with the pressure of the depth, on a physiological as well as on a psychological level. Obviously, a WaterDancer practitioner must be fully in tune with the receiver, gauging intuitively how long it is appropriate to hold the inversion. At the beginning of a session, inversions should not be used. Later on, inversions can be repeated, so that the receiver can get deeper into the experience. Some people need to have a moment of rest after inversions or be guided with other moves before going underwater again, especially if they had some emotional reactions.

Inversions can be seen in the inverted fetus as well as the two-leg over shoulder.

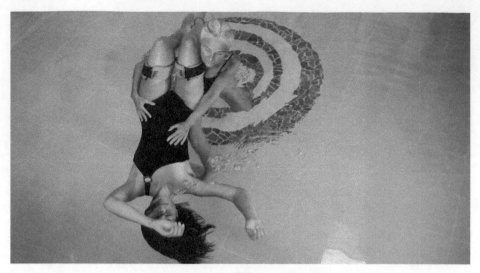

Figure 11.8: Two-leg over shoulder

(We thank Alexander George, founder of Healing Dance, and Minakshi for their support in describing the categories of movement.)

WaterDance in clinical practice

One of the main areas that WaterDance can be of benefit to clients within a clinical practice is its ability to target the breath and in turn improve vagal tone. We know that the benefits of improving vagal tone through breath-holding can ultimately break up compensatory muscular holding, improve the depth and quality of respiration and decrease stress responses. We also understand that full water immersion can provide equal pressure on sensory systems in the body that better organize individuals with sensory challenges like autism as well as penetrating high tone patterns in clients with neurological disorders. In addition, the breath is of key importance to populations that are experiencing the effects of post-traumatic stress disorders.

Clinical areas that may benefit from WaterDance therapy include:

- Fibromyalgia
- Arthritis
- Autism
- Post-traumatic stress disorder
- Neurological disorders
- Pain disorders
- Musculoskeletal disorders
- Gastrointestinal disorders.

Special considerations for WaterDance treatment

When we screen clients to see if full immersion is appropriate we want to fully understand and know their water history. Knowing if they have had any traumatic events in their past like drowning or an accident related to themselves or to others is of great importance. We also want to make sure that there is not a cardiac concern that would preclude them from going underwater.

WaterDance trainings as a holistic and integral approach to aquatic bodywork

In the context of WaterDance aquatic therapy and holistic and integral meaning, we are engaging the whole person on a physical, emotional, mental and spiritual level. This is why we work in WaterDance trainings with the four elements (earth, water, air and fire). Different exercises during land classes are used to encourage students to connect on both an external and internal level with the four elements (consciously or sometimes unconsciously):

- Earth as their body
- Water as their emotions
- Air as their mind
- Fire as (their) energy.

It may seem surprising to give so much importance to all four elements in WaterDance, and not only to water. However, over the years teaching WATSU and WaterDance classes, I found that consciously including the other three elements in our work helps counterbalance and re-harmonize the dissolving and melting qualities of the practice in warm water. Spending eight hours (or more) a day in water, in combination with learning a lot of new material, may cause over-flooding emotions and trigger childhood traumas. I have witnessed students losing their center and grounding by simply spending too many hours a day in water. As with everything in life, having too much of one thing brings us out of balance.

As a matter of fact, I usually teach half of the training hours in the pool and the other half on land. If possible, I start the class before breakfast with a meditation, a yoga and *pranayama* practice, or an outdoor activity. After breakfast, I teach three to four hours in the pool. Following a two-hour lunch break, we then spend time in the group room and one afternoon is for grounding in nature. The evenings are reserved for WaterDance practice with the assistants.

During land sessions, a sacred wheel is placed in the middle of a circle of people, symbolically holding space for all four elements (and cardinal directions), while honoring and inviting them at the same time.

For the water

This is the place of all beginnings and rebirth. In this element, we can embody our childlike nature; we are invited to experience the world through our senses rather than our mind. This way, we can come to recognize our innocence, playfulness, profound connection to nature, and sometimes deep sadness and loneliness (of the abandoned child). By caring and welcoming the archetype of the inner child, we learn to recognize and acknowledge another person's inner child, which occurs quite often in warm water sessions. In the element water reside the *emotions*. With WaterDance, we touch and welcome deep emotions in ourselves and in the people we carry in our arms. We practice compassion and acceptance.

For the earth

This is the place of deep introspection. It is the element that invites us to meet the parts of ourselves that we do not want to see. It is through confronting the darkness and struggles within that we can move into the depths of our therapeutic and healing work, and recognize how our shadows offer us insights into who we are. In this element, we meet our individuality and personality, our color and our perfume. In the earth, we have moved from childhood to adulthood; we are willing to take responsibility for ourselves, for our family and children, as well as for our clients and patients. Here resides the *body*. In WaterDance trainings, we take care of our body by doing bodywork, by eating healthily and consciously, by grounding, and by connecting with Mother Earth.

For the air

This is the place of our greatest gifts. It is the element of maturity, the place of the elders. Here, we know and embrace who we are as we grow into what we have to offer to the world. In this place, we practice and understand responsibility and leadership. We are willing to take care of a community (e.g., for a WaterDance class as a teacher) and we contribute to society in our own uniquely meaningful way. In the air resides the *mind*. By practicing and/or teaching WaterDance, we become aware and conscious of the holistic and integral learning and growing process in ourselves, as well as in our students or clients. Breathing exercises (both gentle and strong) help us connect in a deep way with the air element as well as with the breath.

For the fire

This is the place of transformation, of death and rebirth. It is largely linked to the dawn of the day, the most spiritual and awakened moments, where darkness turns to light and everything comes to life. It invites us to embrace our deepest nature by connecting with our divine part, and therefore with our ability to create our reality. It is there that we can understand who we truly are: beings of light and love. In the fire reside the *soul* and the *vision*. When we are active in this element, we are practicing awakening, connecting with the vibration of different energies of music, dancing and singing, nourishing our inner fire and creating a strong bond among the participants.

In that sense, the sacred wheel connects all things visible and invisible, while the center of the wheel represents the *aether, the fifth and transpersonal element*. Aether is the name given to "the material" that is believed to fill the universe beyond the terrestrial sphere, the substance that fills the invisible space. Aether is pure consciousness, pure awareness, which is the spirit, which is the divine. Reconnecting with this fifth element brings about a feeling of openness, inner peace, stillness, and ultimately oneness.

I find that the intimacy and gentle bonding that a group creates in water opens the door to authentic exchanges on "dry land" as well. It is beautiful to see how participants learn to trust the healing process that the group is gradually creating, and how they bring it out of the water into the sharing circles.

Shamans have been making associations between all sorts of things in life and in nature for thousands of years, partly because of the belief that all things are connected and interconnected. The cardinal directions are a characteristic of the divine universe that connects us all with nature and spirit.

Water ecology

In conclusion, I would like to address two issues: working in *chlorinated versus natural pools* and *conventional versus sustainable heating systems* of the water.

Most aquatic bodywork is practiced and taught in standard pools using chemicals like *chlorine* or *chlorine-related products* as a quick and simple way to kill bacteria and germs, control organic debris from perspiration and body oils, and prevent algae growth. Although this sounds good, it is highly debatable. Chlorine's job is to promote the health of people, but while it may prevent exposure to harmful bacteria, it comes with its own slew of hazards for our long-term health. The long-term effects of chlorine on us are relatively unknown, although the Centers for Disease Control in the US have cited negative effects of chlorine overexposure on a person's health. Among the most alarming ones are blurred vision, respiratory issues and asthma. Less serious and far more common complications of chlorine exposure include eye and nose irritations, dried-out skin and hair and premature wrinkles. Many studies are inconclusive, and we can't yet be sure what will happen long term.

As aquatic bodyworkers, when we work in chlorinated water, the chemicals are absorbed into our skin, and overexposure can happen quicker than we think. For some of us, it might take years of regular work in chlorinated waters, and for others, it might only take one training...

The unpredictability and uncertainty of long-term exposure to chlorine is a real problem. On one side, we offer wonderful and powerful therapeutic work, and on the other side, this actually happens in toxic, even carcinogenic water. This is a contradiction, which has been a challenge for me for many years.

Israel is a country known for many innovative things, but one of the highlights that it offered to me was the discovery of *two natural pools*, heated to 35° C. What an amazing feeling to work in such a pool! These natural pools have *zero chemicals*. Instead, they mimic the human body by utilizing bacteria and microbes to stay clean and healthy. I am not an expert for this kind of technology but obviously natural pools are a much safer alternative, as the installed plant-life acts as a natural filtration system. Moreover, sensitivity to aquatic plants is quite uncommon.

According to Larry Carnes (natural pool expert and owner of Reflections Water Gardens), natural pools have *fewer harmful effects on the environment as well*, contrary to the chlorine used in swimming pools. Chlorine plays a significant role in contributing to global warming, acid rain and ozone layer depletion. Chlorine must be generated by a system to sanitize and oxidize the pool water, and the energy used for this generator itself also has a significant negative impact on the environment. Natural pools have little to no environmental impact.

It seems a challenge to heat a natural pool up to 35° C and keep the filtering and cleansing plants alive. Nevertheless, I have seen these two beautiful natural pools in Israel. They both functioned for many years, and served practitioners and clients for aquatic bodywork sessions. The very first natural pool worldwide was in Rishpon, near Tel Aviv. It functioned for seven years without any chemicals until the Health Ministry decided that it was too dangerous and mandated the owners to switch to a salt chlorine system. However, the other private and heated pool that I discovered, located in Eilat, in the south of Israel, has been functioning in a completely natural way for eight years now. These heated natural pools were invented by Yael Ben Zvi (Israel).

Another topic I wish to touch on is *the heating systems* generally used to prepare water for our needs. I was the owner of a pool myself for 12 years in Belgium, and I have heated the water in summer and winter for teaching and practicing aquatic bodywork. We used a conventional swimming pool heater that worked with fuel oil. All that hot water and heating our home was therefore contributing to climate breakdown and the cost was a major downer as well.

In warm countries, *solar pool heating* is the most eco-friendly and inexpensive way to heat a pool. It is very effective given the high numbers of hours of direct sunlight per day. Still, according to Energy Star reports, *geothermal heating* is the most environmentally friendly and efficient way to heat pools.

However, this requires an upfront investment in a geothermal heating system, which can be costly.

This contradiction—to contribute with our work to the healing of humanity and thus of the planet also contributes massively to the destruction of it—creates an inner discrepancy, which becomes increasingly burdensome.

Clearly, there's an urgent need to transform these obsolete systems into sustainable and ecological heating and cleansing systems for our work and play places. Although WATSU, WaterDance and all other forms of aquatic bodywork have existed for several decades now, these methods are still pioneering forms of therapy and are little recognized in medical circles or even known in public. As pioneers, we know about the great potential that this work has but we are still trying to overcome great challenges. Our work needs more investigations and scientific studies and better working conditions in healthy and ecological pools and environments.

Vision and mission

It is therefore a dream of many aquatic bodyworkers from both the younger and older generations to develop autonomous, decentralized and interconnected communities, where all those who once stood against each other as competitors are reconciled and work together. Imagine a system of self-sufficient communities, healing centers and villages that research and model a new planetary culture, aligned with the universal patterns of life, in cooperation with animals and nature. And so we all have a wish and a duty to contribute to creating a suitable environment to nurture this.

I would like to end this chapter on WaterDance with the words of Dieter Duhm (sociologist, psychoanalyst, art historian and author, and one of the co-founders of Tamera, a peace research center in southwestern Portugal). Combining findings from cybernetics, system theory, holography and other disciplines of modern sciences, Dieter Duhm developed his Political Theory in the 1980s. It shows why and how healing biotopes can become globally effective.

To put it briefly, life evolves through "morphogenetic fields." These are pervasive informational patterns that store the collective physiological, psychological and mental habits of each species. Life doesn't evolve gradually, but through evolutionary leaps. A breakthrough in one or a few places generates a new field that changes everything. After the steam engine was developed in the 18th century, the Industrial Revolution spread worldwide. After the personal computer came on the market in the 1970s, the digital revolution began to transform the world.[3] The same principle applies to freeing our world from war.

A morphogenetic field of fear and violence currently dominates humanity, as can be seen in the catastrophes around the world. Yet, we all also carry a different pattern within us, which makes us breathe, digest, heal and love. We call it the *sacred matrix*—it is inherent to all that lives. Neither fear nor violence exists within the sacred matrix, as it is the matrix in which all beings are interconnected.

If there are even just a few societal prototypes on Earth that embody the sacred matrix in sufficient complexity and depth, we're likely to see an effective morphogenetic field of peace emerge to eventually replace the current field of violence. Wars will end because people will no longer be able to carry out violent acts in this field. Once we awaken from the hypnosis of fear, we can see this possibility. To become our reality, it needs our will, intelligence and action. (Duhm n.d.)

References

Chödrön, P. (2001). *Start Where You Are: A Guide to Compassionate Living*. Boulder, CO: Shambhala.

Dispenza, J. (2014). *You Are the Placebo: Making Your Mind Matter*. London: Hay House.

Duhm, D. (n.d.). Tamera Peace Research & Education Center in Portugal. www.tamera.org.

Gallego, J., Nsegbe, E. & Durand, E. (2001). Learning in respiratory control. *Behavior Modifications*, 25(4): 495–512. doi: 10.1177/0145445501254002. PMID: 11530713.

Schröter, A. & Brunschwiler, A. (1990). *WasserTanzen: Aquatische Körperarbeit Aurum*. Braunschweig: Aurum Verlag.

Sovik, R. (2000). The science of breathing—the yogic view. *Progress in Brain Research*, 122: 491–505. doi: 10.1016/s0079-6123(08)62159-7. PMID: 10737079.

Velkumary, S. & Madanmohan. (2004). Effect of short-term practice of breathing exercises on autonomic functions in normal human volunteers. *Indian Journal of Medical Research*, 120(2): 115–121. PMID: 15347862.

---

3   Note from Arjana: after WATSU had been created, WaterDance, Healing Dance, Jahara and all the other aquatic bodywork methods sprouted all over the world.

Chapter 12

The Neuroscience of Relating and Mirroring in Healing Dance Practice

ALEXANDER GEORGE

The origins of Healing Dance

In 1990, while being a resident at Harbin Hot Springs in northern California, I studied WATSU from its founder, Harold Dull. Following the course, I began experimenting and improvising in the Harbin warm pool. I was influenced not only by my professional background in ballet and Trager work, but also by the ways in which the body and water interact in movement. After studying Water-Dance in 1993 from Arjana Brunschwiler, I found that a new spaciousness and three-dimensionality appeared in my experimental moves. By then, I had created a flowing and dancing side branch of WATSU. Healing Dance was born and I continue to refine this form of aquatic bodywork with the sheer joy of movement to discover its full therapeutic potential. Since 1999, Inika Sati Spence has collaborated closely with me in defining and growing the work into a distinct technique. Since 2007, Kathrin George's perspectives as a physical therapist, practitioner and teacher have advanced the technique tremendously. The application of the Spiraldynamik teaching of Christian Larsen has brought further refinements.

Healing Dance in practice

Healing Dance (HD) is a form of aquatic bodywork practiced in 35° C warm water. Because it offers a profound level of relaxation, pleasure and refreshment, HD has appeal as a wellness treatment in hot springs and resorts. In private practice, an HD practitioner may also have clients who are coming primarily for the emotional benefits experienced in a single session or over time. Practitioners with additional qualifications in massage therapy, physical therapy, dance therapy, art therapy or psychology are able to integrate the skills of their field into water sessions to work clinically toward specific goals. Such a synergistic union of HD with other therapy forms can produce marked benefits. All practitioners take care not to exceed their competencies by suggesting interpretations or otherwise guiding the receiver in processes that are not within their current scope of practice. If invited, the practitioner can share pictures or impressions afterwards at the wall but without interpretations, always with a view to support the client in arriving at his or her own understandings. What we have found over the years training therapists around the world to incorporate HD into their current practice is that Healing Dance has similar therapeutic benefits for special needs populations as its ancestors WATSU and WaterDance. However, the focus of this chapter will be on the unique neuroscience of *relating and mirroring* in Healing Dance practice.

The history of mirroring in Healing Dance

Back in the early 1990s, when my warm pool experimentations were coalescing into an exotic offshoot of WATSU, anything resembling mirroring was absent, with the exception of the Water Breath Dance. Mirroring was simply not part of Healing Dance's DNA. As with the other forms of aquatic bodywork at that time, it was also innocently unencumbered by technique. So long as the nose stayed out of the water, what could go wrong? It was an era of discovery and we were in the business of imparting movement. My initial fascination was with choreography, creativity and improvisation, rather than with responsiveness and sensitivity to the well-being of the client.

However, after 2000 when Healing Dance was reaching its maturity as a technique, I and the other instructors discovered that the waves, spirals and gentle holdings of the sequence were leading clients into their own movement expression. We had always given time to our version of WATSU's Follow Movement, but it was more of a shared dance than truly sensing and accompanying the receiver's movement. As we began encouraging our clients to allow their movement impulses, we were evolving an approach to accompany them. The creation of the course, Relating & Mirroring, in collaboration with other instructors Inika Spence and Kathrin George, was a natural development of this shifting emphasis. The principles we formulated and the exercises to practice them brought clarity to our exploration of how best to support clients in their self-expression. It was the beginning of a process with further refinements yet to come.

In writing this chapter, I discovered that mirroring was more pervasive in the technique than I had thought. It was there not only when we mirrored the breath and the spontaneous movement impulses of clients, but also in the verbal interactions, in the bodywork and in the technique itself throughout the sequence. So, why take the trouble to write this, to delve a little deeper? For me, the answer is to be able to give better sessions and to advance the work on behalf of our clients today and in the future. Healing Dance needs to stay contemporary and relevant, to keep up with the advancements being made in other therapeutic forms, which hopefully this update in theory will accomplish. I will refer to my client as she/her throughout this chapter.

Let's now take a brief look at the origins of mirroring in human life and its role in our development. We will learn how mirror neurons function in the brain and see how prevalent mirroring is in our everyday life. Then we will consider the relation between mirroring and Healing Dance, starting with the experience of mirroring and being mirrored, then continuing on to the different forms mirroring takes during a session. Next, we will examine how the five principles of Hakomi provide an ideal framework for relating in our work. To finish, we will take a closer look at the phenomenon of empathy and how it relates to mirroring in Healing Dance.

What is mirroring?

Can you solve this riddle? What is hardwired into our brains from birth, but can be developed through experience over a lifetime? What is both external and internal, conscious and unconscious? What is operative when we see, when we listen, when we read and when we imagine? What allows us to learn, to form our initial sense of self, to empathize, and to navigate through the complexities of our social existence? The answer, in every case, is mirroring.

Developmental origins

Did you know that in its first hour of life a newborn can already mimic gestures and facial expressions (Iacoboni 2009, p.48)? This pre-cognitive ability to mirror only gets stronger with practice. And a lot of practice there is, as parents and babies are constantly sharing smiles and laughter, initiated by one or the other, establishing their life-long bond. Mirroring comes naturally to infants as shown by their delight in games involving imitation, and later when toddlers play together, they will unconsciously mirror each other's actions (Iacoboni 2009, p.49). When babies mimic the actions, sounds and facial expressions of their parents they are learning to empathize and understand another person's emotions. When parents mirror their baby's facial expression and vocalize the emotion, the baby can learn to associate the emotion with the expression and feel validated in having the feeling. On the practical side, mommy knows that when she opens her mouth wide, so will baby, and she can land that spoonful of porridge inside.

Examples of mirroring in everyday life

Here is a scenario you may be familiar with: imagine you are taking a Healing Dance training and the teacher is demonstrating body mechanics at the side of the pool. At first you only watch, then you start to copy her movements. This is an example of conscious mirroring, imitating what someone is doing based on observation. It is the oldest form of learning, pre-dating language. Why does it work so well? You are not only performing an external action while watching; something else is happening internally, in your brain. In the part of the brain known as the premotor cortex a particular group of brain cells, or neurons, are firing that enable the specific actions you are doing as you imitate the teacher. But here's the catch, they were also firing at the start of the demo while you were only watching, "pretending" to do the action you witnessed, a sort of rehearsal before trying out the movements (Iacoboni 2009, p.55).

This is the way the brain works: the same cells are responsible for both perception and action. These "mirror neurons" were identified in the brains of Macaque monkeys in the 1990s by a team of four Italian neuroscientists working in Parma, Italy. Thousands of subsequent experiments with humans worldwide using magnetic imaging have confirmed that our brains behave in the same way as the brains of the Macaque monkeys. However, the existence of individual mirror neurons in humans has not yet been proven conclusively, as the method of experimentation necessary, attaching electrodes through the skull into the brain, would be unethical (as if doing it to monkeys is not).[1]

Still imagining you are in a Healing Dance class, it is lunchtime. After eating, you meet a fellow participant in the hotel cafe to drink a coffee. Sitting together at the little round table and sipping your lattes, you notice that your body postures are exactly mirroring each other. This kind of unconscious mirroring occurs all the time, especially if people like each other. Your premotor cortex activates, just as if you yourself were in the position of your companion across the table from you, and without an inhibiting check to close the gate into action, your body assumes the same position (Keysers 2011, p.65). "Look," you say, "we're mirroring each other," and share a chuckle. This kind of mirroring is the glue of our social world. To quote Marco Iacoboni, "We read the world," constantly assessing and unconsciously imitating the actions, expressions and subtle body signals of those we meet. When we mirror each other it strengthens our sense of rapport and connection.

Still working those lattes, you listen as your friend reveals some disturbing

---

1   Limited research has been done with epileptic patients who, for medical reasons, have electrodes implanted into their brains. This allowed, with their consent, the stimulation of single cells responsible for specific actions. The results supported the existence of mirror neurons in human beings (Iacoboni 2009, p.23).

details of his relationship. Unbeknown to both of you, another instance of mirroring is taking place inside you. The speech motor area in your brain is activated, corresponding to the words you are hearing. It is as if you are speaking what you hear (Iacoboni 2009, p.104). Who would have thought it, that his partner snores?

Since you have been sitting so long, you notice you fancy some dessert. Opening the menu, you look for something tasty—sweet, but not too filling. As you settle on the double chocolate blackout brownie, it has happened again. It turns out that reading is not a simple perceptual activity (Iacoboni 2009, p.93). The menu tantalizes you with a description of how you won't be able to resist taking the brownie, bringing it to your mouth and biting into it. As you read, mirror neurons in the premotor cortex of your brain are again firing just as if you were snatching the brownie from its plate, conveying it to your mouth and chewing it. Why are we so easy to manipulate?

Well, there's a bit of time before the afternoon land session begins, so back in your room you lie down and go over the material you learned in the morning. As you close your eyes and imagine doing the moves, the premotor cortex is again activated, firing the same neurons you would use to execute the movements (Keysers 2011, p.66). This is a technique ballet dancers use, by the way. They have lengthy choreographies to memorize, so to help the process they visualize doing the steps before sleeping and directly before performances. Just keep that in mind the next time you're inclined to complain about how long the sequence is, okay?

Let's continue in the story. The afternoon land session begins and you take your place in the circle. One by one the participants check in and share what is going on for them. As one woman starts to speak, she is overcome with emotion. Tears stream down her face as she recounts how she was triggered in the water. Everyone in the circle is quiet and focused on her. The person next to her gently offers a tissue. Your mirror neurons are allowing you and the rest of the group to feel what she is feeling. Looking at her face you unconsciously mirror the sadness visible in her features. A part of your brain has activated that is responsible for making this facial expression. This part is connected to a structure called the insula which mediates to the limbic system, the seat of emotion in the brain. Research shows that as all three areas activate, you are able to empathize, to feel what others are feeling (Iacoboni 2009, p.118). This pattern of reacting began very early in life when you copied the gestures and expressions of your parents, learning to understand them and an ever-widening social circle, making it possible to navigate your way through the human landscape.

The experience of mirroring and being mirrored

In the context of a Healing Dance session, mirroring is a volitional act of the practitioner in relation to the client. It is not the simple imitation of body signals, facial expressions and actions; we practice a more sophisticated concept of mirroring that allows the client to feel heard, seen and felt. Mirroring, as we define it, consists of a broad set of skills designed to evoke these reactions in the client and to facilitate her flow of movement expression. Research has shown that our own motor skills affect how we perceive (Keysers 2011, p.54). That means that if we have in our own bodies experienced spontaneous, authentic movement expression, there will be much more mirror activity in our brains as we accompany a client doing similar movements. The assumption can be made that we will understand the movements better and more easily mirror them than if they were unfamiliar.

Mirroring comes most intensely into play when the receiver enters a phase of self-generated movement. Especially in such moments, mirroring can be both meaningful and fascinating for the practitioner. He focuses all of his attention on facilitating a very personal opening and journey for the receiver. An awareness of having related respectfully and ethically, even in phases characterized by sensuality, can enhance his sense of self-worth. He may feel enriched as he comes into contact with the non-ordinary state of consciousness in which the receiver is moving. He may also feel deeply fulfilled to have been accompanying his receiver in a state of empathetic self-forgetfulness for the better part of an hour. Seeing the joy in his receiver's face, he cannot help but feel it too, smiling as she smiles. Additionally, the witnessing at close quarters of another's personal truth can be very nurturing. In short, it is an alluring and uplifting experience when the client is caught up in her movement expression and the practitioner facilitates her, applying the principles of *relating and mirroring*.

To be mirrored is trust-inspiring and comforting, and at the same time natural and liberating. Our client is symbolically receiving the "yes" from life that encourages her to express herself, that unlocks her personal dance. The client senses she is seen and can let go of vigilance, knowing that someone is present with her, keeping her safe. Particularly in phases of self-generated movement, it may feel so amazing that it leaves her unable to describe her experience. When each gesture, turn of the head, arch of the back or other movement impulse is acknowledged and supported, there may be little in her life to which she can compare it. It may be that the last time anyone paid such complete attention to her was in childhood, accounting for a reminiscent quality to the joy some clients feel when being mirrored. Mirroring has the potential to take some clients back to the forgotten wonder days of infancy when the world was bright and fresh, and love was in every face, voice and touch. Of course, the opposite may be the case, that a client is reminded of how she lacked such loving attention. Becoming aware of a deep hole in the soul can trigger feelings of loss and sadness, and at the same time provide the opportunity to receive the love and nurturing that was so poignantly absent.

To be mirrored may evoke not only a joyous association with infancy; the receiver may feel instead as if she is in the arms of an ideal dance partner, or lover, or a divine being when the giver's empathic presence and mirroring so perfectly correspond to her impulses that she loses sight of how she is creating the movement and the practitioner is only following. Transference and counter-transference are never far away in such situations, which call for all of our ethical clarity on behalf of the client, ourselves and the profession.

Mirroring in a Healing Dance session: The pre-session intake

Mirroring occurs in all phases of a session: during the pre-session talk and medical intake, in the session itself and afterwards at the wall during the closing verbal exchange. In the pre-session medical intake, it is key that we meet our client where she is. Every detail of voice and body that we can notice will be mirrored in the corresponding area of our brain, providing us with a basis for understanding and empathizing with the person who is before us. We are forming impressions that will guide us in the session. Paying attention to subtle signals of body language, we adjust our own in order to be appropriately present, for instance finding the right distance between us, orienting ourselves toward her or angled slightly away, and if we are in the water already, not towering over her, but sinking democratically to the same level, eye to eye. Research has shown that maintaining good eye contact allows a person to remember better what you are saying (Otteson & Otteson 1980, p.50). While mirroring the eyes with eye contact and nodding in response to her statements might in general be the best recipe for the receiver to feel felt, too much of this could make the shy client uncomfortable. And even as with some clients we may be natural and friendly, feeling connection and openness, others will be more at ease if we are strictly professional and not too personal, letting them break the ice when they are ready. As our client shares details of her state of body and mind, it may be appropriate to practice verbal mirroring, either reflecting her statements word for word or paraphrasing them. Either way, the goal is that the client feels heard and you learn what you need to take into consideration to prepare for the session. Following your intuition, you will vary how you explain the nature of the session, laying emphasis on the physical, emotional or spiritual aspects of the work as seems right. On occasion, it is necessary to gracefully cut short the client's storytelling of irrelevant details, perhaps by reminding her that she is free to continue, but that it takes away from the allotted time in the water. On the other hand, in the case of the impatient client who is eager to start, we need to insist on giving a few important details, perhaps letting them know we sense they would like to begin but a bit more explanation will enhance their experience. We need to keep in mind that when we empower our client, she will feel more at ease and be more likely to surrender and let go during the session. We can do this by placing decisions in her hands, as in "Would you like to start with the head pillow and noodle or go directly into my arm support?" and "Would you like to begin now?" In summary, mirroring is an excellent tool to get you through that sometimes gnarly thicket of communication before the session.

Mirroring in the pick-up

Following the pre-session medical intake, we find ourselves in the water standing opposite our receiver and inviting her to stand as we are standing, in horse stance. We extend our hands palm up to her and see how she takes them. Looking into the receiver's eyes we draw her attention to how she is breathing and invite her to feel the support of the water. Eventually we indicate she may close her eyes and go into her own inner space. Either before or after she closes her eyes, we begin to mirror her breath. Did you notice that in this preliminary upright phase of the session there are already three mirrorings going on? When the client sees our horse stance and assumes it herself, she is mirroring us at our invitation. Such reciprocal mimicking of body positions can already be establishing rapport. When we next mirror the receiver's gaze, not only are we giving her a feeling of being understood and validated, we are engaging in a pastime familiar since infancy. Studies show that infants smile more and cry less when adult eye contact is increased (Samuels 1985, pp.105–114; Lohaus, Keller & Voelker 2001, pp.542–548). Direct gazing increases their face recognition, as well (Farroni, Johnson & Csibra 2004, pp.1320–1326). A final bit of science is most interesting: according to researchers at the University of Paris a person is far more aware of what is going on in his body when someone else makes eye contact than when they do not. So looking into our receiver's eyes can actually help her to focus on herself.[2]

As practitioners, we have probably experienced how this initial simultaneous communication of looking into the eyes can create a powerful attunement.[3]

---

2   https://theartofcharm.com/art-of-dating/science-eye-contact-attraction.
3   If you don't know what co-counseling is, imagine something like Relating & Mirroring but in the realm of speaking and listening. Two people sit opposite each other. One speaks uninterrupted for an agreed length of time while the other only listens. Then the roles reverse. When the listener holds the gaze, synchronizes his breath and is fully present, there arises a flow of self-expression in the speaker not unlike what we reach non-verbally in movement in the water.

Our gaze should be open and accepting, making no demands, giving us a chance to practice unconditional positive regard, literally. And yet, as beautiful as that can be, it is not suitable for everyone. Whereas some clients need time looking back into our eyes to feel trust and safety, others find it too intimate and immediately shut their eyes. Moreover, there are those receivers who want to "do it right" and not make any mistakes. In the absence of clear guidelines from our side, and without healthy boundaries, they may continue returning our gaze, even if it is awkward for them. Sensing such a reaction we need to promptly give them permission to close their eyes.

Mirroring the breath

The third mirroring we do facing our partner in the pick-up is of her breath rhythm. We continue doing it in mirroring the breath, the first figure in the Healing Dance I sequence. Floating the receiver in first position before us, she can palpably feel the mirroring as we countertraction the pelvis away from the head on the in-breath, lengthening the pelvis slightly away on a diagonal footwards, then allowing the pelvis to sink on the out-breath, accompanying it down with neutral contact. It is mainly through the receiver's tactile sensation of this rising and sinking of the pelvis that the mirroring registers in her awareness. If we perform it correctly, she will feel neither rushed nor delayed. The receiver is aware not only of the union of her breath and the movement of her body, but that the giver is creating this mirroring. She may marvel that someone, a stranger, is noticing her breath and moving her exactly in its rhythm. To receive such attention can make a strong impression on a receiver for whom such intimate regard is unfamiliar. It can send the message "You are important." For other receivers, this joining with the breath may be too personal. For this reason, we need to observe how our receiver is reacting and be ready to move on if it makes her uncomfortable. We must meet our clients where they are and not burden them with too much presence in service of an ideology. Another reason for aborting the mirroring the breath exercise is that it can be so subtle that some clients don't notice that anything is happening and become impatient for the session to begin. When once you have had a client interrupt your meditative mirroring of the breath with the question "When are you going to start?" you will be sure in the future to notice any signs of antsiness.

During a session, we are also literally mirroring the breath; that is, breathing in sync with the receiver's rhythm. We engage with the breath not like a metronome, mechanically, but sensing the quality of the breath, really "breathing with." We connect our breath to the receiver's breath in order to stay attuned to her, able to empathize with her and intuitively make the right decisions as the session unfolds. Normally we would be giving plenty of space to our receiver, holding her out away from us in the dance frame, but depending on the circumstances, there might be contact between our chest and her near side, so that our breath rhythm transmits directly to her. Another technique of bringing our mirroring of the breath to the receiver's awareness is to breathe audibly, though this can be experienced as invasive and should be used sparingly and only when we are sure it is appropriate.

Mirroring the breath through the sequence

Moving on into the body of a surface session, we continue to read the breath so that we can offer certain movements in harmony with the breath. This is particularly important when the trunk is folding into flexion, then opening into extension. The power accordion in Figure 12.1 is a good example.

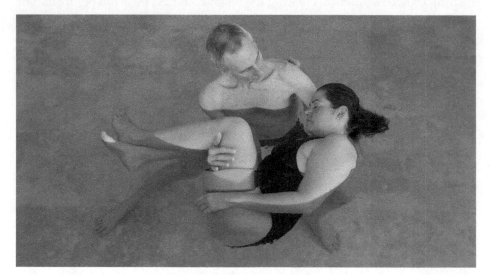

Figure 12.1: Power accordion

The thighs come toward the chest in the fold together, compressing the abdominal contents and diaphragm upward against the lungs, and causing an exhale. As we open the body in the power accordion the pressure on the abdomen stops and the body naturally breathes in again. Mis-timing the movement in relation to the breath will hinder the movement and cause discomfort for the receiver. The hip wave also follows this pattern.

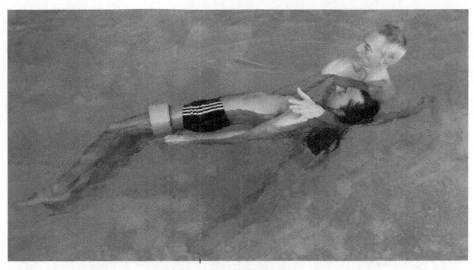

Figure 12.2: Hip wave

In the rounding/flexion phase, the reduced space in the chest dictates that it happens timed with the out-breath; in the lengthening/extension phase the lungs can fill up more easily in the expanded internal space of the ribcage.

A second category of movement requiring us to coordinate with the breath is when the body ascends and descends in the water, as its buoyancy increases and decreases. In this case, the air entering the lungs in the inhale assists the upswing by making the body feel lighter, while the air leaving the lungs on the exhale facilitates the down-stroke by making the body seemingly heavier. The pegasus wave from Healing Dance II illustrates this dynamic well.

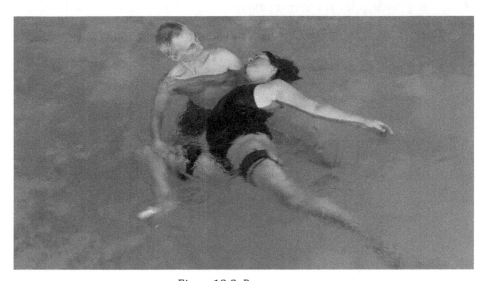

Figure 12.3: Pegasus wave

Holding the near leg, we pull the body up to the surface into a back arching on the inhale, then pull it down toward the bottom of the circling wave on the exhale. Ascending or descending out of sync with the breath cycle will feel wrong for the receiver and cause the giver to strain.

Quiet positional sanctuaries later on in the sequence, such as the safe harbor, hara hug and the fan, are ideal for mirroring the breath.

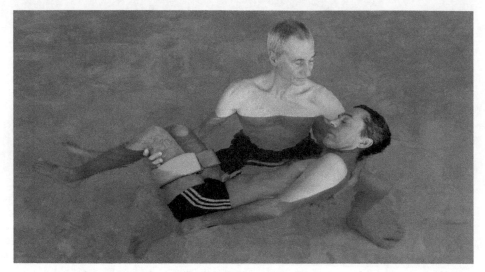

Figure 12.4: The safe harbor

We can find the breath more easily than when the body is in motion and there is no occasion for confusion, as in mirroring the breath at the beginning, about what is happening. The receiver is enjoying the stillness to integrate the effects of the movement and can better appreciate having her breath mirrored.

In Healing Dance, we have the concept of the "usable breath," meaning that the receiver's breath rhythm is one that harmonizes well with the rhythm of a movement. When the breath is calm and long, as happens when the dive reflex activates, its rhythm is too slow to provide a basis for movement, so we simply move in an appropriate rhythm. Likewise, when the breath is so rapid that mirroring it in movement would not make sense, we might coordinate with every other breath or again find a moderate rhythm. In this last example of a too fast "unusable" breath rhythm, the tendency of the receiver to entrain her breath to our slower rhythm can serve to calm her down.

Mirroring the breath in underwater sessions
Mirroring the breath is fundamental to the technique of Healing Dance's underwater work. We are constantly reading the breath so as to impeccably

time the different actions involved in a submerging to exactly the right moment in the breath cycle. We give the signal to submerge into the out-breath, not too close to its end, to give the receiver enough warning that she may consciously take one more breath before going under. We make sure that her last in-breath is complete before initiating the takedown. We track the length of the receiver's breath hold underwater over successive dives to know how much time to give her before surfacing. And arriving at the surface we are mindful of any stresses in the breath to gauge how much time she needs before being ready to go under again. Because the receiver has an activated dive reflex and is taking fewer breaths than we are, we can mirror her breath with our breath only at the moments of submerging and surfacing.

Mirroring the body in motion

Mirroring is not only breathing with the receiver and moving her in harmony with her breath rhythm. It is also a sensitivity to her body's unique quality of movement as it surrenders to the flow. Several factors contribute to what we could call *kinetic mirroring*, and these include its size, shape, flexibility, specific gravity and hydrodynamic qualities. Taking these into account, we adjust our holds, timing and body mechanics to bring out the maximum of grace in any given movement. Applying the principle of ideokinesis first developed by Lulu Schweigard, all we have to do is visualize the movement in its fullness and beauty, and our nervous system will execute this directive without our conscious mind knowing exactly how. What we have is a conscious intention translating into an unconscious execution. By reading the moment-to-moment subtle sensations of the receiver's body in motion we can automatically convert this information into the hand placement, footwork, use of weight and timing that creates the vision we have imagined. We are visualizing and mirroring to arrive at an ideal, the full potential of grace for our receiver; not just what would be acceptable, but what could be.

The hip wave makes an excellent move to analyze.

Our intention is to create a long, graceful wave that is spacious and articulated in both the rounding and extension phases. Knowledge of all the points of technique assists us in visualizing the ideal. Notice if the leg flotation allows the body to descend gradually from head to feet and if the near leg suspends below the far leg, where it should be. Sense the amount of weight in the hip hand and the interplay between this hand and the hand palming the shoulder to set the 45° angle orientation of the trunk. Have we caught the occipital curve in our elbow crook in order to be able to traction well and are we swinging our partner out away and behind us for the "Best in Show" effect? Are we leaning back, especially with the step on the foot-foot? Can we use our weight more?

Can we slow down the wave and still travel it well? Most importantly, are we feeling the receiver's body in motion? Does it have an ideal rhythm of oscillation? How much drag, how much buoyancy? Is there a little more length, a little more grace to be had?

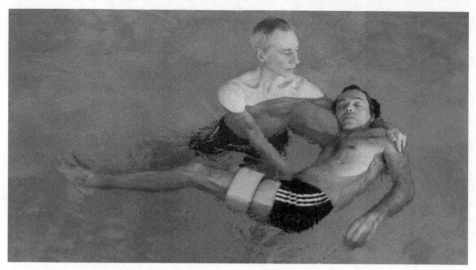

Figure 12.5: Hip wave

Kinetic mirroring, in which we are refining and adapting the set moves of the sequence to our receiver, is not the only form of mirroring we practice in a session. We are also making dozens of decisions and small adjustments to enhance the receiver's comfort, reflect her wishes and honor her limits. Here are a few internal monologues you may have had:

"All right, she wants to throw her head back in an arch. Fine, but I'll just keep supporting under the occiput and see what happens."

"There's some tension coming into the body; I need to slow these waves down."

"This wave doesn't seem right now; maybe time for some stillness…"

"Hmm, something big is going on in this pose; good to stay longer…"

"Uh oh, doesn't feel like she's comfortable anymore in this embrace. Let's move out of it right away."

"Her shoulder's loosened up from the massage. I'll come back to that later."

"Good, some more flexibility coming into the body; maybe time to try a bit stronger stretch…"

"She's starting to roll her head into the water. I guess I should offer the nose clip and skip the second side of the warm-up."

"Well, she kept her mouth closed for over five seconds after surfacing. The next dive can be longer."

"Wow, that's a big smile after the dolphin! Let's repeat it on the other side right now!"

Mirroring the tissue

It is possible to mirror not only the body's movement, but the body itself, its cellular structure. More specifically, we are relating to the cells of the soft tissues; that is, the skin, connective tissue and muscles. It is through touch, massage and stretches that we are able to do this, each practitioner drawing on their own bodywork background. When we calibrate our quality of touch, the pressure of our massage and the intensity of our stretches to the client's wishes and what her body is telling us, we are meeting the body, mirroring its needs.

Touch

One way of understanding touch is to see it in a range from yin to yang. Yin touch is characterized by sensitivity, respect, nurture and listening. The most yin touch is used in energy work, simply laying the hands softly onto the body in still positions such as the heart sandwich or hara hold. We let them melt into the body as they sense the quality of the tissue, the temperature, the pulse of circulation and energy, and the person.

Yang touch is more matter of fact, firm and robust, giving clear guidance, and "speaking" rather than listening. Our hand on the back heart in pegasus is a prime example, bringing the upper back into delicious extension and sweeping the body across in front of us. Our grips in macarena and the vortex are similarly forceful.

The strong dynamic of these moves calls for this yang quality of touch.

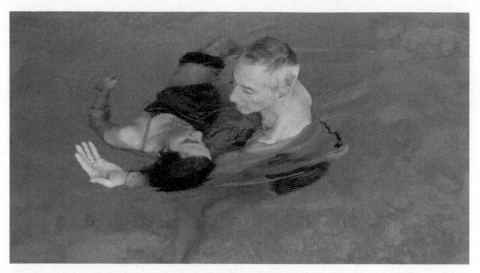

Figure 12.6: Macarena

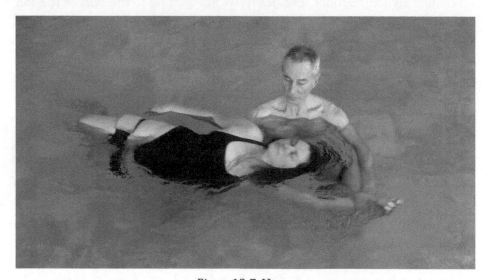

Figure 12.7: Vortex

Many of the dynamic traveling dives of shape and space, such as the dolphin, the parachute and the shark rodeo, feature such holds, as well.

Another way of seeing touch is along a continuum between closeness and spaciousness. It is permissible in a Healing Dance session, more so than in a land massage, to bring not only our hands in contact with the receiver, but the cheek, shoulder, arms, chest and thighs. This fuller, more encompassing touch is possible on account of the spatial juxtaposition of giver and receiver and because the giver is supporting the receiver, having become the table, so to speak. Healing Dance has many examples of such embracing touch, touch that provides containment. The safe harbor, hara hug, accordion offering and klimt come to mind.

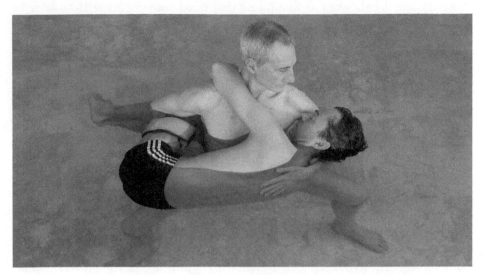

Figure 12.8: Klimt

On the opposite end of the continuum is touch that is minimalized, disappearing and giving space. When we wave the receiver with one arm alone in the silk wave or pull her in head pull and head wave, cradling under the occiput, the body experiences maximum freedom with minimum contact.

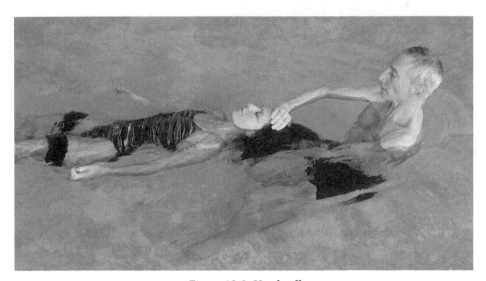

Figure 12.9: Head pull

Massage

Before the session when a receiver mentions a sore neck or back that would like massage it behooves us to address that need sooner rather than later in the session. Do this and you have won the client over, showing that you are reliable. It also demonstrates to the receiver that she has been heard and that expressing a need is okay. Massage speaks to the specific part of the body involved, telling it that it matters. Moreover, massage toward the beginning of a session can serve as an icebreaker, generating trust and surrender.

Another way of mirroring the receiver's needs and getting it just right is to ask! Before the session we might ask how she likes her pressure or stretches: light, medium or strong? "And would you like a feedback system during the session of saying '5' if it is just right, '4' if it is not quite strong enough and '6' if too strong?"

We come across quite a range of body types in aquatic bodywork: from the tiny flexible ladies to enormous stiff guys. Regardless of who we are floating, our hands are sensing the degree of muscle tonus and adjusting the pressure of our massage. The hyper-flexible woman with hypotonus in the muscles would not be a candidate for strong massage. Whereas the man tending toward inflexibility and hypertonus would more likely enjoy a deeper pressure that would break up contracture, move out metabolites and improve circulation. How fortunate that the warmth, buoyancy and pressure of the water all serve to enhance massage—softening, relaxing and favoring circulation in the muscles. Of course, we pay attention to the receiver's appreciative sighs of relief or protective tensing up to further guide us.

Stretching

We mirror the tissue when stretching by sensing it through our hands and adjusting the intensity of the stretch accordingly. It is even possible to sense how the body stretches as it meets water resistance in movement to give us information. If we keep with the two body types just given as examples, the woman who is flexible, perhaps hypermobile in her joints, might enjoy the feel of a stretch, but not really need it. For her, a "psychological" stretch would be in order, one that is pleasurable but not held long enough to have a lasting effect. The same would apply to tractions for her: we would want to avoid destabilizing her joints with too strong a pull. For the man in our example, the opposite would be the case: we could use stronger tractions and stretches to good effect. A "physiological" stretch might be the right thing for him, one that is held longer in order to create a real shift in the tissues.

The principles of relating and mirroring

The most important thing to remember about relating and mirroring is that it is all about responsiveness, not creativity. When we facilitate a receiver in her kinetic self-expression, it is not about concocting some amazing moves out of our imagination. Nor are we entering into a glorious dance that will delight her beyond her dreams. When we attend strictly to responding to the movement impulses of our client, there may indeed emerge some beautiful moves that have never before seen the light of day, and observed from the poolside, your interaction may have the appearance of a dance such as one could hardly imagine. Yet, it is not about us; it is about noticing as many of the receiver's signals and impulses as possible and responding appropriately to them.

The principles of relating and mirroring fall into two categories. The first group has to do directly with mirroring. The second group supports this mirroring, facilitating the process in different ways. As they are part of the training Relating & Mirroring, we will not be describing them here; they must be studied and practiced in order to be fully understood. Simply reading about them would not do them justice. As we fully disclose in Chapter 1 and the chapters that follow, proper hands-on training and certification are paramount and required.

Underwater relating and mirroring

As Healing Dancer practitioners, we need to be ready to relate and mirror not only in surface sessions but also in those which go underwater. Here are a few thoughts and guidelines to approach this aspect of aquatic bodywork.

It can be that your receiver is surrendered and receiving the movement on the surface, but after the signal and submerging becomes active to a lesser or greater degree. We need to be able to accept this and shift gears to drop any plans as the "doer" and instead embrace an auxiliary role.

Your receiver may actively submerge herself, choosing the moment and manner that suits her, then continue her own movement underwater. That's okay and it may require us to react quickly as the receiver's submerging could be sudden and the length of time spent on the surface between dives could be brief.

Kinetic self-expression underwater can range from gentle to very dynamic movement. Some receivers may be seeking stillness; others are wanting to move. Our job is to keep accompanying whatever they are doing and support them in it, even if it is not what we "want" or would most enjoy.

Receivers who become active underwater do not usually have as long a breath as passively receiving ones. We need to anticipate that they will have to come up sooner.

Our responsibility is to be vigilant for our partner and bring her to the surface when she needs or wants to come up. We must constantly observe her when she is underwater, noticing any signal indicating discomfort or the wish to surface.

Some receivers in their enthusiasm and fantasy may initiate movements that would bring them into contact with the pool bottom or a wall—their eyes are closed and they are not noticing. We must redirect them in this case. We must also steer our clients clear of other carbon-based lifeforms in the pool.

The advantage of underwater relating and mirroring over that on the surface is that we may release our client completely and allow her to enjoy the totality of moving in a three-dimensional space. Setting movement impulses and releasing the body generally works quite well for the subaquatic dancers.

Receivers who are releasing energy or feelings may become quite loud or even violent in their movement. Depending on whether you are working in a public space or a private one, it falls to you to curtail such behavior when it is inappropriate. And you need never place yourself in danger of being injured.

Relating in Healing Dance

Even though the theme of this chapter is mirroring, any explanation of theory meant to accompany relating and mirroring would not be complete without exploring relating, as well. Relating and mirroring are not distinct from each other; the line between them is often blurred. Mirroring is a way of relating; relating can take the form of mirroring. As we have shown above, mirroring is causal to empathy, and empathy can in turn increase the capacity to mirror.

The mirroring that we do in the Relating & Mirroring course is an intensification of the mirroring that occurs all through a session. By way of contrast, the relating that we do in Relating & Mirroring phases of a session is the same as in the rest of the session; it does not differ in any way. Our inner attitude determines our outer relating. There is a tendency to see relating as synonymous with empathy, but relating is more than empathy alone, composed of a constellation of inner intentions, practiced attitudes and beliefs. Imagine if practitioners were each to make a personal list of inspirations and attitudes that guide their approach. No doubt love, gratitude, humility, patience, compassion, forgiveness and openness would find a place on many of their lists.

Although we will look more closely at empathy later, what I wish to present to you first are the five principles of Hakomi. Since the early days of aquatic bodywork they have been making an impact on WATSU, which is not surprising, considering that both WATSU and Hakomi share roots in Zen Buddhism. Healing Dance is also indebted to Hakomi, not just for the strategies of "setting impulses" and "taking over," which we translated into mirroring techniques, but for these foundation principles, which are so universal that they can be applied to all holistic bodywork approaches.

The five principles of Hakomi

Organicity

The first principle of Hakomi recognizes that people are living systems, organisms. They maintain themselves, procreate and evolve. They are sensitive to their environment and interact with it. A living system is not a machine, which can break and then needs to be repaired; a living system has the ability to heal itself. Think of how a wound naturally heals. Our self-healing capacity extends to the psyche, as well. When we have faith in the principle of organicity, we know that by allowing natural processes to unfold, a person is moving toward healing their emotional wounds. As practitioners then, we do not put pressure on ourselves to "fix" the receiver. We need only hold a space for her self-healing to operate, whatever that may look like. A receiver's timing is her own, not known to us.

Mindfulness

Our beliefs define the "field" in a session, the range of the possible for the receiver. Practicing mindfulness, we are believing in the transformative power of awareness. We notice all that we can, feeling no pressure to react or act. It is okay for things to happen by themselves. Nor do we need to judge or even understand what we perceive. We remain focused in the present moment, open and willfully passive. We take care with our quality of touch, noticing how the body moves and how our client reacts. Our awareness is not focused solely on the receiver; we also pay attention to what is going on inside us: our feelings, projections and associations. However, our self-awareness should not be at the expense of staying adequately present with the receiver. A certain amount of our attention must go to the surroundings, as well, specifically how close the wall is and where other people are in the pool. If we are working in a spa or hotel pool there are occasions when others will heedlessly stray into our space, in which case a warning glance, an evasive maneuver or a ward-off hand on the offending bather's back will avert a collision. Our mindfulness is diminished to the extent that we daydream, going over our shopping list, deciding on our Netflix entertainment for the evening, and so on.

Non-violence

In its simplest form, violence is forcing, showing an insensitivity to the receiver's boundaries. The stretch that is too strong, the massage pressure that is too deep, the embracing hold that is too close are all forcing, generating the natural reaction—resistance. When the giver practices nonviolence, he shows respect for the receiver's limits and behaviors, not labeling them negatively as "defenses." Pushing process, in which the giver purposely takes a person over their limits in order to trigger them into catharsis, is the most unethical example of violence that comes to mind. Subtler examples are thinking one knows better and following an agenda rather than the signals from the receiver. Trust in the internal intelligence of the receiver is the antidote, creating a supportive environment that unlocks her self-healing potential. This implies a therapeutic relationship in which teamwork, listening and problem-solving have a place. This may even include empowering the receiver to express her wishes at any time, even directing the course of the session if she desires.[4]

Body-mind holism

According to this Hakomi principle, the body and mind are parts of an integrated whole, encompassing the physical, emotional, mental and spiritual. The realm of thoughts, memories and beliefs can be accessed through the body, just as our mental life can manifest in the body as images, sensations and emotions. In massage school our instructor told us, "The issues are in the tissues." Massaging deep into the body, for instance, may cause memories of an unresolved trauma to surface. Working from the other direction, a shift in a core belief can cause a shift in the physical body. At the interface between body and mind, either realm can be accessed through the other. Dance therapy, body psychotherapy and psychosomatic medicine are among the many other disciplines utilizing this connection.

Unity

The principle of unity places each of us in ever-widening systems, beginning with the family, expanding to the community, nation, humanity as a whole and ultimately the universe. It affirms our belongingness to the whole and our interconnectedness. After a warm contact with a friend or neighbor, or time spent in nature, one feels, "I am home, this is life." Unity within an individual arises through communication and harmony between his constituent elements: conscious and unconscious, masculine and feminine, human self and Higher Self. This paves the way toward wholeness and healing. And when the giver sees himself as not so different from his receiver, on the same level, then there can be oneness in this relation as well, rather than duality. Unity arises in our work through the sharing of a session with our receiver, looking past our differences and affirming our commonality in a healing interaction characterized by empathy, openness and trust.

---

4   We do this in trainings on land, calling it the "request massage," in which the receiver is stating her wishes and the giver is following them. A colleague recently told me of a water session in which she encouraged the receiver to verbally express her wishes. This she did, asking for an intense enveloping pressure (as in the womb), involving the use of the wall and permission to lay her head on a nurturing breast and hear the heartbeat. Aquatic bodywork is ideally suited to provide such a visceral experience of re-parenting.

The science of empathy

As infants, we learn what we are feeling and what others are feeling through unconscious mirroring. As we become aware of our own feelings and start to understand the feelings of others, we acquire the rudiments of empathy. And who better to learn from than our parents? Maternal empathy creates such a powerful attunement, it has hardly an equal in the universe. Our mothers spent endless hours looking into our eyes, mirroring our expressions, sounds and slightest gestures. They awoke out of deep sleep when we cried. They taught us to love. They forged a bond strong enough to last a lifetime, even unto death, as the young soldier or the dying octogenarian calls out to his mother.

Healing Dance practitioners who are parents may have an advantage over others in the ease with which they can empathize, having for years of their lives practiced mirroring on a daily basis with their children. They may find that relating and mirroring come naturally to them. People in professions which are hands-on and involve some non-verbal relating may also have well-developed empathic skills. These include, but are not limited to, nurses, veterinarians, pediatricians, psychologists, physical therapists, and any kind of bodyworker, including ourselves—aquatic bodyworkers.

Mothers may have another practical advantage over non-parents when it comes to relating and mirroring. One study (Iacoboni 2009, pp.127–128) showed that when mothers viewed pictures of their own babies they had strong responses not only in the mirror neuron areas simulating the babies' expressions, but also in the pre-supplementary motor area of the brain, which is responsible for complex motor planning and putting together sequences of actions. It was as if the mothers were not only empathizing, but rehearsing a subsequent interaction with their baby. Dare we suppose that a strongly empathic giver has an easier time arriving at a response to his receiver's flow of movement expression?

Research indicates that we tend to like more those who imitate us (Iacoboni 2009, p.117). Likewise, people tend to imitate those whom they like. Could we make the leap to wonder if sharing a session strengthens a reciprocal bond between giver and receiver?

One of the most frequent corrections I give in class is "Watch the face." Students need to check the water level of the head, look for any hyperextension in the neck, and search the facial features for signs of discomfort or feeling. As explained earlier, when emotion is reflected in the face, we unconsciously mirror it, caused by an activation in the premotor cortex. This part of the brain connects to the emotional centers of the limbic system via the insula, allowing us to understand and feel what the receiver feels. As surprising as it seems, empathy is set in motion through the visual witnessing of feeling. Science is telling us that meditating on the face is an effective means to stay in contact with our receiver.

If empathy means "feeling into," how can we do this if we do not know exactly what a receiver is feeling? Much of what transpires within her will not be apparent in her features, not at all visible in her trance state. And when there is an emotion to witness, we cannot precisely identify it, whether it be happiness, fear, anger or sorrow. All we can do is to get a taste of the receiver's inner state and be mindfully present. We are not commiserating; we do not join the receiver in her despair or anger, but rather hold an open, accepting space that can contain such feelings without judgment. We allow ourselves to be touched by a feeling, but do not merge with it.

Another aspect of empathy associated with mirroring was discovered by Christian Keysers. He found that in his experiments dating back to 2006, which established how the same neurons activate when viewing an action as when performing it, a detail had been overlooked. Not only were the mirroring areas of the premotor cortex and parietal cortex activated, as to be expected, but the most posterior area of the parietal cortex, the primary somatosensory cortex, also consistently showed activity (Keysers 2011, p.134). This part of the brain has to do with the feeling in the body as it moves and touches objects. This implies that as we mirror our receiver, we are both simulating her action and how it feels. I can imagine this resonates for those of you who have already done some relating and mirroring. This allows us to access a rounder, more sensual appreciation of what the receiver is experiencing. Not only are we able to "inhabit" each body position and the changing tonus in her muscles as she moves, we can vicariously feel the resistance of the water and its warm, tingling flow over her skin, even what the contact of our hands must feel like to her.

Summary

Mirroring is pervasive in present-day Healing Dance. It is the underlying reality in the technique, applied in the verbal exchanges of a session, in looking into the eyes of the receiver, in synchronizing with the receiver's breath rhythm whenever possible, in creating the figures in a way that best corresponds to the receiver's unique qualities of movement, in responding to subtle body signals and adjusting dozens of minute details of technique, in adapting our touch, massage and stretches to the preferences of the receiver, and in phases of self-generated movement applying the mirroring principles.

Although inner unconscious mirroring (the activity of mirror neurons) and outer unconscious mirroring (imitating of the receiver's expressions in order to empathize) are present in Healing Dance sessions as in everyday life, we have evolved a type of mirroring that is conscious and imparts to the receiver in her own movement expression the feeling of being seen and felt.

The close fit that the liberating movements and non-invasive holdings of Healing Dance are to the human body and psyche opened the way to a higher dimension of aquatic bodywork. An approach came into existence that allowed the spontaneous movement impulses of receivers to find full expression in freedom and safety. This was enabled by the development of refined body mechanics and ways to minimize the hands, allowing maximum freedom to the body whether passively surrendered or in self-created movement. The care with which closer holds are adapted to the receiver's boundaries is the counterpoint to the many ways we discovered to lever and guide the body in motion. At last, not only feeling states but movement expression can be truly mirrored.

The techniques and principles of relating and mirroring reflect the maturity of Healing Dance. Our approach is multifaceted, effective and growing. It is natural and empathic while at the same time client-centered and supported by science. The Healing Dance mode of relating, honoring its indebtedness to the Hakomi method, is clean and without confusion, having taken pains to evolve and embrace a high ideal of presence.

References

Farroni, T., Johnson, M.H. & Csibra, G. (2004). Mechanisms of eye gaze perception during infancy. *Journal of Cognitive Neuroscience*, 16(8): 1320–1326. doi:10.1162/089892904230 4787. PMID 15509381.

Iacoboni, M. (2009). *Mirroring People: The Science of Empathy and How We Connect with Others*. New York, NY: Picador.

Keysers, C. (2011). *The Empathic Brain*. Createspace Independent Publishing Platform.

Lohaus, A., Keller, H. & Voelker, S. (2001). Relationships between eye contact, maternal sensitivity, and infant crying. *International Journal of Behavioral Development*, 25(6): 542–548. doi:10.1080/01650250042000528.

Otteson, J.D. & Otteson, C.R. (1980). Effect of teacher's gaze on children's story recall. *Perceptual and Motor Skills*, 50: 35–42.

Samuels, C.A. (August 1985). Attention to eye contact opportunity and facial motion by three-month-old infants. *Journal of Experimental Child Psychology*, 40(1): 105–114. doi:10.101 6/0022-0965(85)90067-0. PMID 4031786.

Chapter 13

Aquatic Integration™ and Eastern Medicine

CAMERON WEST

History and development of Aquatic Integration

As the founder of Aquatic Integration (AI), I believe it is important to explore its history in order to provide a basis of knowledge and understanding of its validity and relationship to the clinical/complementary arena.

Thirty-five years ago, I began my search for a technique that would help merge my adaptive physical education background and love of Tai Chi with my clinical massage therapy practice. During this time, I came across an article about WATSU.

I was immediately intrigued by the description of this form: using thermo-neutral body temperature water, implementing stretching, the idea of "being" vs "doing," accessing the meridians, and using nature as the model for treatment.

Soon after, I attended a class in San Jose. I had never observed or experienced a WATSU session before. I was so inspired by WATSU that it changed my entire approach to my professional practice.

As with most things that are alive, change is inevitable. Loving both clinical and complementary modalities, my clients had been teaching me that there was no one technique that fits all beings. Thus, with the practice of WATSU and Tai Chi, combined with my clinical training, I began to blend and morph these modalities. Over time, Aquatic Integration was born into my practice.

AI is a warm water, holistic therapy that encourages sensory integration through touch, communication, stillness and movement. Rooted in WATSU and neurosomatic assessment, AI bridges Eastern and Western approaches in healing. It is an effective treatment for sensory neurological re-patterning as a result of physical and emotional trauma.

Utilizing deep listening and the natural elements of water, it invites the receiver to enter into an intuitive, reflective state of awareness. This can support a greater potential for movement, ease and synchronicity. AI cultivates an atmosphere through which curiosity and gentle inquiry is nourished within a safe, fluid environment.

The AI practitioner views the body as a natural landscape and understands that, like nature, a state of balance is dynamic and adaptive, rather than static or fixed. Tailored to the needs of the individual, each session is a unique, organic response to the receiver's physical and emotional state of being. Aquatic Integration facilitates greater access to the receiver's positive resources within, promoting a healthy, more integrated self.

Concepts and principles of AI

Acceptance, allow, educate: these are three terms that describe the essence of AI.

In *acceptance*, there is no plan of action, but to accept where, how and what evolves, with curiosity and no expectations. An AI practitioner stays with what is happening or not happening in the moment and uses an open door of inquiry through movement, touch, energy and sensations.

While in this state of acceptance, the ability to have patience develops, and this way, we *allow* the client's body to have a chance to respond or not respond. Both are learning experiences.

Educate is a result of accepting and allowing as the client's body and entire system receive an invitation to experience awareness. This can happen on any level: physical tissue, muscles, bones and emotionally, energetically.

Within an AI session, it is helpful to establish a breath/rhythm connection early on. This is accomplished by pure listening, being present and trusting in the personal rhythm and tempo of your receiver. It is essential to take the necessary time for this unfolding. It is your dual breath patterns that will bring you both into this connection. Breath connection will continuously advise and inform you throughout the entire session.

Rhythmic mirroring is a concept where the establishing of rapport happens between practitioner and receiver. There is a non-verbal communication of acceptance, caring and consideration through thoughtful observation. It allows for the rhythm of both parties to get "in sync." This relationship of trust allows each to be in the moment of movement. A dimensional presence is established, enveloping the session in a deep sense of peace. The practitioner has become a natural channel for information to flow and the receiver is able to feel secure and safe.

In order to ensure natural shifting during a session, the principle of respectful pacing is implemented through relevant invitation. As practitioners, we must remember that the psyche and body are not separate entities, and whatever has caused a shift in structure, muscle, bone, mood, behavior, belief has a direct effect on the whole organism. These shifts will show up in the physical form as holding patterns or habituated postures. Introducing any change in rhythm and tempo needs to be at a pace that your receiver can handle and integrate.

Finding a well-matched rhythm with a receiver is the basis of bridging to compatibility. As practitioners, we need to understand that energy translates through the body in physical form, as different sized movements, waves, spirals, rolls and patterns. Within these patterns lie frequency, vibration and their relationship to the whole being. Finding a compatible rhythm establishes an entry into the dialogue for change. Variations in rhythm will result in positive outcomes if they are not forced or felt as mechanical.

Even though they sound alike, there is a dichotomy between the concepts of "weighting" and "waiting" used in AI which results in two entirely different, yet correlated intentions. Utilizing your senses as a practitioner, it reflects initially how much "weight" you place on any given area of the body. Then, to follow, it requires the willingness to pause and "wait," giving time for the tissue, fascia and cells to respond to touch, invitation and subtle energetic cues.

Holding patterns have a frequency and vibration that can be keyed into by matching and then varying tempo and pace. Therapeutic chaos, a palpable change in rhythm, disrupts existing frequency and can invite change. This invites the receiver to slide into any kind of shift, breaking up what has been and empowering them to direct themselves in a new way.

A human system's balance can be more easily maintained in a warm water environment, anywhere from 94 to 96° F, with a PH of 7.3, and is the closest our bodies can get to reaching homeostasis. This is a state where the body and mind equilibrium is met and supported.

All the above principles provide structure for each and every session. Drawing from a protocol or framework of moves typically allows the practitioner to respond in a fluid and continually adaptive way to any situation or condition, with an increasing alertness, awareness, ease and poise.

Kinesiology in water

In AI, our understanding of kinetics is applied through the development of correct alignment and attention to movement progression. The dynamics for learning these two essential elements of safe postures and movement in AI have been strongly influenced by the Jahara technique and WATSU.

Through learning and an understanding of core stabilization, the physiology of movement, and observation and practice, a healthy relationship between the head, torso and feet develops. We are able to create an internal barometer for assessing and coordinating the balance needed to perform simple movement patterns with a receiver.

The base for human movement is rooted in the feet, accelerated by the legs, controlled by the waist and hips and conducted along the spine. This movement is translated through the eyes/head, knees and toes, assisting us to turn in the desired direction. This fluid synchronization of movement is called applied kinetics.

One of the most vital coordinations of movement is shifting the weight and turning the waist simultaneously. In AI, we pay particular attention to the posture as a whole entity. For example, if a foot is not in correct alignment to the progression of movement, the move can be stunted and balance may be compromised.

There are five fundamental forces of movement: *inward*, *outward*, *rise*, *descent* and *rotation*. The human body is a miniature solar system, with the ability to move around its own axis (spine) utilizing all these forces. It is essential to be able to sense and use inner awareness in detecting direction of movement which then allows for follow-through action.

In AI, we are not bound by particular or set moves and foot patterns, we evolve a session through the integrity of coordinated safe movements. To enhance understanding of balanced moves it is essential to understand correct foot mechanics.

Healthy foot mechanics is an integral part of the overall body's postures. It is the base for stability and balance of each and every AI move. This is similar in how stability must be directed through the core and therapeutic touch through the hands. Fluidity in the move is translated through well-balanced feet.

The base foot that leads the movement can go forward, backward or laterally. The base foot takes on the primary amount of weight (about 70%) and is always in flat position, toes pointing in the direction your body is facing. The balance foot holds the (counter) balance of your weight. The base foot and balance foot can be either the forward or back foot.

In each AI session, balance postures and alignment will organically evolve into any movement pattern the practitioner is led into by the receiver. The most essential elements of a session are staying focused, utilizing good core awareness and maintaining an understanding of continual movement. Movement patterns are rarely static, thus it is imperative that each move smoothly transitions into the next.

AI therapeutic application and assessment

As a holistic paradigm for treatment, AI strives to engage all parts of a person to move with synchronistic harmony. Assessment is based on listening, viewing and an understanding of bio geometry. This translates into a practitioner seeing each human system as a unique, moving sculpture or landscape.

As explained above, an AI practitioner understands that alignment and balance are dynamic and adaptive, not static and fixed. Thus, the emphasis is to educate our receiver in recognizing their patterns of pain and holding. This does not mean identifying postural "faults" which may place limits on both the practitioner's thinking and the receiver's empowerment. Instead, it means that we pay more attention to the spirals and functional movement as opposed to a static postural stance.

Once this "rhythm of relationship" is established, several treatment methods can be utilized to help resolve a pattern. It is important to fit your technique to your receiver, not your receiver to your technique. This progressive unfolding ultimately creates a path towards continuity and a sense of dimensional balance.

The AI process of visual assessment and treatment below are modeled after a Shiatsu therapy and clinical-based intake. It is imperative to orient your receiver at the start of each session.

The utilization of a generalized info sheet that is shared with your receiver before their first session can be one option. It can also happen through an initial consultation or conversation. This may help to ease any confusion or anxiety if they have never received an aquatic session before. It can establish the length of their session, thus creating a sense of safety in knowing what they can expect and what things might be unpredictable.

Outlined below are some of the tried and true aspects of assessment that promote a successful beginning for further treatment. It is written in second person to allow *you*, the practitioner, to sink into the essence of this process. These aspects remain helpful for both initial and ongoing sessions.

Assessment strategies

1. It is important to establish connection, through verbal, visual and touch cues. This can be done by a simultaneous progression of: look, listen, sense, feel.
2. Early in the session, inquire about sense of safety, where/if they feel safe inside (their body) and outside (their environment). Perhaps this is with a friend, loved one, an animal or a place. Establish a resource of safety and also an intention for the session. If your client seems to be in overwhelm, just notice the body language and do not overload them with too many questions. You can use the warm water itself as a resource.

3. Remember that assessment can be accomplished through the art of presence, the sensory system, intuition, alignment and education. Allow the receiver's verbal and body language to inform you. This will reflect when and how they choose to participate. This is done both in a "vertical" and "horizontal" orientation and is continuous throughout the session.

4. Ask yourself what the receiver's landscape is revealing to you. Is there a rounded convex/hill (*jitsu* or full) presenting or a hidden concave/valley (*kyo* or empty) coming through in their body patterns? It is important to accept what the receiver brings, either verbally or non-verbally, without judgment or projection. Allow for a healthy relationship to develop, linking practitioner to receiver.

5. Minimize expectations for yourself and your receiver.

6. Observe your receiver's rhythm keenly. This means that you invite change through mirroring, bridging, weighting/waiting and (if needed) the use of creative therapeutic chaos. Guide your receiver towards pathways they are not traversing. Allow them to complete the polar phases of contraction and expansion. Pause and wait for any reactions that may assist in your choreography, such as movement or stillness.

7. Bring clarity to mind and technique to each of your sessions to enhance your ability to respond in a fluid and agile way. This will offer more long-lasting results.

8. Continue to inspire expression (you may provide homework to increase participation), observe reaction and respond, until the strength of dominant patterns dissipates and new expressions of harmony and balance are shared.

9. At the end of each session, reflect and reframe your receiver's observations. This allows for a description of what is different, what might work, what might not.

10. Consider using some sort of scale to determine pain/flexibility at the beginning and at the end, as this will help to qualify and quantify your session.

11. Chart your receiver's treatment and progress to maintain continuity and progression of treatment, and promote validity of technique. In some facilities you will be required to chart, so be sure to utilize the correct names of moves, techniques and types of massage so that clarity and integrity are maintained.

In the practice of Shiatsu and Aquatic Integration, there are parallels in the make-up of each session. Different aspects in each technique/form bring the particular progression into light. In the beginning of each session, there is a period of collecting information, with no analysis or interpretation. Slowly, there is a building of rapport, using inquiry language that may lead to change. There is always a need to work within the capacity of the receiver, no more, no less. At some point, there may be a time to reach out with a "nudge" or intention. If this is done with respect and gentleness, change will have the opportunity to evolve within a safe container.

Anatomy of an AI session

- Breath/Rhythm connection
- Rhythmic mirroring
- Bridging to compatibility
- Respectful pacing
- Therapeutic chaos—balance.

Aquatic Integration summary

In summary, Aquatic Integration as a form has evolved through years of experience and coursework. There is no tried and true method of treatment; each session evolves from a place of noticing what is happening and not happening, and being willing "to be" with whatever shows up. Covert patterns are just as important to give attention to as those that are obvious and overt. They all tell us a story of the individual in our care. The most necessary elements for an AI practitioner are a willingness to be educated through training, staying open to possibilities, as well as remaining neutral, patient, curious and creative throughout each session and ongoing treatment process.

Further reading

Barstow, C. (2005). *Right Use of Power*. Boulder, CO: Many Realms Publishing.

Calais-Germain, B. (1991). *Anatomy of Movement*. Seattle, WA: Eastland Press.

Calais-Germain, B. (2006). *Anatomy of Breathing*. Seattle, WA: Eastland Press.

Dull, H. (2010). *WATSU Basic and Explore Paths*. Middletown, CA: Watsu Publishing.

Duncan, A.D. & Kain, K. (2019). *The TAO of TRAUMA*. Berkeley, CA: North Atlantic Books.

Franklin, E.N. (1998). *Dynamic Alignment Through Imagery*. Champaign, IL: Human Kinetics.

Gach, M.R. (2005). Acupressure Charts. Acupressure Institute.

Hanna, T. (1988). *Somatics*. Cambridge, MA: Perseus Books.

Levine, P. (1997). *Waking the Tiger*. Berkeley, CA: North Atlantic Books.

McHose, C. & Frank, K. (2006). *How Life Moves*. Berkeley, CA: North Atlantic Books.

Myers, T.W. (2001). *Anatomy Trains Myofascial Meridians for Manual & Movement Therapists*. New York, NY: Churchill Livingstone.

Reichstein, G. (1998). *Wood Becomes Water: Chinese Medicine in Everyday Life*. New York, NY: Kodansha America.

Rothschild, B. (2000). *The Body Remembers*. New York, NY: W.W. Norton & Company.

Sarno, J.E. (1991). *Healing Back Pain: The Mind Body Connection*. New York, NY: Warner Books.

Sawyer, D. (1999). *Birthing the Self*. Boulder, CO: David Sawyer.

Sova, R. with Konno, J. (1999). *Ai Chi: Balance Harmony & Healing*. Port Washington, WI: Port Publications.

Taylor, K. (1995). *The Ethics of Caring*. Santa Cruz, CA: Hanford Mead.

van der Kolk, B. (2015). *The Body Keeps the Score*. New York, NY: Penguin Books.

Wooten, S. (1995). *Touching the Body, Reaching the Soul*. Santa Fe, NM: Taos Mountain Press.

Chapter 14

The Anatomy of an AMNION® Aquatic Session

KAREN DAVID AND MARY SEAMSTER

AMNION

There is an early longing wired in all infants to be seen, to be felt, and to have our involution validated by another. (Involution = inner evolution of the heart, mind and soul. Involution helps us attain self-understanding and self-mastery.) When our personal experience is empathically held, contained and allowed, we come to a natural place of rest and relaxation in our whole being. What is love, really, other than fully allowing the other to be who they are, for their experience to be what it is, and to offer the gift of presence to their unique experience?

By offering the gift of space, we do not interfere with the unfolding of their heart and majestic inner process. We do not pathologize their experience or demand that they be different, change, transform, shift or "heal" in order for us to love them. If sadness is there, or fear, or despair, or shame, or depression, or profound grief, we will infuse their inner knowingness with validation and presence. We will be there for them, but only if they need us. We will not engulf them with the projections of our own unlived life, nor will we unload on them our own requirements and hopes and fears. Instead, we will hold with neutrality allowing the inner *light* to shine forth from the obscuration of the *shadow*.

There is an intimacy that is experienced in water. The water holds and caresses our whole body and surrounding field. Our individual hairs are stroked, and our fluid bodies are immersed in a fluid field. Look below for further discussion on the earliest development of the sense of touch (McGlone, Wessberg & Olaussof 2014). We are held in the arms of another. We are skin-to-skin, and heart beating to resonant heartbeat. There is a sense of our being held—by the beloved—who is none other than your own miraculous nervous system, heart and somatic brilliance. In our own stories, we may not have experienced this awe infusing miracle of being held, being seen and being felt. In time and in the kindness of the water with an attuned practitioner we can come to trust that it is unfolding according to a unique blueprint which is emerging out of the unseen hand of love.

The unique quality of this modality, AMNION therapy, is that you are in a morphogenetic presence of the ancestors long before you realize that you have floated into this field. Rupert Sheldrake postulated that there is a field of habitual patterns that links all people, that influences and is influenced by the habits of all people. The more people have a habit pattern—whether of knowledge, perception or behavior—the stronger it is in the field, and the more easily it replicates in a new person. In fact, it seems that such fields exist for other entities too—for birds, plants, even crystals. Sheldrake named these phenomena *morphogenetic fields*—fields that influence the pattern or form of things. Look up Rupert Sheldrake on YouTube for more information.

We can extrapolate that the field of her mother and her grandmother affected the egg in your mother's womb. Each contains a built-in memory given by self-resonance with a morphic unit's own past and by morphic resonance with all previously similar systems. This memory is cumulative. The more often particular patterns of activity are repeated, the more habitual they tend to become.

Within an AMNION session the water creates such safety and unconscious agreement that you find yourself falling into implicit positive memory. Implicit memory is sometimes referred to as unconscious memory or automatic memory. It is often described as being pre-verbal and it can originate in the person's embryonic time. Implicit memory uses past experiences to remember things without thinking about them. The performance of implicit memory is enabled by previous experiences, no matter how long ago those experiences occurred. Sometimes traumatic memories arrive from those pre-verbal times when a traumatic event is "remembered" without words, and is not experienced as memory. These non-verbal physical and emotional memory states do not "carry with them the internal sensation that something is being recalled… We act, feel, and imagine without recognition of the influence of past experience on our present reality" (Siegel 1999).

The receivers are not led; they are invited to come into their deepest psychic space. This can only come from creating a field that has a resonance that stimulates longing and remembering. We can remember our earliest imprints when placed in a warm fluid embrace. Where they go with it is up to them. Interventions from the therapists are only meant to steer a person closer to themselves, not to steer the client where the practitioner thinks the client should go. Subtle, you say; yes, this is so subtle that you may not notice that you have come to an internal place to which you have never been. More radiant, more self, more seen, most of all more embodied. We, as practitioners, need only sit back and amplify the field so it becomes apparent to the witnessing aspect of the client. We sit, we wait and we follow. The client already knows where they want to go, and who they are. We only wait and hold a mirror to themselves, on which they cast longing glances. Looking deeply into oneself takes willingness and perseverance. Many of us have no choice but to let go and let the glory of "who we are" come into us.

History of AMNION therapy (by Mary Seamster)

This is the story of how AMNION was conceived and who helped me get here. When students ask how I came to WATSU and AMNION, this is the story I tell. In 1994, I gave my husband Bill Carroll a gift certificate for a "Couples WATSU" at Ten Thousand Waves. That was the stepping off point for all the training in water. We were running a retreat center in northern Washington state at the time and both of us had numerous trainings in the body and body-centered psychology. In 1996, Bill decided to go to Harbin and he took WATSU 1 and 2 with Harold, Minakshi, Alexander George and Michelle Chilenza. He came back to the retreat center raving about his experience, and we instantly decided to put in a 24-foot pool. Alexander came in 1997 to teach and it all took off from there. After taking and assisting several WaterDance classes I began to notice something else was informing and directing the sessions. One of our students suggested studying with David Sawyer LPC, a therapist who blended his study with William Emerson and his Integrative Body Psychotherapy, and WaterDance. The work was profound, and I will always be indebted for David taking me to a new level of curiosity. The question arose: What are we seeing in bodies in water when there is no outside intervention, no mind, no judgments, and only pre-trauma health? I realized from both my personal experience of losing my twin brother, and what I was palpating with clients, that I needed more training. This took me on the lengthy journey of studying with Ray of Castellino Training, the Chittys at the Colorado School of Energy Studies, and Jane Peterson at the Human Systems Institute. This last family constellation training with Jane Peterson allowed me to explore the generational themes that we see in most of our clients. We are hardwired to keep repeating the same pattern of our ancestral trauma until we make sense of it within our own bodies.

Anatomy of a session

The anatomy of the session lies in the ten-page intake form that is sent out after scheduling the first session. The intake form was created collaboratively by

Karen David, Wendy Hodsdon ND and Mary Seamster as part of Karen's Degree of Master of Science in Integrative Medicine Research. We jointly spent months reviewing and discussing the pros and cons of each intake form that we came across for our inspection. We gathered intake forms from naturopathic doctors, cranial sacral practitioners, pre- and perinatal somatic psychology therapists and attachment-based therapists to name but a few. We added questions from the adverse childhood experiences (ACEs) questionnaires, exploring the ways these experiences have been linked to a variety of adult conditions, ranging from increased headaches to depression and heart disease. The ACEs quiz[1] is described in Chapter 4, The Imprint of Trauma, and covers questions such as: "Did an adult often or very often: swear at you, insult you, humiliate you, push, grab or slap you?" It goes on to ask about whether you had enough to eat, or were your parents too drunk or high that you were neglected.

With the intake, we wanted to find a way to gather information that would help the practitioner orient themselves to the subtle intentions underlying the reason for the session. We incorporated questions about whether the client was seeing more than one practitioner for their concern, the history of childhood medical interventions and their birth history.

By the time the client has started filling out the form they are fully in a pre-event session. Clients often say that when filling out the form, they have the experience of traveling back over time and gathering pertinent data. They describe the actual act of unlocking some hidden memories, of distant and pre-verbal recollections that have been stored in their liminal archives.

Some clients are actually able to interview their living parents and grandparents. They can get stories/histories that help create the foundation for a solid session. In other situations, more confusion is generated as family secrets get in the way of the truth. As practitioners, we have found it enlightening to be able to read information passed down from the previous generations that does not match the felt sense experience of the client in front of us. The body always tells the truth, but stories handed down by the family are not always accurate.

Bert Hellinger's family constellations

The Hellinger Institute of Northern California website writes about Hellinger's dedication to the work of studying families. He observed that many family members will take on the familial pattern of anxiety, depression, loneliness, alcoholism, rage, guilt and "even illness as a way of 'belonging.'" "Bonded by a deep love, a child will often sacrifice his own best interests in a vain attempt to ease the suffering of a parent or other family member." We have noticed

---

1   https://americanspcc.org/take-the-aces-quiz

when treating clients that the secrets the family kept/keep from each other are often the unconscious driving force that organizes around a "trauma vortex." A "trauma vortex" is a metaphor that describes the whirlpool of chaos in trauma's aftermath. The imagery of a black hole is often used to describe the effect of a trauma vortex. The force of the vortex can impact clients, so that they are unable to control their sensations, images, feelings, thoughts and behaviors. To quote Jennifer Jabalay (2009), "Secrets are like stars. They blaze inside the heart and ultimately could be explosive. But there are two types of secrets. Small secrets, like small stars, will eventually burn out... But big secrets, grow stronger...eventually...become a black hole."

Start of a session in the pool

The first hour of the initial session is spent standing or sitting in the warm water. The warm water acts as a protective field, a comforting cloak that allows the client to settle. The salt water can hearken back to the experience of being in utero surrounded by the amniotic fluid. We want them to be vertical for this aspect of the session. When they are vertical, they are more in their prefrontal cortex. We can better assess their ability to accurately articulate sequence of events, consistently stay at the edge of activation and know what their resources are in present time.

We spend approximately an hour delving more deeply into the intake form. We are able to traverse the unfolding of deeper held secrets. This phase of the session is where safety is created. We pay attention to the pacing, to the interplay of practitioner and client, not too slow and not too fast. We track: micro expressions (à la Paul Ekman), skin color, breath and repeated whole body movements. Paul Ekman's work is used extensively by law enforcement agencies to track involuntary micro facial expressions of a suspect being interviewed (Ekman & Friesen 2003). As practitioners we are detectives looking for subtle signs that reinforce the needs underlying the actions.

We can mirror the client's movement allowing for a deepening into attunement that can be described as a kinesthetic and emotional sensing of others, knowing their rhythm, affect and experience by metaphorically being in their skin. Attunement is a key word in the study of working with babies and small children. Attunement of caregivers with the baby is the foundation for secure attachment. Our clients come because their close personal relationships have fallen apart, their lives are disintegrating around them. Rewiring the original breach of their attachment to self and parent is what much of the work of AMNION is about.

The horizontal session ensues once the relational practitioner/client piece is fully interwoven. The water, the field around the client, the voices of the ancestors all come together to make an easy flow of unfolding the body in water. Clients, once they stand back to vertical and have taken some time to integrate, will say something like: "I can feel safe in my body for the first time," "I know that I am seen, attuned with and protected," "I know I exist," "I know somewhere in my past, maybe not in this lifetime, my ancestors made compromises for me to be here." Mainly they feel as if they have a purpose and calmness to find the way forward.

Water by itself floats, supports and surrounds us as if we are being embraced in a dream. A dream that seems as real as waking reality. If you add presence of the practitioner and a gentle touch, one could hypothesize that by bringing an adult body into the same felt sense as being in the womb one could evoke the very sacred threshold we experienced prior to and at birth.

This quote from the article "Discriminative and affective touch: Sensing and feeling" (McGlone *et al.* 2014) has brought together years of curiosity about the origins of touch:

We propose that one explanation for the early development of the sense of touch is that the affective architecture of the social brain is primed by activation of skin receptors, C-tactile afferents, via massaging by the amniotic fluid during the prenatal period. K. Bystrova [2009] has hypothesized a mechanism for human fetal growth regulation whereby the repeated oscillations of lanugo hairs during fetal movements in the amniotic fluid stimulate CT afferents, the function of which is to activate brain regions such as the hypothalamus and insular cortex. Indeed, it has been proposed that the developing social brain—and hence the sense of body self—is primed during gestation.

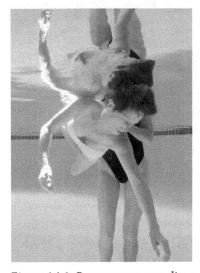

Figure 14.1: Post-mastectomy client

Themes taken from Karen David's master's studies

AMNION is a somatic therapy, which takes place in a warm salt-water pool. A prospective case report explored the changes in a variety of qualitative and quantitative outcomes in a person who sought treatment from a private practitioner of AMNION. A 48-year-old female accessed this therapy in May 2015 after years of treatment for chronic pain and discomfort. She was referred by her acupuncturist to Mary Seamster, who has over 40 years of experience doing bodywork and WATSU. Mary created AMNION as a way of working with clients' somatic experience in the water. Mary utilizes a biodynamic craniosacral approach in a therapy session allowing the client to initiate movement during the session. The natural movement of the body in the water allows for ease and expression that is not as accessible on land (table or chair).

AMNION sessions are conducted in a 24-foot circular pool with 96-degree salt water. Sessions commence with a verbal intake period between the practitioner and client to assess what might be pertinent to the treatment time. The practitioner provides flotation devices for the legs to support the client to float comfortably in the water. Ear and nose protection are used during the sessions. Sessions are unique to each client. A session may involve quiet floating at the surface of the water; body movements include swim-like motions, pushing against the edges of the pool or moving under the water with a nose clip. When a session is complete, the client is gently settled against the pool wall and allowed space and time to integrate their experience. The practitioner checks in with the client and conducts a verbal debrief appropriate to the client's experience. Each session is one and a half to two hours in length and the practitioner documents any pertinent verbal exchange and notable session experiences. The client received therapy sessions on three consecutive days, lasting up to two hours each day.

Qualitative and quantitative measures were collected and analyzed to elucidate what changes occur when someone experiences a somatic therapy.

The Patient-Related Outcome Measure (PROMIS-43) quality of life scale includes categories of pain, daily living, social interactions, anxiety and sleep. The Scale of Body Connection (SBC) body awareness scale compares body awareness and body dissociation. The Experience of Close Relationship (ECR) attachment scale looks at relationships with parents, partner, friends and therapist, providing a standardized score, which detects secure from insecure attachment, categorized as either avoidant or anxious/ambivalent.

Thirteen semi-structured interview questions were formulated by the researcher and practitioner to understand the client's experience of their AMNION session. Interview questions were very general in nature and designed to prompt the client to report her own experience in her own words. The interviews addressed her experience with the therapy, the water and the practitioner, and how her life might have changed in the ensuing weeks. The researcher conducted the interviews, which were recorded and transcribed verbatim for coding and analysis. The transcribed narrative of the interviews was read and coded by the researcher and four other individuals unfamiliar with the client. The four individuals included researchers with doctorates in psychology and rehabilitation sciences, a naturopathic physician and a graduate student in integrative medical research. Words and phrases were underlined by each coder, who then assigned these words and phrases to codes selected by the researcher. The coders assigned all selected narratives to a list of themes mutually agreed on. The three main themes were identified when unanimously selected by all four coders. A narrative was deemed "supportive" when identified by four out of five coder selections. These themes related to the overall question of what changes occurred in this client as a result of this water-based somatic therapy. Using these themes as the lens, the case analysis consisted of combining the various sources of data, including the impressions of the practitioner and input from the subject's other clinicians, to explore what changed as a result of this therapy.

Following three AMNION sessions the client in this case report was less anxious and more joyful than before the treatment, as indicated by both the quantitative and qualitative data. Prior to treatment, the client scored in the normal range in most every category of quantitative scales, yet following treatment, she experienced improvement in the areas of anxiety, social interactions and body dissociation, and reported a slightly more secure attachment experience with her mother and father relationships, even though her mother was no longer living. While the quantitative results alone were relatively unremarkable, they supported and correlated with the qualitative narrative. The client remarked on the success of this work, as she experienced many inner bodily changes as well as cognitive awareness. These results corroborate the client's personal experience post-treatment in her daily life. They also support the theme of a perception shift in implicit memories regarding her relationship with her mother and her father.

The changes experienced by the client in this case report provide a sequence of events that may be inherent and important to the effectiveness of somatic therapies. The researchers saw that 1) the client needed to feel safe within the client/practitioner relationship, 2) the client needed to go to the body in order to access implicit memories, and 3) the subsequent movements that arose led to a change in the perception of her life and story. This change in perception provided a source of integration and internal resources to carry forward in her life. The measurable outcomes were an improvement in some parameters of her quality of life.

The client/practitioner relationship and safety

The client/practitioner relationship is essential for creating a sense of safety in any therapy, as we all carry implicit memories and attachments. If a client enters therapy with insecure attachment or an experience of trauma, there may be difficulty in trying to form a safe attachment to a therapist. However, when a therapist encourages exploration with an open, curious attitude rather than providing interpretations of the person's internal experiences, a sense of safety can be created. It becomes a different experience for a person who is used to having experiences of childhood trauma replicated. In this case report, the client's perception of safety allowed her body to express movements and sensations (theme 1: physical sensations) that exposed awareness of implicit memories: fear was being held in her body in the form of contractions and compressions. She expressed trust and safety with the practitioner and recognized the importance of that relationship for her treatment. The client showed evidence of probable insecure attachment to her early caregivers, giving rise to the question of how well she would respond to a therapy involving such close, physical work.

Training of somatic therapy practitioners requires helping them learn to "hold the edge"—show compassion and empathy without intruding on the client's process. When a practitioner can successfully hold an edge with a client, it allows them to feel, experience and express their sensations and feelings. This expression can feel like a pushing against, a pulling away, a reaching out or a drawing inward. The ability of the practitioner to provide safety, support and freedom is a critical function that allows a client to do their work. The modalities of biodynamic craniosacral therapy and AMNION are unique somatic therapies that offer such open, non-judgmental experiences. The practitioner is holding the client's attachment history as well as his or her own so that the skills of staying neutral and grounded are important.

Immersion in water and the element of touch are inherent safety issues with AMNION. Many times, a participant of AMNION will become completely immersed in the water, so advance preparation by the practitioner regarding the possibility of that event and proper equipment will improve the client's experience and comfort. Touch is utilized as an important technique for teaching awareness of a client's body sensations—their "felt sense." During a therapeutic experience without physical touch, a person can maintain a mostly cognitive orientation, cut off from much of their experience. Touch, therefore, can help clients develop a sense of their inner sensory world, and thereby develop kinesthetic and body ego. Touch is used in AMNION to support the body in the water and also to offer resistance: a feeling of being met that is sometimes necessary when a client is experiencing sympathetic nervous system activation.

Perceptions and integration of implicit memories

Much of the narrative from the client in this case report involved the feelings and sensations of her experience in this therapy. She expressed a profound knowledge of emotions being attached to bodily sensations. The movement of her body in the water allowed an integration of these implicit memories with the awareness of an "expansive place," "a huge shift," a "quiet presence," and an "absence of fear" (theme 2: perceptions). These phrases and words became a vocabulary that was consistent throughout her post-treatment narrative, indicating that this experience allowed her to change her perception of her life and story, particularly concerning fear manifesting as the contracted state in her body. Intuitive beliefs or implicit memories are non-verbal; they are a felt-sense rather than a thought. They guide our actions, so they are truly beliefs. The myths a person lives by are available to their consciousness, but they haven't been mindfully examined. Without being verbalized, they can't be questioned or doubted. When they are unavailable for doubt, they are unavailable for change. Words can be doubted, so beliefs must be brought into consciousness and verbalized to change. States of wonder and mindfulness are not intellectual states; they are states in which our contact with pure experience is unyielding (Salzberg 2015). A person may have a "felt sense" that nobody loved them, for example, arriving with grief too heavy to bear. AMNION aquatics therapy is a way to help people access those altered states of consciousness, even if prenatal or birthing traumas are informing their physical sensations. Once accessed, they can process what has come up. If mindfulness is present, they can also notice how they are being affected by what happens, which is the experience of this client as she discovered that fear was running her life and was no longer useful. These implicit memories can even arise before our birth, as we are already making adaptive choices to meet the unmet needs of our parents and taking on self-identity roles in the family (Chamberlain 2013).

A more multidimensional view of body awareness has emerged in recent years, which focuses on modes of attention such as thinking about the body and presence in the body. Humans have a capacity to think about physical symptoms and be aware of a perceptual presence in the body, often labeled as mindfulness. Body awareness can be defined as:

> the sensory awareness that originates from the body's physiological states, processes (including pain and emotion), and actions (including movement) and functions as an interactive process that includes a person's appraisal. This process is shaped by attitudes, beliefs, and experience in their social and cultural context. (Mehling *et al.* 2012)

Similar to cited work, the client in this case report had an awareness of a "boundary rupture" on the left side of her body (theme 1: physical sensations). When eased by slow movements in the warm water, this physical experience became a new awareness of an internal experience. Somatic Experiencing protocols use this process of titration and pendulation as a way to slowly, mindfully touch on sensitive areas, allowing integration of trauma into the present moment (Levine 1997). There is potential clinical importance in the use of measurement of body awareness in response to somatic therapies as a mediator for painful conditions, as well as linking intervention-related changes in body awareness or dissociation to clinical outcomes. The perceptual changes reported by this client support new findings in neuroscience research that reveal more information about how trauma is processed in the body, and how it is often not integrated with cognitive processes (Payne, Levine & Crane-Godreau 2015; van der Kolk 2015). Peter Levine, the founder of Somatic Experiencing, shows the importance of body awareness in the successful treatment of trauma (Levine 1997). Finally, more recent studies have shown the efficacy of a trauma-sensitive yoga practice in patients with complex PTSD (Emerson & Hopper 2011).

Growth of internal resource

AMNION puts the client's somatic experience at the center of the healing process, yet also requires the integration of sensation with cognition, affect and behavior. Therefore, finding the balance between focusing on the body and a client's narrative story can be especially difficult. There is a Hakomi imperative to "stop the story and make contact," and we saw how this client's story often took her away from the present moment (Hakomi Institute n.d.). Allan Schore's (2003a) synthesis of research finds that the best modalities for healing attachment wounds include body-based therapies. In other words, the body needs to feel the return of safe, secure attachment in a deeply physical way—as well as emotionally—so that the new corrective experiences of healthy relating can eventually override original negative wounding. The challenge is that attachment patterning happens so early, beginning in the womb. Schore recommends that a practitioner develops skills to work pre-verbally, with bottom-up processing as well as top-down processing, to educate and help integrate healing at the end of a therapeutic session.

The client in this case report said a "huge shift" occurred in her outlook on life and her past. She gained a sense of joy and well-being that translated into decreased anxiety and improved social relationships following this treatment. These feelings of safety and improvement in the quality of life provided her with internal resources as further stresses arose in her life (theme 3: changes/internal resources). The client expressed that her "birth information no longer informed her life" and this was one of the biggest changes that occurred to her following her AMNION session. Not only had her perception of her birth and life story changed, but she also had a very different internal experience of her relationship with her parents, particularly her mother who was deceased.

She informally offered that she knew her parents "had done the best they could" and she no longer felt such a "charge of feelings" about her childhood with them. She reported "more ease" and "calmness" in her communication with her father following her AMNION session and had even spent more time with him than before. The possibility of altering one's internal experience of attachment to early caregivers is an important outcome that may inform future study.

The changes the client gleaned from these sessions and her other therapies were translated into actions in her external life. She was able to write emails without fear of internal shame or external judgment and experienced an increased ease in many of her social relationships. An informal connection with the client at eight months post-treatment revealed that she continued to experience an increased feeling of well-being and ease in her relationships with her family and friends. Most notable at this time was that head pain was "not forefront anymore."

The attention to bodily sensations and awareness of how feelings can affect physical sensations in this case report also supports studies on how mindfulness therapy has shown to improve functional flexibility in many areas of disease or mental health states. Functional flexibility is a term used in Acceptance and Commitment Therapy (ACT) to describe improved quality of life in people with no medical diagnoses (Desrosiers *et al.* 2013).

These results support the value of qualitative narrative in somatic therapy research design and the current neurobiology of trauma therapy.

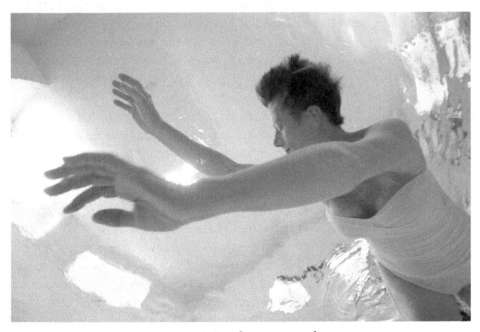

Figure 14.2: Post-breast cancer client

End the session with attunement/attachment theory

Polyvagal theory describes neurobiologically why "meeting a client" is so critical. The theory describes the inclusion of a social branch of the autonomic nervous system (Porges 2007). The autonomic nervous system (ANS) regulates fight and flight but also connection with others (Porges identifies the social nervous system through the vagus nerve). Connections between people and the role of the vagus nerve is an important basis for mind-body medicine. Stephen Porges has described polyvagal theory to explain what is happening physiologically in the different parts of the vagus nerve and how people respond to connection. The vagus nerve acts bi-directionally by giving and receiving information about safety and connection, or "neuroception" (Porges & Furman 2011). The nerve is comprised of 20 percent motor neurons and 80 percent sensory neurons, providing us with continual information about what is happening in the body, as well as controlling body functions. The more ancient branch of the vagus nerve innervates the regions below the diaphragm and comes into play with sympathetic nervous system activation. A myelinated, more modern branch of the vagus nerve system innervates the striated muscles of the face, heart, ears and throat (voice). Porges refers to "neuroception" as the intrinsic, unconsciously operating brain circuitry that registers danger through a variety of perceptual cues. Examples of such cues include auditory stimuli, discernment of the facial expressions of others, and tonal quality of other people's voices—areas innervated by the myelinated vagus nerve branch (Porges 2009). One can activate the parasympathetic nervous system to freeze (primitive, unmyelinated portion), but also to connect with others (modern, myelinated portion of the vagus nerve). People need each other. When something unexpected or threatening happens, people will look around and see how other people are responding to the potential threat. Babies do this all the time, and if the caregiver is calm, the baby will learn to be calm too. This regulation happens by using the neuro-regulation of the face and other structures at and above the heart in response to a threat. A person will turn to social interactions to monitor stress and transition to calmness or action. If a person is left alone or overpowered, their nervous system turns to more primitive methods of reaction, and either flees or shuts down. This primitive system comes online only when the modern system (social nervous system) is not present or perceives a threat. Connecting socially with others is a neurological response that helps humans manage stressors and supports resilience. Listening and witnessing is a part of reciprocal behavior. When a person feels safe, they are accessing parts of the brain not available when activated in fight, flight or freeze. A person can then be creative and bold. This state of having the social nervous system engaged and being connected to others becomes a resource because a person knows they can use social behavior to calm themselves. When a person is in this state, they are receptive to kindness and understanding in the eyes, faces and speech of others.

Attachment

People develop their social behaviors initially with their primary caregiver as they form their early attachment relationships. The state of the primary caregiver's nervous system and brain has a powerful imprint on the child's brain patterning. Early attachment can also affect how a child will begin to self-regulate (Schore 2003b). Because attachment and implicit memories are linked, regulatory patterns of various types of bonding become etched in our bodies and brains. When a child (or any person) is present with someone, they are taking in a great deal of information through mirror neurons and resonance circuitry (Rizzolatti 2005). A person will hear the tone of voice, see a face, notice body language—all senses that assist a person in internalizing another. This concept becomes crucial when clinicians are working with clients. In the area of mind-body work, a practitioner must be conscious of the ability of the client's body to reflect self-knowledge and regulation of health and well-being. If a client has no memory of a safe person in their past, it will be difficult for them to get better without experiencing a safe, trusting relationship (van der Kolk 2002). A goal of therapy becomes providing kind, compassionate care; when a practitioner provides calm attunement, the client has a chance of rewiring old neurobiology and creating new stories and perceptions. Daniel Siegel (2015) suggests that the creation of new neural circuits happens through a variety of types of psychotherapy and the autonomic nervous system has an inherent capacity to self-regulate.

Follow-up to the session

In the case study, Karen did two follow-up phone interviews with the subject. Thirteen semi-structured interview questions were formulated by Karen and Mary to understand the client's experience of an AMNION session. Interview questions were designed to inquire about how the client's presenting problems might have changed as a result of her AMNION session and how her overall life might have changed. The client did not review the interview questions before the two-week post-treatment interview, but she did have online access to the questions 24 hours before the six-week post-treatment interview. Karen conducted the interviews and Mary was available to answer any further questions from the client. These phone interviews were recorded and transcribed verbatim for coding and analysis. The transcribed narrative of the interviews was read and coded by the researcher and four other individuals unfamiliar with the client.

Both researcher and practitioner felt that this follow-up contact allowed the client to tell their story (moving the experience into the prefrontal cortex). In the retelling of their stories, new memories surfaced that were out of the client's awareness. Making sense of these and coming to new understanding can take time.

This chapter has been a labor of love between two colleagues who traveled a protracted journey starting in 2015. The research for Karen's thesis took us on many long hikes. As we walked, we talked, and Karen figured out how to follow a prescribed research method for case studies. Working in warm water can create many uncontrollable issues, such as variances in water temperature, consistent noise and smell levels. We regularly used ourselves as guinea pigs. We gathered heart rate variability data by the side of the pool and we also monitored ourselves each morning for over a month. Several years have passed and our lives have changed, and we now find ourselves reconnecting over this book. Thank you to the editor for bringing us back to our original journey.

One final quote from a client: "I was reaching out to the edges of the womb, I felt like the Leonardo da Vinci man with outstretched arms and legs. My very fingertips traced the boundaries of the womb."

References

Bystrova, K. (2009). Novel mechanism of human fetal growth regulation: A potential role of lanugo, vernix caseosa and a second tactile system of unmyelinated low-threshold C-afferents. *Medical Hypotheses*, 72(2): 143–146. https://doi.org/10.1016/j.mehy.2008.09.033.

Chamberlain, D. (2013). *Windows to the Womb: Revealing the Conscious Baby from Conception to Birth*. Berkeley, CA: North Atlantic Books.

Desrosiers, A., Vine, V., Klemanski, D.H. & Nolen-Hoeksema, S. (2013). Mindfulness and emotion regulation in depression and anxiety: Common and distinct mechanisms of action. *Depression and Anxiety*, 30(7): 654–661. doi:10.1002/da.22124.

Ekman, P. & Friesen, W.V. (2003). *Unmasking the Face: A Guide to Recognizing Emotions from Facial Clues*. Los Altos, CA: Malor Books.

Emerson, D. & Hopper, E. (2011). *Overcoming Trauma through Yoga*. Berkeley, CA: North Atlantic Books.

Hakomi Institute (n.d.). Hakomi Method, Mindful, Body Centered, Somatic, Experiential Therapy. https://hakomiinstitute.com.

Jabalay, J. (2009). *Lipstick Apology*. New York, NY: Razorbill.

Levine, P. (1997). *Waking the Tiger*. Berkeley, CA: North Atlantic Books.

McGlone, F., Wessberg, J. & Olaussof, H. (2014). Discriminative and affective touch: Sensing and feeling. *Neuron*, 82(4): 737–755.

Mehling, W.E. *et al.* (2012). The Multidimensional Assessment of Internal Awareness (MAIA). *PLoS One*, 7(11): 1–22.

Payne, P., Levine, P.A. & Crane-Godreau, M.A. (2015). Somatic experiencing: Using interoception and proprioception as core elements of trauma therapy. *Frontiers in Psychology*, 6: 93. doi:10.3389/fpsyg.2015.00093.

Porges, S.W. (2007). The polyvagal perspective. *Biological Psychology*, 74(2): 116–143. doi:10.1016/j.biopsycho.2006.06.009.

Porges, S.W. (2009). The polyvagal theory: New insights into adaptive reactions of the autonomic nervous system. *Cleveland Clinic Journal of Medicine*, 76(2): S86–S90. doi:10.3949/ccjm.76. s2.17.

Porges, S.W. & Furman, S.A. (2011). The early development of the autonomic nervous system provides a neural platform for social behavior: A polyvagal perspective. *Infant Child Development*, 20(1): 106–118. doi:10.1002/icd.688.

Rizzolatti, G. (2005). The mirror neuron system and its function in humans. *Anatomy and Embryology*, 210(5–6): 419–421.

Salzberg, S. (2015). What Does Mindfulness Really Mean Anyway? On Being. https://onbeing. org/blog/what-does-mindfulness-really-mean-anyway.

Schore, A. (2003a). *Affect Regulation and the Repair of the Self*. New York, NY: W.W. Norton & Company.

Schore, A. (2003b). *Affect Dysregulation and Disorders of the Self*. New York, NY: W.W. Norton & Company.

Siegel, D. (1999). *The Developing Mind: Toward a Neurobiology of Interpersonal Experience*. New York, NY: Guilford Press.

Siegel, D. (2015). *The Developing Mind* (second edition). New York, NY: Guilford Press.

van der Kolk, B.A. (2002). Beyond the Talking Cure: Somatic Experience, Subcortical Imprints and the Treatment of PTSD. In F. Shapiro (ed.), *EMDR as an Integrative Psychotherapy Approach: Experts of Diverse Orientations Explore the Paradigm Prism* (pp.57–83). Washington, DC: American Psychological Association.

van der Kolk, B.A. (2015). *The Body Keeps the Score*. New York, NY: Penguin Books.

Chapter 15

Watsupath-Craniosacral Therapy in Water™

Fascia as a System

ELISA MUÑOZ BLANCO

Chapter objectives

- To present clinicians with the anatomical, physiological, and biomechanical foundations of Craniosacral Therapy in Water, based on the state-of-the-art craniosacral and fascial systems.
- To change the paradigm of considering WATSU and Craniosacral Therapy in Water passive forms of aquatic therapy, using the emerging scientific evidence.
- To consider Craniosacral Therapy in Water in aquatic therapy practice by describing treatment principles and application techniques, specific indications, and contraindications.

Background

Craniosacral Therapy in Water is a subtle and profound concept that aims to promote the proper functioning of the craniosacral system (CSS), release the restrictions of the fascial system, and recover the hydrodynamic balance of the body, taking advantage of the thermal and mechanical properties of the aquatic environment.

It is based on the existence of a subtle rhythmic pulse that emerges in the tissues and fluids of the core of the body, the craniosacral rhythm (CSR). This rhythm can be perceived as a wave or a tide, a subtle respiratory movement in all the structures that compose the craniosacral system (brain, spinal cord, meninges, cranial bones, pelvis, and sacrum), and is transmitted to all the organs and tissues in the body.

The CSS has the vital role of maintaining the proper environment for the central nervous system (CNS). Knowing that brain and spinal cord are parts of the CNS, the CSS has a strong influence on a wide variety of functions in the body.

With a slight contact, a trained therapist can feel the pulsations of the CSR transmitted to the whole body through the fascial system. As every organ, every muscle, every vessel, nerve, bone, and so on is also part of this unique fascia, a restriction in them can alter the structure and its function.

Our therapeutic approach consists of helping the patient to restore the normal flow of movement through the attenuation or disappearance of these local or systemic restrictions, encouraging a better global state of health and balance.

Introduction
History
Craniosacral therapy was based on three laws described by Andrew Taylor Still, father of the osteopathic method: the unity and self-healing capacity of the body, and reciprocity between structure and function.

The craniosacral treatment method was developed in the early 1930s by William Garner Sutherland (1873–1954), father of cranial osteopathy. He focused his attention on the fluid components of the body, especially the cerebrospinal fluid (CSF), and observed that even the subtlest impulses on the fluids were able to remove dysfunctions of the most solid structures (Güeita Rodríguez et al. 2020). In the 1970s, craniosacral therapy was developed and structured by the osteopathic physician Dr. John E. Upledger, from his findings, and based on the discoveries of Dr. Sutherland (Upledger Institute International 2021b).

In 2002, I was working in the Canary Islands, Spain, as a physical therapist and spa manager in a Thalasso Center there. We had a flotation tank in which I started flirting with the application of craniosacral therapy in the water while beginning my training with Upledger Institute.

It was also when I first experienced WATSU. A German therapist came to the spa, and with me as receiver and him giving a demonstration, I completely fell in love with WATSU. At that moment, I knew that was my path.

In February 2005, I had a severe car accident and that was the final trigger to start my WATSU training. It was also the moment I really deepened into Vipassana meditation practice and came back to yoga. One year later I took a flight to India and started my WATSU training at WATSU Goa.

I became a WATSU practitioner in 2008 and started giving sessions in a beautiful and deep pool. I'm not a tall person, 1.65m tall, and this pool was 1.40m deep. This fact forced me to bring more and more craniosacral therapy into my sessions. Amazingly, it became natural that both WATSU and CST melded together, and this new reality brought my practice to the next level.

In 2009, CST in Water was introduced as part of the program in the Expertise of Aquatic Physical Therapy at the European University of Madrid, and in 2010 at the Expertise of Aquatic Therapy of Rey Juan Carlos University of Madrid, which continues today. By that time, the Worldwide Aquatic Bodywork Association (WABA) credited CST in Water as a continuing education program, so I developed a full training path and also started teaching abroad.

That made me decide to register the contents with the Registry of Intellectual Property, which I presented in 2010 and was granted in 2011. It was the year I became a Basic WATSU instructor.

CST in Water was growing as a dynamic concept, and in 2012 the Watsupath-CST in Water trademark was created!

In 2014, the same year that Watsupath was registered as a credited training institute, the Education Standards Advisory Committee approved CST in Water as an elective class under WABA, and that opened the spectrum beyond limits.

In January 2015, I was asked to include a chapter about CST in Water in the book *Aquatic Therapy. Approaches from Physiotherapy and Occupational Therapy in the Aquatic Environment* and again for the second edition in October 2020 (Güeita Rodríguez *et al.* 2020). This was an important step in the practice being seen by health practitioners as a specific method of aquatic therapy intervention in raising its profile in the international arena.

During these years I continued my trainings both on land and in water. I was certified in other disciplines, and it was fun to observe how the awareness of the subtleness of all fluids in the body were incorporated into my practice.

It was also in 2015 that I started working as physical therapist in a special education school, both on land and in water. It was something new for me, as until that moment I had never worked before with cerebral palsy (CP) patients or other neuromotor disorders.

These children, their families, and the professionals I worked with completely changed my life. They taught me how to speak a deeper language of understanding, compassion, and unconditional support.

In 2016, I enrolled in a Master of Science in Pediatrics course to gather more tools to help them. The final project, which was conducted at the school, aimed to describe the experience of children and youth with CP participating in an aquatic therapy program within a special education school, with consideration given to their educational and therapeutic perspectives. A qualitative descriptive case study was developed. It was a powerful team effort and we learned so much from it. I will always be thankful for everyone involved in it, but specially to the children and families who opened themselves up to me and the water (Muñoz Blanco *et al.* 2020).

The Watsupath and CST in Water Training Program is now available in Hungary, Czech Republic, UK, Germany, Italy, France, Portugal, Argentina, Costa Rica, Mexico, and the United States, and it is a specific intervention method of reference in the field of aquatic therapy.

Due to all these events, I now see in my body, mind, heart, and soul that CST in Water transcends me and was meant to happen, so this chapter is evidence of that, and is why I am presenting the facts as you are reading them now.

Definition

Craniosacral Therapy in Water was born as a concept in 2010, as the result of my years of study, research, and clinical practice. I used to define it as a "powerful and subtle method, designed to balance the CSR and release restrictions of the connective tissue throughout the body, taking advantage of mechanical and thermal properties of the aquatic media" (Muñoz Blanco 2010).

As there weren't sessions equal to another and no recipes nor magic formula could be given to students, I soon realized that rather than a method it should be understood and integrated as a concept on which patients, students, practitioners, and instructors could rely.

Based on the application of WATSU therapy, craniosacral therapy (CST), manual therapy, and Myofascial Induction Therapy (MIT)® in the aquatic environment, CST in Water facilitates interoception, and produces local and systemic effects aimed at improving and restoring the overall health of the patient. This concept aims to promote the proper functioning of the craniosacral system, release the restrictions of connective tissue, and recover the hydrodynamic balance of the body.

CST in Water brings CST techniques with WATSU tools flowing as a continuum, a unique and inward shared journey for patient and therapist (Güeita Rodríguez *et al.* 2020). Both WATSU and CST are based on common principles: listening to the subtlest physiological rhythms, facilitating spontaneous movements and body tendencies, observing the needs, respecting the limits, and framing the therapeutic intervention from an attitude of *being* with the patient, and not *doing* to the patient (Muñoz Blanco 2010), as Sutherland used to name *complete emptiness* (Sutherland 1962).

WATSU provides constant elongation, symmetry, and alignment of the head through support, fluidity in transitions, correct positioning, and body management in all dimensions, while the therapist remains aligned, invisible, alert, and connected.

CST in Water gives us the facilitation by an intentioned light touch of the therapist and the mechanical and thermal stimuli, constant in the aquatic milieu. The application of the deeper techniques makes the reorganization of the tissue acquire a three-dimensional character, without the limits found on land (Güeita Rodríguez 2020). Interoceptive awareness of the patient, suspended and surrounded by water, guides the process, and is followed by the therapist's facilitation.

All these factors create the ideal frame for correction, allowing the homeostasis of the body to occur, in an environment of real listening and presence in which the patient can surrender and trust.

Principles in the therapeutic approach
The therapist's attitude

The already accepted Tensegrity Model (Liem 2006) as a human body model presented the body as a three-dimensional structure expanding from cellular to extracellular level. In this model of biotensegrity, liquid elements were not taken into consideration. By integrating solid and liquid fascia, we are now considering the fascial continuum with the lymph and blood in a new model.

The name given to this new model is Rapid Adaptability of Internal Network (RAIN). Bodily fluids are silent witnesses to mechanotransductive (Pilat 2022) information, allowing adaptation and life, transporting biochemical and hormonal signals. While the solid fascial tissue divides, supports, and connects the different parts of the body system, the liquid fascial tissue feeds and transports messages for the solid fascia (Bordoni, Lintonbon, & Morabito 2018).

On the other hand, knowing that every part of physical body, mind, soul, and the emotions are interconnected and interacting, the biopsychosocial model is inadequate, as it is often applied in a fragmented manner, and through that, although unintentionally, perpetuates dualistic and reductionist beliefs. Considering the limitations of the pain theories, an enactive approach to pain has been explored as an alternative big picture framework.

Informed by established theory and research by phenomenologists and cognitive scientists, pain was described as: embodied, embedded, enacted, emotive, and extended. Overall, with an enactive approach, pain does not reside in a mysterious immaterial mind, nor is it entirely to be found in the blood, brain, or other bodily tissues. Instead, it is a relational and emergent process of sense-making through a lived body that is inseparable from the world that we shape and that shapes us (Stilwell & Harman 2019).

Throughout all these concepts, I am guiding you here to understand the importance of treating craniosacral and fascial systems.

Our gentle approach helps to normalize the craniosacral system and allows the body to self-correct. By unraveling pain and dysfunction at the source, we naturally help eliminate stress, strengthen resistance to disease, and enhance health in every dimension. Applying CST in the water multiplies its therapeutic effects in this state of decreased gravity where hydrostatic pressure awakes corrective movement in the body.

CST in Water is the best form of treatment for the fascial system because in the suppression of gravity the underlying traumatic pattern can be better expressed. In addition, water as a great facilitator aids the learning process of the explorer and the sensitivity of palpation needed to feel the craniosacral rhythm, the life breath (Muñoz Blanco 2010).

Especially when we are beginners it is essential to remain relaxed and not try too hard. Any tension in the therapist's body will be reflected in the patient's body, so find a posture that is stable, clear, alert, and energetically aligned. Remind yourself that the patient comes for help in the self-healing process, not for "curing" in the sense that the therapist "fixes" her (Muñoz Blanco 2010).

CST in Water attempts to maximize the patient's responsibility for their overall well-being, freeing the patient from dependence on any type of health-care provider. Constantly scan yourself, making sure that your physical and mental attitudes are appropriate.

Interoception

Transpersonal psychology uses seven levels of the experiential scale to move from felt sensation to self-awareness, through the process of experiencing in the body, by focusing and unveiling, and the creation of meaning (Gendlin 1975, 1997, 1999a, 1999b). I found this process very similar to what our patients experience with CST in Water, or what we achieve with Vipassana meditation, and I was fascinated to find out how more and more evidence was supporting these ideas.

While working with people suffering from various conditions over the years, including psychosomatic, orthopedic, musculoskeletal, vascular, and neuro-logical, I could witness their life-changing processes through the work, just by experiencing their bodies in warm water while they were being sustained, listened to, encountered, and facilitated in a very specific way.

How could WATSU or CST in Water be considered passive forms of aquatic bodywork if there were all these learning processes occurring during and after the sessions? Studying the latest research about interoception (the perception of the body's internal state) and interoceptive awareness has allowed me to understand better the complex mechanisms of the body and start to explain how WATSU and CST in Water are not passive forms of aquatic therapy as the scientific community was insisting.

Many mindfulness practices involve sustained attention to interoceptive sensations of respiration or bodily sensation, designed to improve the stability and frequency with which one perceives the transitory nature of human experience.

Neuroplasticity research has focused predominantly on attention to external stimuli, when findings suggest that the development of interoceptive attention (IA) may be one foundation by which mindfulness training (MT) promotes cognitive change (Farb, Segal, & Anderson 2013).

In anatomically partitioned analyses of insula activity, MT predicted greater IA-related activity in anterior dysgranular insula regions, consistent with greater integration of interoceptive sensation with external context.

Research indicates that interoceptive training modulates task-specific cortical recruitment, analogous to training-related plasticity observed in the external senses. Further, modulation of IA networks may be an important mechanism by which MT alters information processing in the brain, increasing the contribution of interoception to perceptual experience (Farb *et al.* 2013).

It has been suggested that individual differences in interoception can be divided into three distinct dimensions: interoceptive accuracy (performance on objective tests of interoceptive accuracy), interoceptive sensibility (self-reported beliefs concerning one's own interoception) and interoceptive awareness (a metacognitive measure indexed by the correspondence between interoceptive accuracy and interoceptive sensibility) (Murphy, Catmur, & Bird 2019).

An accurate perception and interpretation of autonomic changes may lead to emotional experiences that are easy to understand and to regulate, whereas an inaccurate perception and interpretation of autonomic changes may lead to emotional experiences that are difficult to understand and to regulate. Individuals who are more accurate in interoception are generally more efficient in the regulation of their emotional experiences, regardless of whether they re-interpret the emotional experience via reappraisal strategies or inhibit the emotional experience via suppression strategies (Murphy *et al.* 2019).

This is very important for us to know and be aware of while holding our patients in water, while listening to their body tendencies as well as the way we use therapeutic dialogue either before, during, or after the session.

In recent research, while interoceptive training resulted in significant enhancement of interoceptive accuracy scores and significant reductions in somatic symptom and state anxiety scores, in contrast, it did not cause significant changes in decision-making indices (Sugawara 2020). This indicates that the relationship between interoception and emotion regulation is far more complex than suggested in other research.

All this supports the view that interoception is essential for both the regulation and experience of emotions (Lischke 2020). The clinical implications of all these investigations support the fact that a patient receiving CST in Water as well as WATSU is not passive at all.

In our therapeutic approach, various mechanisms are occurring that will create permanent changes to the self-image of the body, both for patient and therapist: local modifications in the tissues, changes in conscious and unconscious perception (exteroceptive, proprioceptive, nociceptive, and interoceptive) that modulate pain through central and autonomous nervous systems. Let me discuss all of them step by step.

We as therapists aim to optimize movement and behavior by optimizing efficacy and efficiency, with efficacy referring to the ability of the body to do what it is designed to do, and efficiency to the economy and effort required for the structure and its function.

How do we know that the patient has a balance between effectiveness and efficiency? By listening, sensing, and assessing the various physiological rhythms of the body. Breath, heartbeat, cranial rhythmic impulse (also used to name CSR), lymphatic rhythm, astrocyte calcium waves…all this is happening simultaneously and autonomously in our bodies.

Sensibilization of the system will compromise effectiveness and efficiency as far as more structures are forced to compensate for the energy that needs to be spent. Not only will systemic processes compromise our systems with a big amount of energy and effort, but a dysfunction that is local at first can end up being systemic because of the many locals met in the evolution of the disease, dysfunction, or crisis.

The "neutral state" of the therapist, according to Jim Jealous, founder of Biodynamic Osteopathy, is comparable with a concert in which the different instruments of the orchestra come together to create music; the reciprocal tensions in the body and the aspects of the body, mind, and spirit are united in the "neutral state," forming a homogeneous body-mind-spirit unity. In this state, the patient's globality is particularly accessible and receptive.

Thus, the so-called "breath of life" can enter in the most effective way into interaction with the patient, and a direct reaction of the patient to the forces of the so-called tidal movements is facilitated. This state creates the easiest possible conditions for healing and transforming dysfunctional models (Liem 2009).

The "neutral state" requires the therapist to provide the least amount of strength to put a technique into practice. In addition, the amount of force to be applied to carry out a technique and the time at which the end of the technique has been reached is most clearly perceived.

The negative consequences of a treatment are minimized and the patient himself perceives the changes in his body. In some rare cases, the neutral state is not reached. This usually occurs after loss of consciousness or extreme violence, resulting in an extreme dissociation between body, mind, and spirit. According to Jealous, the indication in these cases is the application of the Compression of the IV Ventricle (CV-4) technique, which I will describe later.

Palpation—the power of touch

Palpation is a mechanical induction (with perpendicular or tangential pressure) towards a static (solid) and hydrostatic (liquid) tissue, within a specific period. It is an important part of the physical examination, a manual exploration of the tactile perception (Bordoni & Simonelli 2018).

When first approaching the craniosacral system, place your hands on the body as quietly as possible. Begin with your hands on rather than in the tissue, resting in the interface between the surface of the skin and the atmosphere, between "self" and "not self."

Picture yourself as a water spider perched on the surface tension of the water. Be still and receptive. If you begin your therapeutic interaction with your patient in this way, you will have the wisdom of her body to assist your own. After a short time, the proprioceptive tract will extend itself across your sensorimotor cortex and connect with the motor function (Muñoz Blanco 2010).

Touch has been always regarded as a powerful communication channel, playing a key role in governing our emotional well-being and possibly perception of self. The sense of touch is divided into two major categories: proprioceptive and interoceptive (affective), activated by distinct mechanisms with cerebral correlates in the somatosensory and insular cortex, respectively.

As far as the interoceptive aspect is concerned, the insula is known to be part of the interoceptive/salience neural network; it integrates information from multiple brain regions, processing sensations ranging from physiologically driven motivational states to emotional awareness to somatosensory stimuli, including touch, which serves to maintain interoceptive homeostasis.

Passive and active palpation

The pressure applied in CST in Water is minimal, since this compression stimulus, with only a few grams of pressure, will correspond to a passive palpation, which is necessary to appreciate the physiological movement of the organism in a relatively resting state (Güeita Rodríguez 2020).

Active palpation utilizes the application of digital pressure (Pacinian corpuscles) or movement to assess parameters such as range of motion, pain sensitivity, shape, consistency, and muscle tension, and may induce a response or movement in the subject.

Passive palpation utilizes minimal pressure and movement so that the physiologic motion of the whole organism can be appreciated in a relatively undisturbed state.

In developing appreciation of the CSR and other subtle motions of the organism, passive palpation is the choice. Active palpation used inappropriately may also induce a defensive tension response in the neuromuscular structures of the subject, and this tension will tend to interfere with the tissue's ability to transmit the inherent wave activity accurately. Lastly, motion on the part of the therapist/facilitator involves motor activity of the palpating hand and competes with the perception of the sensory tracts.

The tactile perception system gathers information about the environment using mechanoreceptors and thermoreceptors residing in the skin, as well as the deeper mechanoreceptors located in the myofascial and articular system. The palm of the hand has specific receptors, which permit you to determine the size of the palpated tissue (Meissner corpuscle and Merkel cell complex) and understand the tissue's ability to deform under a rapid or continuous touch (Ruffini and Pacinian corpuscles).

Gentle touch sensation in mammals depends on synaptic transmission from primary sensory cells (Merkel cells) to secondary sensory neurons (Fechner & Goodman 2018). Hoffman *et al.* (2018) identified norepinephrine and b2-adrenergic receptors as the neurotransmitter-receptor pair responsible for sustained touch responses. Results identify both pre- and postsynaptic mechanisms through which Merkel cells excite mechanosensory afferents to encode gentle touch (Fechner & Goodman 2018).

As a sensory-neural organ, skin provides both a protective barrier and an environmental interface that allows organisms to react to changing conditions. Signaling between epithelial cells and somatosensory neurons shapes touch, itch, nociception, and chemoreception. Since their initial description as "touch cells," Merkel cells have served as the archetypical skin cell that mediates somatosensation.

Inspection and palpation activate the superior and inferior parietal lobules in the operator's cortex. The present findings extend this pathway from primary somatosensory cortex (S1) to the insular cortex by prefrontal and posterior parietal areas involved in multisensory integration and attention processes (Rullmann, Preusser, & Pleger 2019).

Palpation is part of a personal experiential memory bank useful to find tissue anomalies, and it is a manual art. As with all arts, the result is not always reproducible in the same way. But this doesn't mean that what you feel isn't real! Sometimes it just means we haven't found the way to measure what we're feeling.

This is exactly what has happened with CST (in water and on land) and myofascial release. It has taken decades to count on the tools and research able to prove our clinical findings, and we're still in the process, but we can't lose our perseverance, curiosity, confidence, and trust!

We are not a soul that can be split from a body, nor is our body superimposed parts, nor are we formed by an intellect inserted in a compendium of muscles, bones and organs, nor are we separated from our own body; on the contrary,

I am not in front of my body, I am in my body, or better, I am my body. Our self is an embodied self. (Barceló 2013, p.273)

State-of-the-art craniosacral system (CSS) and fascial system

I will now look at some consistent and recent findings about the mechanisms that explain this cranial rhythmic impulse. It will help us to understand how our body is constructed in a way that every piece contributes to the system and all the systems work in favor of balance and homeostasis.

The cranial membrane system

Remember that the central nervous system is protected by skeletal elements: the spine and skull; and a system of membranes interposed between the CNS and those elements of bone, the meninges: dura, arachnoid, and pia mater.

The dura mater, the outer meningeal layer, completely envelops the neuro-axis from the vault to the sacral canal, and it is named topographically as the cranial and spinal dura mater. The cranial dura mater is attached to the inside of the skull bones and has extensions or partitions into the cranial cavity to hold in place the different parts of the CNS.

On its continuum, the spinal dura mater completely encloses the spinal cord. The foramen magnum is the place of transition between the cranial and spinal dura. The dura, starting from the cranial vault, is inserted into the fora-men in the vertebral bodies of C2 and C3. It runs freely through the spinal canal to S2 and inserts also at the coccyx.

So, there is a connection between very distal segments in the body such as the cranium and the sacrum that communicate and move together, and this is the foundation of craniosacral therapy. Notice the very relevant places where this dura is firmly attached!

Another important component of this system is the cerebrospinal fluid (CSF), the fluid habitat of the CNS, and a highly specific fluid for the most sensitive organ. It is the role of CSF to provide the environment that is best suited for the survival and proper function of the brain and spinal cord. It is considered the most important center of the activity of the organism (Liem 2009).

The craniosacral system
Primary respiratory mechanism

Sutherland discovered that the bones of the head had some mobility. Over the next 50 years he devoted his life and clinical work to demonstrating the implications that this mobility had for the human body. In the later years of his life, he revealed his most advanced theories, presenting the concept of "breath of life" as the vital force expressed in the human system by the inherent principle of order and healing. It can be perceived as a subtle mobility, or "tide," throughout the body, forming what is called the "primary respiratory mechanism" (Liem 2009).

The primary respiratory mechanism is in some way considered the engine that allows the involuntary subtle movements in the body (Muñoz Blanco 2010). It consists of the following factors:

1. Motility (inherent and independent movement) of the brain and spinal cord.
2. Fluctuation of the cerebrospinal fluid.
3. Mobility of the intracranial and intraspinal membranes.
4. Mobility of the skull bones.
5. Involuntary mobility of the sacrum between the pelvic bones.

We describe craniosacral rhythm as a rhythmic impulse that occurs 6–12 cycles/minute throughout the body, with a flexion phase and an extension phase.

We now know that there are different mechanisms behind CSR, and we still need higher quality studies (Güeita Rodríguez *et al.* 2020). Blood pressure and blood flow velocity present low-frequency rhythmic oscillations related to so-called Traube-Hering-Mayer (THM) oscillations or waves. This theory is consistent with the phenomenon of rhythmic movement of tissues practiced in cranial osteopathy (Güeita Rodríguez *et al.* 2020).

Researchers are discovering that CSR might be also related to the extracellular matrix dynamics, piezoelectricity of collagen, drainage of lymph, cerebrospinal fluid, interstitial, venous, and lymphatic fluid, polymerization and depolymerization of hyaluronic acid, hypothalamic-pituitary-adrenergic axis activity (cortisol, polyvagal theory), and homeostasis and allostasis (Pilat 2022).

I will do my best to synthetize and give a global perspective on how the body works as a system under this biotensegrity model.

The fascial system

Fascia is a colloid, and it was defined as comprising particles of solid material, suspended in fluid. Histologically, connective tissue comprises stationary cells (fibroblasts, telocytes, fasciacytes) and free cells (macrophages and mast cells, engaged in immunity), as well as extracellular matrix (elastin, collagen, reticulin fibers, and fundamental substance). Each one of the specialized components of fascia gives unique and multiple characteristics and functions.

The amount of resistance that colloids offer to load increases proportionally to the velocity of force application. This is the thixotropy property of colloid, which means that the more rapidly force is applied, the more rigidly will the tissue respond.

Chemically it is collagen in the fascia that allows its change. Collagen can change from fluid to solid state and from solid to fluid in response to the force acting on it. With chronic stress the collagen tends to be reduced, shorten, and harden. It won't return to its initial liquid state without external intervention. (Pilat 2003, p.97)

Fascia has a global presence throughout the body; it is involved in almost all aspects of dysfunction and disease, either as an effect or as a cause. It connects structures, providing the scaffolding that permits and enhances transmission and absorption of forces. It also has sensory functions, and on the microscopic level is engaged in individual cell-to-cell communication (Guimberteau, Delage, & Wong 2010).

Ultimately, fascia provides the facility for tissues to slide and glide on each other and offers a means of energy storage, acting in a spring-like manner, via pre-stressed tensegrity structures such as the large tendon and aponeuroses of the leg, during the gait-cycle (Findley & Shalwala 2013).

Physical and chemical communication processes that take place between specialized cells, such as fibroblasts and telocytes, and the soup-like extracellular matrix network in which they function, amazingly result in changes in gene expression and inflammatory responses.

A seamless web of connective tissues that covers, supports, and penetrates the viscera is part of the fascial system. Although the difference between the cells in different tissues is evident, their behavior in the case of mechanical stress is very similar. Cellular deformation makes the cell aware of what happens inside it and in the environment in which it lives, resulting in behaviors that can anticipate the deformation (Boccafoschi *et al.* 2010).

We know all cells present in the liquid and solid fascial system have electromagnetic fields stimulated by membrane deformation. The ions exchanged during an action potentially make a change in the cell volume, causing cell deformation and inducing a transient electromagnetic field. This mechanism creates microwaves, which radiate to other cell membranes influencing the rotation or the orientation of electrons and affecting other electromagnetic fields (Bordoni & Simonelli 2018).

A cell communicates with the other cells by sending and receiving signals; this concept is part of quantum physics, and it is known as quantum entanglement: a physical system cannot be described individually, but only as a juxtaposition of multiple systems, and the measurement of a quantity determines the value for other systems. According to quantum theory, each element has a non-hierarchical form of organization, and it only responds when necessary (mechanical and metabolic stimulation).

This brings me to the last steps of this section.

The primo vascular system

In the early 1960s, one hypothesis was proposed to explain the anatomical basis of the meridians. Over the past ten years, the number of scientific papers that report anatomical and physiological evidence confirming the existence of an anatomical basis for the meridian system has increased.

The primo vascular system (PVS) is a previously unknown system that integrates the features of the cardio-vascular, nervous, immune, and hormonal systems. It also provides a physical substrate for acupuncture points and meridians. Announcements of the morphological architectonics and the function of the PVS fundamentally changed the basic understanding of biology and medicine because the PVS is involved in the development and the functions of living organisms.

This system consists of a dense network of primo vessels (PVs) and primo nodes (PNs) that is distributed throughout the entire body (Stefanov *et al.* 2013; Stefanov & Jungdae 2012). The DNA contained in the primo vascular fluid provides genetic information and it functions as a store of information that can be obtained from the electromagnetic fields of the environment.

The PVS is the communication system between living organisms and the environment and is a "reservoir of life."

Polyvagal theory

Lastly, I'd like to correlate CST in Water with polyvagal theory. In CST in Water, we frequently experience regional unwinding and SomatoEmotional Release (SER®). Spontaneous release by positioning is another concept that comes to us from osteopathy (see Figures 15.1 and 15.2). It serves as a foundation for applications that are profound and have yet to be fully explained.

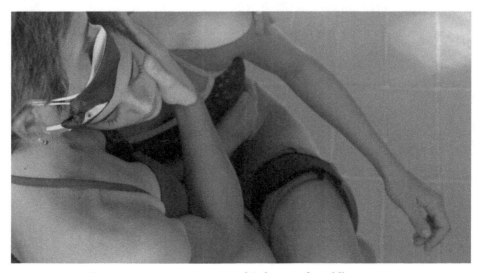

Figure 15.1: SomatoEmotional Release: side saddle position

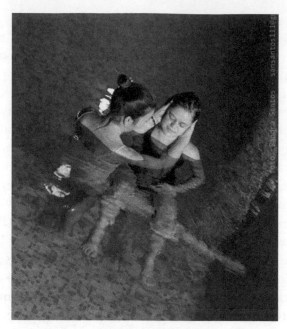

Figure 15.2: SER®

If the trauma has sufficient impact, which may be physical, mental, or emotional, it can become locked into the holding pattern of the tissue. This response is registered into the neurostructure partially as the configuration of body position at the time of impact. If the configuration can be recaptured (or reconjured), the body can be given the chance to release this configuration of holding and free up some autonomic reserve, as illustrated in Figure 15.3.

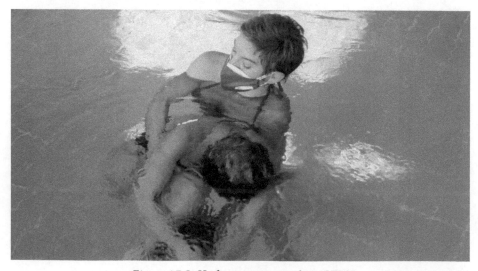

Figure 15.3: Underwater unwinding: SER®

Polyvagal theory basically emphasizes that our nervous system has more than one defense strategy and the selection of whether we use a mobilized fight/flight or an immobilization shutdown defense strategy is not a voluntary decision (Porges 2017).

Our nervous system is continuously evaluating risk in the environment, making judgments, and setting up priorities for behaviors that are adaptive, but not cognitive. For some people, specific physical characteristics of an environmental challenge will trigger a fight/flight behavior, while others may totally shut down in response to the exact same physical features in the environment. And we must understand that it is the response, and not the traumatic event, that is critical.

Appropriate populations/contraindications

By complementing the body's natural healing processes, CST is increasingly used as a preventive health measure for its ability to bolster resistance to disease and for a wide range of medical problems associated with chronic pain and dysfunction, including migraines and tension-type headaches, chronic neck and low back pain, chronic fatigue, fibromyalgia, pelvic girdle pain, and lateral epicondylitis (Haller *et al.* 2020), anxiety and depression, dementia, stress and tension-related disorders, motor-coordination impairments, infant and childhood disorders (Harrison & Page 2011; Gerdner, Hart, & Zimmerman 2008; McManus & Gliksten 2007), multiple sclerosis (Raviv *et al.* 2009), malocclusion and TMJ Syndrome (Green *et al.* 1999), whiplash (Ventegodt *et al.* 2004), learning disabilities, autism, ADD/ADHD (attention deficit and hyperactivity disorder) (Wanveer 2007; Weber & Newmark 2007), post-traumatic stress disorder, scoliosis, orthopedic problems, and many other conditions (Upledger Institute International 2021b).

In the study carried out by Fernández-Pérez *et al.* (2008), in which the suboccipital technique, the CV-4 technique (IV ventricle compression technique), and the deep cervical fascial technique were applied, a decrease in anxiety was observed in the experimental group. Heart rate and systolic blood pressure were modulated during the techniques, and all these effects were maintained for up to 20 minutes after therapy.

Research was developed in 2018 to investigate aquatic myofascial release effects on flexibility and delayed onset muscle soreness after high intensity exercises. It was concluded that it is effective to reduce pain perception and to improve flexibility of the studied population submitted to a high intense exercise session (Lêdo *et al.* 2018).

In 2017, we conducted a qualitative study in our special education school (Muñoz Blanco *et al.* 2020). This study aimed to describe and analyze the impact of an aquatic therapeutic proposal on children with cerebral palsy, on their families, and on professionals with whom they related. The intervention described consisted of Halliwick-Water Specific Therapy, WATSU and CST in Water, depending on the needs of each patient (Güeita Rodríguez *et al.* 2020).

Data was collected via non-participant observation, semi-structured and informal interviews, focus groups, and researcher field notes. A thematic analysis was conducted, revealing the following themes: (a) the connection with the environment; (b) postural improvements and mobility; (c) the opportunity to perform tasks; (d) learning and transfer. Participants described health, learning, and participation benefits. The benefits collected included normalization of tone, decreased spasticity, strengthening, autonomy and self-determination, and increased concentration. The professionals reported minimal risks, numerous benefits, and high adherence.

These findings may enhance understanding regarding the potential benefits of implementing multidisciplinary aquatic therapy programs in specialist school settings. CST in Water always improves movement in all systems throughout the body. Therefore, there are no situations where it should not be applied, except where the results are undesirable for some reason.

Relative contraindications

There are certain situations where application of CST would not be recommended. These include conditions where a variation and/or slight increase in intracranial pressure would cause instability. Acute aneurysm, cerebral hemorrhage, or other pre-existing severe bleeding disorders are examples of conditions that could be affected by small intracranial pressure changes (Upledger Institute International 2021a), and for the same reasons leaks of CSF after epidural anesthesia, or hydrocephalus.

We need to be cautious and respect recovery time for fractures and soft tissue injuries in the acute phase, and open wounds, inflammatory soft tissue states, infectious diseases, and febrile states, as for any other type of aquatic therapy.

In acute circulatory deficiencies, advanced phlebitis, and osteomyelitis, we might not apply this therapy or be very careful with doses, following the important rule: "less is more."

We also take doses into consideration in patients being treated with corticosteroid and anticoagulant therapy, and patients with hemophilia and advanced diabetes, and we are especially careful in periods when their medications are being adjusted. Malignant cancer, leukemia, and Hodgkin lymphoma used to be absolute contraindications. You'll see in testimonials that when haemopoietic levels are balanced, in some cases, when the state of the patient is appropriate, under medical recommendation it can be an indication. We have seen that in clinical practice we can improve health and boost the immune system, and research is starting to go in this direction too.

Osteoporosis in advanced stage, as well as osteosynthesis, is a relative contraindication as we could cause a fracture in the first case and displacement in the second.

Skin hypersensitivity or allergies to components of the water and lack of acceptance by the patient are other considerations.

The application of these techniques is not recommended for elite athletes two or three days before competition, as the profound changes the body is integrating may prevent the athlete reaching their peak performance in the 48–72 hours after the session.

"Pearls for practice" (principles, treatment techniques, and additional indications)

The objectives of the therapy are to increase joint mobility, reduce membranous tension, improve circulation, reduce nerve compromises, and improve the qualities of CSR. The techniques used will have local and global effects and will be aimed at restoring the health and well-being of the patient. We are aware that dysfunction in the craniosacral system may be primary or secondary.

Therefore, depending on the need, direct methods can be applied (where the barrier is reached and we apply a force in the direction of correction), or we can use indirect action techniques (we maintain the neutral position while applying the activation force) or, more frequently, exaggeration methods (in favor of the barrier) (Muñoz Blanco *et al.* 2020).

From the moment we stand in front of our patient in the water, before accompanying him in flotation, we connect with his CSR to evaluate how it is perceived in his forearms or wrists (Güeita Rodríguez *et al.* 2020). We establish the triangle of head support and accompany the patient in flotation. This will be another opportunity to reconnect with the breath and cranial rhythmic impulse, to accompany them and let them express themselves in this new situation.

We both create this long and single move, this continuum. And we, therapists, observe, feel, and perceive all the signals that the inner intelligence of the body is giving us.

WATSU will help us release the most superficial restrictions so that inner spontaneous movements can be expressed, as well as restrictions. Assessment and treatment of the CSS may continue during the session in any part of the body linked to the primary cause.

Balancing the dural tube

This technique is used not only to evaluate, but also to normalize, dural tube dysfunctions. With the patient in flotation, we place one hand on the base of the occipital and the other on the base of the sacrum, as we do "distant stillness," shown in Figure 15.4. We feel the CSR and stimulate a gentle swing between the two, so that, when the sacrum reaches flexion, we will induce it to go a little more to flexion, and when the skull reaches extension, we will induce it to go a little more to extension.

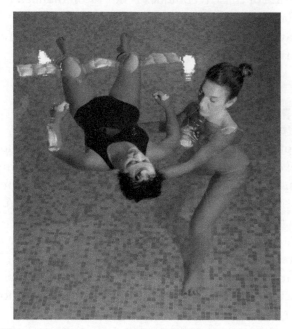

Figure 15.4: Balancing the dural tube from both extremes

The most frequent injury is an anomaly in the tension of the membranes system. Collagen fibers are organized and align in the direction of the tension. This influences its elasticity and affects the tension grade of the membranes on the bones of the skull to which they are attached (Harrison & Page 2011).

The absence of a free movement in any of the bones of the skull indicates a perturbation of the system. Bony restrictions are rigid and produce a lack of movement in the sutures, while membranous restrictions are flexible and are felt as an elastic band.

The release of membranous restriction is achieved through a smooth and sustained traction. As a result of the correction, the physiological movement between the bones of the skull is restored (Harrison & Page 2011).

Some signals we feel in the body while the therapeutic process is taking place are softening and lengthening of the collagen fibers, increase of liquid fluid, increase of energy flow, heat, improved symmetry of CSR, therapeutic pulse, deep breathing (sigh), or changes in the breathing pattern.

Still point induction (Muñoz Blanco 2010)

The still point feels like a "shutting down" of the CSS and can be interpreted as representing a neurologic opportunity for processing autonomic change.

It is appropriate at any phase of treatment but may be induced either near the beginning of treatment, where it serves to encourage receptivity in the patient's nervous system, or at the conclusion of treatment, where it serves to allow the integration of changes elicited in the neurostructure.

Still point on the cranium: CV-4 (Muñoz Blanco 2010)

This could be considered the most interventionist technique and you should not perform it unless you are properly trained. To induce a CV-4 we cradle the head with cupped hands so that mastoid processes rest externally to our thenar eminences and our fingers extend caudally along the neck, as illustrated in Figure 15.5. We touch our thumbs together as we listen for the cranial rhythm.

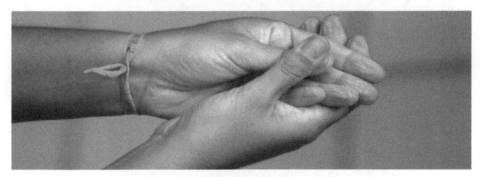

Figure 15.5: Still point on the cranium: CV-4, hand positioning

Indications for CV-4

The CV-4 is used as a technique to balance the CSS. It helps to remove minor restrictions with only a few applications in series and has a profound effect on the ANS, inducing profound relaxation. Any CNS hyperactivity suggests a still point. It also improves the exchange of fluid between body compartments, and increases blood flow by reducing sympathetic tone. It helps with any acute pain, has a cleansing effect of metabolic toxins, and can reduce fever by 1° C or so.

Contraindications for CV-4

- Acute stroke
- Increased intracranial pressure

- Herniated nucleus pulposus
- Skull fractures and recent whiplash
- Cerebral aneurysm
- Leak in the dural tube.

Once the stiffness of the cranial vault has decreased, we can evaluate and treat the base of the skull, and more specifically the sphenobasilar synchondrosis.

The sphenobasilar synchondrosis compression-decompression technique

The sphenoid is the most important bone of the cranial vault and, of course, of the entire craniosacral system (Harrison & Page 2011). The sphenobasilar synchondrosis compression-decompression technique aims to release meningeal stresses and the horizontal membrane system (see Figure 15.6).

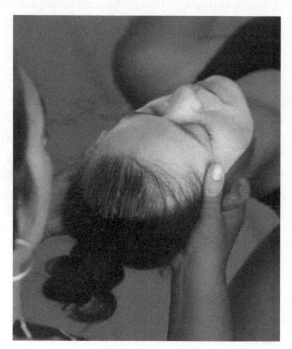

Figure 15.6: Compression-decompression of sphenobasilar synchondrosis

It is necessary to explore and treat the craniofacial complex, due to its important anatomofunctional relationships, as is the case with the temporomandibular joint.

Knowing the strong inserts of the dura, it will be vital to find out if they are free of movement in the three dimensions of space. Some of the cranial base release techniques and sacrolumbar release techniques may be applied until the sensation of change in tissue viscoelasticity is felt.

Occipital cranial base release (Muñoz Blanco 2010)

The occipital cranial base is a region of the body where there are increased cross-oriented myofascial tissues. The occipital articulates with the atlas, and atlas and axis are linked to form a functional unit. Movement between atlas and occipital is primarily flexion and extension, and between atlas and axis is mostly rotation.

From the point of view of their structural connection, myodural bridges constitute the most important relay of intracranial and extracranial tissues. It is a tissue that directly joins the suboccipital musculature (posterior rectus major, posterior rectum minor, and inferior oblique muscles) with the dura mater in the space between the occipital and the first cervical vertebra. Remember that it is at this cervical level where the transmission of neurological impulses from the brain to the rest of the body is carried out, connecting to the peripheral nervous system (Güeita Rodríguez *et al.* 2020).

Ideally, we apply this technique while slowly walking backwards so we maintain a drag that facilitates alignment and traction, although it can also be applied with the therapist resting at the wall as shown in Figure 15.7.

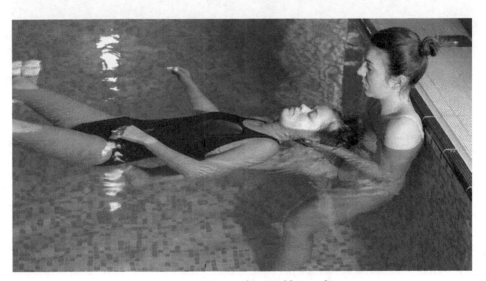

Figure 15.7: Occipital cranial base release

Indications:

- Cranial nerves IX, X, XI (glossopharyngeal, vagus, spinal accessory)
- Hyperkinesis

- Dyslexia
- Increased sympathetic tone
- Headache
- Headache and irrigation problems related to decreased blood flow
- Sacrum shock
- Sixth and seventh chakras.

Fascia and diaphragms

The orientation of the strong connective tissue in its depth is especially dense and cross-sectional in the feet, pelvic diaphragm, respiratory diaphragm, thoracic entrance, hyoid bone, and cranial base. Each of the restrictions on these body vortices can be treated to improve symmetry in the reciprocal tension membrane system.

Neutralizing these diaphragms minimizes their influence on the dysfunction of the craniosacral system. Figure 15.8 shows the hyoid bone diaphragm release.

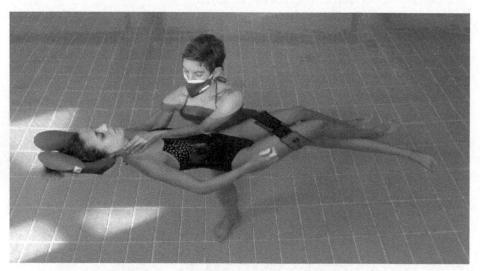

Figure 15.8: Fascia and diaphragms: hyoid bone

The sensitive hand melds with the patient, so that they become the same skin, applying the same amount of presence and contact to the entire surface of the hand. We avoid sliding, especially if the body area we are currently touching is covered by the swimsuit. With more reason, we will turn our attention inside, moving with the fascia.

The movement occurs spontaneously after about 90–120 seconds and is always three-dimensional. The first restriction barrier is dissolved with a relatively long application. Later, the passage between one barrier and the other can be made with short stops in consecutive barriers or through continuous movement. There is often a sinking sensation of the hands inside the patient's body (Güeita Rodríguez *et al.* 2020).

Patient's experience after the session

The mind needs time to receive, interpret, and establish the new body sensations. It is important that after receiving we take some time to integrate, in silence, and both stillness and movement, and to keep hydrated and aware of sensations in the body so that the CNS integrates the changes that occurred during the session.

The body needs a day or two to settle into its new pattern and orientation, so it is relevant to keep a good alignment in all positions.

Small worsening of pain may occur, which usually lasts a few hours (48–72 hours), so it is relevant to keep an open channel of communication with the patient. This constant communication right before, maybe during, and immediately after the session once they are back in vertical position (see Figure 15.9), and when they are back home, will allow us to set the goals, plan the treatment, ensure adequate doses, change patterns, establish new ones, and in the end enable change, learning, and health.

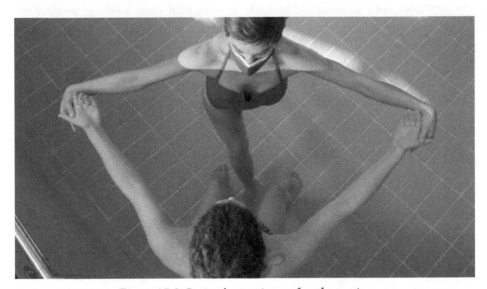

Figure 15.9: Patient's experience after the session

A great gift you can give someone is the space to be themselves, without the threat of you leaving. We want to maximize their independency but also we want them to feel heard and supported, to know that they are not alone in their process, that we are with them.

CASE STUDY

My back had been alerting for quite some time since I worked for many years as a TV camera operator and, at that time, they were bulky and excessively heavy devices.

I had been treated with traditional medicine, which always led to tests and medication with acupuncture, which worked well, although there were occasions when, during the sessions, I noticed a lot of discomfort.

I also had physiotherapy, with different professionals, which was sometimes effective, but later I did not have effective or lasting results until I found the person who could understand what my body needed, and the sessions were much more effective and not painful at all.

My first experience as a receiver was about eight years ago. I was encouraged by Ana, my partner, and Javier, the physical therapist who treated me at that time, and to whom I will be eternally grateful for insisting that I attend my first appointment.

The experience was really revealing, my body received therapy that didn't involve any kind of pain; moreover, the feeling at the end was different from everything I had experienced before.

It gave me a generalized and infinite relaxation; days went by, weeks went by, and I still felt that the work Elisa had done with my muscles, my joints, and my limbs persisted, it was still there.

This therapy has taught me that I can take care of both body and mind, I can unify the physical part of work on my own body with consciousness, with the mind, recognizing the peace that this entails. It has taught me to be able to surrender to another body to move, immerse me, stretch, shrink me, surprise me, make me fly in the water, and I am confident that everything will be fine.

I would like to highlight the importance this therapy has had for me at times of my life when the levels of stress or the concerns generated by personal situations were great. It has helped me enormously to relativize, understand, accept, and overcome.

I have had Hodgkin lymphoma and I have tried to attend my sessions whenever my immune system has allowed me. Now as a survivor, I can say that it has helped me reduce the effects of chemotherapy on a physical level, such as stiffness in the muscles, heaviness in the extremities, and a feeling of shortening in certain areas of the body.

On a mental level, some of the benefits it has brought me have been tranquility in what I have had to go through, calm to face every piece of news or test, the dream of healing for several days without noticing the effects of corticosteroids, and a feeling of being able, being balanced. I believe this is due to the learning my body and mind gained after each session.

My experience with this therapy does not end when I leave the pool after each session but stays with me and leaves physical and psychological memories that teach me wonderful things. It's magic in the water.

Noelia Doblas Miquel

Conclusions

CST in Water is a valuable tool for therapists committed to the support and facilitation of people with various pathologies in the aquatic environment. It is the best form of treatment for the fascial system because in the suppression of gravity the traumatic pattern can be better expressed.

Its practice involves extensive study, an appropriate attitude, and, above all, a constant and persistent practice with appropriate training by a certified Craniosacral Therapy in Water instructor.

A CST in Water session is a life-changing experience in which all systems in the body are brought into communication for the benefit of the entire system. Our stimuli remodel the extracellular matrix, modifying the physical characteristics of the tissues. The patient's perception and the afferent impulse in the spinal cord created by our stimuli reach central and autonomous nervous systems, modulating pain and enhancing interoceptive awareness, changing the patient's body image.

All these factors create the ideal frame for correction, allowing homeostasis of the body, and therefore in an environment of real listening and presence the patient can actively surrender, trust, learn, and heal.

References

Barceló, T. (2013). *La sabiduría interior: Pinceladas de filosofía experiencial*. Bilbao: Desclèe de Brouwer.

Boccafoschi, F., Bosetti, M., Sandra, P.M., Leigheb, M., & Cannas, M. (2010). Effects of mechanical stress on cell adhesion. *Cell Adhesion & Migration*, 4(1): 19–25.

Bordoni, B., Lintonbon, D., & Morabito, B. (2018). Meaning of the solid and liquid fascia to reconsider the model of biotensegrity. *Cureus*, 10(7): e2922.

Bordoni, B. & Simonelli, M. (2018). The awareness of the fascial system. *Cureus*, 10(10): e3397.

Farb, N.A.S., Segal, Z.V., & Anderson, A.K. (2013). Mindfulness meditation training alters cortical representations of interoceptive attention. *Social, Cognitive and Affective Neuroscience*, 8(1): 15–26.

Fechner, S. & Goodman, M.B. (2018). Synaptic communication upon gentle touch. *Neuron*, 100(6): 1272–1274.

Fernández-Pérez, A.M., Peralta-Ramírez, M.I., Pilat, A. & Villaverde, C. (2008). Effects of myofascial induction techniques on physiologic and psychologic parameters: a randomized controlled trial. *Journal of Alternative Complementary Medicine*, 14(7):807–11.

Findley, T. & Shalwala, M. (2013). Fascia research congress evidence from the 100-year perspective of Andrew Taylor Still. *Journal of Bodywork and Movement Therapies*, 17(3): 356–364.

Gendlin, E.T. (1975). The Newer Therapies. In S. Arieti (ed.), *American Handbook of Psychiatry* (second edition), *Volume V: Treatment*, pp.269–289. New York, NY: Basic Books.

Gendlin, E.T. (1997). The Use of Focusing on Therapy. In J.K. Zeig (ed.), *The Evolution of Psychotherapy: The Third Conference*, pp.197–210. New York, NY: Brunner/Mazel.

Gendlin, E.T. (1999a). A new model. *Journal of Consciousness Studies*, 6(2–3): 232–237.

Gendlin, E.T. (1999b). The first step of focusing provides a superior stress-reduction method. *The Folio*, 18(1): 178.

Gerdner, L.A., Hart, L.K., & Zimmerman, M.B. (2008). Craniosacral still point technique: Exploring its effects in individuals with dementia. *Journal of Gerontological Nursing*, 34: 36–45.

Green, C., Martin, C.W., Bassett, K., & Kazanjian, A. (1999). A systematic review of craniosacral therapy: Biological plausibility, assessment reliability and clinical effectiveness. *Complementary Therapies in Medicine*, 7(4): 201–207.

Güeita Rodríguez, J., Alonso Fraile, M., & Fernández de las Peñas, C. (2020). *Aquatic Therapy. Approaches from Physiotherapy and Occupational Therapy in the Aquatic Environment* (second edition). Spain: Elsevier.

Guimberteau, J.C., Delage, J.P., & Wong, J. (2010). The role and mechanical behavior of the connective tissue in tendon sliding. *Chirurgie de la Main*, 29: 155–166.

Haller, H. *et al.* (2020). Craniosacral therapy for chronic pain: A systematic review and meta-analysis of randomized controlled trials. *BMC Musculoskeletal Disorders*, 21: 1.

Harrison, R.E. & Page, J.S. (2011). Multipractitioner Upledger CranioSacral Therapy: Descriptive outcome study 2007–2008. *Journal of Alternative and Complementary Medicine*, 17: 13–17.

Hoffman, B.U. *et al.* (2018). Merkel cells activate sensory neural pathways through adrenergic synapses. *Neuron*, 100: 1401–1413.

Lêdo, C. *et al.* (2018). Aquatic myofascial release applied after high intensity exercise increases flexibility and decreases pain. *Journal of Bodywork and Movement Therapies*, 22(1): 97–104.

Liem, T. (2006). *Praxis de la Osteopatía Craneosacra*. Badalona: Paidotribo.

Liem, T. (2009). *La Osteopatía Craneosacra* (fourth edition). Badalona: Paidotribo.

Lischke, A., Pahnke, R., Mau-Moeller, A., Jacksteit, R., & Weippert, M. (2020). Sex-specific relationships between interoceptive accuracy and emotion regulation. *Frontiers in Behavioral Neuroscience*, 14: 67.

McManus, V. & Gliksten, M. (2007). The use of craniosacral therapy in a physically impaired population in a disability service in southern Ireland. *Journal of Alternative and Complementary Medicine*, 13: 929–930.

Muñoz Blanco, E. (2010). *Course Manual CranioSacral Therapy in Water™. Module 1*. Registry of Intellectual Property held on 12 July 2011, with number M-010363/201, being presented on 29 December 2010.

Muñoz Blanco, E. *et al.* (2020). Influence of aquatic therapy in children and youth with cerebral palsy: A qualitative case study in a special education school. *International Journal of Environmental Research and Public Health*, 17(10): 3690.

Murphy, J., Catmur, C., & Bird, G. (2019). Classifying individual differences in interoception: Implications for the measurement of interoceptive awareness. *Psychonomic Bulletin & Review*, 26(5): 1467–1471.

Pilat, A. (2003). *Terapias miofasciales: Inducción miofascial*. Madrid: McGraw Hill Interamericana.

Pilat, A. (2022). *Myofascial Induction: An Anatomical Approach to the Treatment of Fascial Dysfunction*. London: Handspring Publishing.

Porges, S.W. (2017). *The Pocket Guide to the Polyvagal Theory: The Transformative Power of Feeling Safe*. New York, NY: W.W. Norton & Company.

Raviv, G., Shefi, S., Nizani, D., & Achiron, A. (2009). Effect of craniosacral therapy on lower urinary tract signs and symptoms in multiple sclerosis. *Complementary Therapies in Clinical Practice*, 15: 72–75.

Rullmann, M., Preusser, S., & Pleger, B. (2019). Prefrontal and posterior parietal contributions to the perceptual awareness of touch. *Scientific Reports*, 9: 16981.

Stefanov, M. *et al.* (2013). The primo vascular system as a new anatomical system. *Journal of Acupuncture and Meridian Studies*, 6(6): 331e338.

Stefanov, M. & Jungdae, K. (2012). Primo vascular system as a new morphofunctional integrated system. *Journal of Acupuncture and Meridian Studies*, 5(5): 193e200.

Stilwell, P. & Harman, K. (2019). An enactive approach to pain: Beyond the biopsychosocial model. *Phenomenology and the Cognitive Science*, 18: 637–665. https://doi.org/10.1007/s11097-019-09624-7.

Sugawara, A., Terasawa, Y., Katsunuma, R., & Sekiguchi, A. (2020). Effects of interoceptive training on decision making, anxiety, and somatic symptoms. *BioPsychoSocial Medicine*, 14(1): 7.

Sutherland, A.S. (1962). *With Thinking Fingers*. Indianapolis, IN: The Cranial Academy.

Upledger Institute International (2021a). About CranioSacral Therapy. Palm Beach Gardens, FL: Upledger Institute International. www.upledger.com/therapies/faq.php.

Upledger Institute International (2021b). Research, articles, and case studies. Palm Beach Gardens, FL: Upledger Institute International. www.upledger.com/therapies/articles.php.

Ventegodt, S. *et al.* (2004). A combination of Gestalt Therapy, Rosen Body Work, and Cranio Sacral Therapy did not help in chronic Whiplash-Associated Disorders (WAD): Results of a randomized clinical trial. *The Scientific World Journal*, 4: 1055–1068.

Wanveer, T. (2007). Autism spectrum disorder: How craniosacral therapy can help. *Massage Today*, 7(7): 1–4.

Weber, W. & Newmark, S. (2007). Complementary and alternative medical therapies for attention-deficit/hyperactivity disorder and autism. *Pediatric Clinics of North America*, 54: 983–1006.

Chapter 16

Myofascial Release in Water (MRW®)

TOMASZ ZAGORSKI

The sources of Myofascial Release in Water

Myofascial Release in Water (MRW) was born in 2013, when I met my colleague, a structural integration practitioner, at my WATSU class. He highlighted the possibility of using some WATSU positions and moves to influence specific myofascial connections and to adapt some techniques from the therapeutic table to the session in the water. He encouraged me to use my experience and background in the manual therapy field to create a water myofascial release concept. I am very grateful for his inspiration. The MRW concept was presented for the first time in 2013 at the Fascia Summer School in Ulm, Germany. The first presentation in the Polish language took place in 2014 at a conference on movement activities for disabled children and youth in Biala Podlaska. Since then, MRW has been presented at many international conferences and events, including the 2015 Fascia Research Congress in Washington. The first international training took place in 2017, in Yilan, Taiwan.

Concepts in MRW

The MRW concept explains the myofascial connections in the body and provides us with practical tools for changing the structure and function of the locomotor system on land, as well as the unique possibilities and benefits of applying this work to the water. When we understand the connections inside the body, we can see the paths of possible force transmission during static postures and dynamic movements. We can create a map or maps of connections and force transmissions which will help us to understand posture and movement patterns and identify them as optimal for the needs of each person, or as dysfunctional and needing improvement. In MRW, we learn specific myofascial release techniques on land and in the water. Water has been known for its healing properties for years (Becker & Cole 2010; Cameron 2013). Rolfing, structural integration or any other myofascial release on land have proved to be effective and have been applied all over the world for many years. MRW extends this work to the water environment, utilizing water's benefits for diagnostic and therapeutic processes. It connects two different worlds—the field of fascia research and aquatic therapy—in a harmonious and graceful way.

Fascia: The Cinderella of tissue continuity

Clinicians and researchers in the field of manual and movement therapy have been studying primarily muscular tissue, bones and joints for hundreds of years in order to improve the function and structure of the human body. However, connective tissue (fascia) in its different forms and how it presents in the body was beyond their interest (Schleip *et al.* 2012). Within the origins of modern anatomy and methodology, they have found that fascia is almost everywhere in the body. To find the origins and insertions of the muscles and ligaments or to describe the structure of the joint, the anatomist had to go through the layers of superficial connective tissue and cut them off to see the muscles. If someone mentioned the fascia, it was usually associated with a specific structure, like the *plantar fascia* or the *fascia lata*. When the muscle was cleaned from other tissues, the anatomist could describe exact connections to the bones, the shape and tract of the muscle, the supply to the nerves and vessels. This gave the basis for describing the biomechanics of movement of the skeleton. If something was placed in front of the joint, it was a flexor, and at the back of the joint it was an extensor; diagonal structures were associated with rotations, and so on. These are the fundamental rules for classical anatomy and biomechanics, which have been taught for centuries in universities and schools. They are very useful for didactic reasons. Students can pull the body apart into hundreds of pieces, learn the details of each of them and put them back together into a picture of the whole functioning body.

The complexity of the human body is so vast that once students had learned all the anatomical content they did not ask further questions. The teachers were satisfied with the students' completion of the material, and they were not interested in additional research or complicating an already complex content. What works for the learning process does not necessarily work for the living body's physiology. The brain does not see the sum of parts doing their work separately. The brain sees the whole body and its functions as a continuous network. The brain uses proprioception and interoception to take information about the pieces thanks to mechanoreceptors (golgi, pacini, ruffini, interstitial—free nerve endings) located mostly in fascia and, because of continuous connections with neighbor structures, the information does not stop or end at the muscle attachment point (Schleip *et al.* 2012). The brain sees the small parts in relation to each other and to gravity and networks. These parts are connected to the same and opposite lines or planes of force transmission. The image of a network seems to represent the physiology of our locomotor system. At the beginning of the 21st century, research started to highlight the importance of connective tissue, and fascia started to be first on the list of interests of researchers and clinicians (Schultz & Feitis 1996; Fukashiro, Hay & Nagano 2006; Gracovetsky 2008; Schleip *et al.* 2012; Chaitow 2014; Bordoni & Simonelli 2018). The hideous waste that covers the muscles transforms into a lovely Cinderella, shedding new light on the body and its functions (Guimberteau & Amstrong 2015; Stecco 2015).

Biotensegrity

The Cinderella transformation could not happen without biotensegrity, the architecture of the body's structure (Scarr 2014). This structure is the tensional network that keeps the integrity of structures built of solid, hard elements like bones together with the light, tensile elements of soft tissues. Classical architecture is based on the concept of bricks lined one on another, each layer giving more compression to lower layers and, together, creating the stability and the integrity of the whole structure. This gives very strong integrity and minimal mobility. Most of our houses are built according to this concept. Some more challenging structures, for instance long bridges, require another approach. The base is built in a traditional manner, and the rest of the structures are supported by a number of ropes, the tension of which gives the structure its integrity. If just one rope is severed, the entire structure may collapse. Here we still have a lot of integrity and a bigger amount of mobility, depending on how much tension there is in the ropes. The body is an even more challenging structure because it requires a certain amount of stability and a lot of mobility, and both are variable according to current environmental and voluntary demands. In the body, we can find representatives of both bricks and ropes. The bricks are the bones which float in a tensional network of ropes represented by muscles, tendons, ligaments and other soft tissues. The bones bear the load and push the network from the inside out, and the soft tissues keep the bones together by creating tension transmitted between neighboring structures and all over the network. They maintain a constant dynamic balance while dealing with gravity's challenges and the activities of daily life. The authors of this concept are Buckminster Fuller and Kenneth Snelson. Recently, Bruno Bordoni and others added blood and lymph to this concept. According to them, liquid fascia is another element of discontinuous compression inside the biotensegritive myofascial model (Bordoni *et al.* 2018). All the above considerations describe the behavior of the body in gravitational conditions. I hope that exploring this knowledge in the water will give more input and create a bigger picture.

A historical look at fascia

Andreas Vesalius (1515–1564) was a progenitor of describing the fascial connections in the body. Even if he is considered as the father of anatomy in a classical way, his drawings strongly suggest connections between the structures. In 1947, the French physiotherapist Françoise Mézières developed a concept of treating the spine by releasing the tension of the whole muscular chain at the back of the body. Herman Kabat, the creator of the proprioceptive neuromuscular facilitation (PNF), emphasized the importance of including weak muscles in treatment chains in the 1950s. Godelieve Denys-Struyf was one of the first people who described the chains around the whole body. For her, psychological factors played a significant role in the development of dominant muscular chains. French osteopaths Leopold Busquet and Paul Chauffour in the 1980s also described the muscular chains and their cranial and visceral connections. Andry Vleeming, researching thoraco-lumbar fascia, described X-shape connections starting from this region and reaching to the opposite limbs (Vleeming *et al.* 2007). In 2004, Luigi Stecco and his children, Carla and Antonio, developed an interesting fascial manipulation concept based on their medical background and anatomical research (Stecco 2004). They described myofascial units, sequences and spirals. Science is constantly bringing us new evidence and there will be new information about myofascial connections in the body in the future.

Visual assessment

The body is a highly specialized, super-intelligent machine, adapted to living on our planet at extreme levels. Our locomotor system is based on biotensegrity, with the bones floating inside the surface of the soft tissues and gracefully dealing with gravity, which presents us with numerous challenges, particularly when it comes to movement. Our locomotor system is a tool for dealing with these challenges. Therefore, we need to look closely at the quality of it. First, we should see the body in a static position. The posture becomes upright in order to see better, and only humans can sustain the upright position for a longer time. When we think of the body as a series of blocks (feet, lower legs, knees, upper legs, pelvis, lumbar spine, chest, neck, head), the upright position appears to be optimal for balancing the tension of the soft tissues that hold the whole thing together. When something is out of alignment, there is more tension in the myofascial ropes and more energy needs to be spent on static work against gravity. As a result, our posture serves as a starting point for evaluating the quality of our movement machine, acting as a kind of baseline. It gets even more complicated if we bring the body into movement, where we have a whole interplay of soft tissue chains trying to keep the integrity of a series of blocks in gravity with ground reaction forces and movement goals. On top of that, we have internal limitations in terms of energy potential, external obstacles and motivational input. There are so many factors that influence the body and its shape in relation to movement that it is easy to get lost in the body's assessment of movement, especially for inexperienced therapists.

I recommend starting from the baseline and assessing the posture first, before assessing the movements. Visual assessment has its own specific methodology, which is carefully explained during MRW training, where we learn to see the small details of seeing the whole body. It is critical to be guided in looking at the body at first, with a step-by-step explanation of what to look for. It becomes easier and faster with time and practice, and you only need an eye blink to see many important details. With knowledge and experience, you can achieve the mastery level. The visual assessment is an art. Correct visual assessment is a base for creating optimal strategy in therapy. The effectiveness of our work is directly influenced by an effective visual assessment.

In MRW training, our work is enhanced by warm water, where gravity is reduced, as well as muscle tone, which results in the appearance of true fascial restriction patterns (Zagorski 2014). On land, where the body works against gravity even if sitting relaxed or lying down, the postural muscle tension often compensates for connective tissue restrictions, and it is difficult to see all the details, or to determine which restriction is primary or compensatory. In water, when the body goes into even a small relaxation state, we can see the primary patterns due to the unwinding of the body. This gives us additional information, often impossible to obtain in land assessment, that helps us in the decision-making process. There is another benefit for those who decide to get wet and bring the client into the water. We can assess the passive movement of the body in three dimensions, which is not possible on land. And this evaluation frequently leads directly to treatment, where we can apply restriction releases and encourage desired movement patterns. In MRW sessions, we utilize both land and water assessment for clinical reasoning to build the therapy strategy.

Passive techniques

The body shapes itself according to external demands during a certain period of time. If our main work is sitting at the table, and we drive one or two hours in the car to get to and from work, and after work we sit and watch TV when we rest, the sitting position is the main demand for the body, which shapes itself to adapt to this position. The hip flexors have shortened, while the opposing gluteus muscles have grown longer and are usually weaker. When we sit at the computer, our pecs shorten, our rhomboids lengthen, and we have shoulder protraction around the back. Such situations create a series of compensatory patterns: deeper lumbar lordosis, protraction of the head, different force distribution patterns in the lower limbs, which may result in back pain or even injuries. When we combine a lack of physical activity with sitting for many hours a day, we can see such an adaptation effect in a couple of months, which is long enough for connective tissue to make the necessary adaptations that manifest as the aforementioned dysfunctions.

However, the good news about the plasticity of the fascia is that we can create a change in a positive direction and develop desired changes in the soft tissue within the locomotor system. We can literally shape the body using our hands, as an artist does with a sculpture. These changes stay for a short time when there is no demand for new arrangements, so we need to create such a demand by regular application of compensatory movement and repeating manual intervention from time to time (Schwind 2006; Earls & Myers 2010). When we understand the pathological pattern in global aspects, we can break it down into small pieces and address very specific structures of the global chain. Usually, we start by elongating the shortened parts where there are the biggest restrictions. Often, the first intervention is located far from the place where the patient is complaining about it. And, in many cases, such distal intervention results in pain relief or a change in postural pattern in the original area. The previously described biotensegrity rules explain these remarkable outcomes. MRW passive techniques learned on land and in water are the main tools for creating local changes in specific structures, which in turn change global patterns and create a new shape in the fascial system.

Active techniques

Ida Rolf, the originator of Rolfing and the mother of other related concepts, used to say: "Put it where it belongs, and call for a movement." This sentence is the essence of structural work. Creating a local structural change or a series of changes is not enough to achieve sustained results. We need to put this change into the context of the movement on different levels. First, with local tissue movement, where different layers of the tissue glide and slide against each other. Or, at the very least, they should, because immobility, such as a long sitting position, causes an increase in the local activity of fibroblasts and the production of collagen fibers arranged in a chaotic manner, which, on the macro level, can manifest in movement restrictions or even as a form of adhesion if the situation persists for an extended period of time (Schleip & Muller 2013). If something is not moving, something else needs to move more.

As a compensation for the movement restriction, we can have a hypermobile area, which is not good for body mechanics because it can cause an overload of the involved joint or a series of joints. Injury of the area creates forced hypomobility, and again, collagen fibers may create adhesions in other places. The situation is complicated further by unconscious transfer of forces away from the site of injury, which may result in the distal area overloading (Magnusson, Langberg & Kjaer 2010). As a result, we must also look for global movement patterns and distal compensation for local constraints. Besides seeing the movement restrictions, we may use our hands to feel the tissue and how it moves. When we can guide the tissue in a desired way, encouraging movement in restricted areas and slowing down in hypermobile areas, this deep tissue listening can seamlessly transform into a therapeutic touch. This kind of proprioceptive facilitation of movement, called Active Myofascial Release (AMR), is a soft re-education of the tissue, sometimes enough to create a desired change in movement and posture. AMR techniques are used during MRW active techniques training, both on land and in water, together with other aspects of movement related to connective tissue, including applications in sports medicine.

Open positions

In the MRW session, we use two kinds of positions for the client in the water— open and supported. An open position provides full access to the body from all sides and gives a lot of freedom in technique application. We support the head with a special pillow and the legs with standard WATSU floats or specific noodles. Sometimes there is additional support for the pelvis. This position is the easiest for an assessment to be done and to apply the biggest number of techniques, but the limitation is the lack of strong resistance, so we cannot use a lot of force. Another limitation is the head support, which has to be adjusted often.

Supported positions

Supported positions adapt support from WATSU, which is optimal for supporting the head and the spine. Basic position, saddle and under head are the most commonly used. This position allows us to apply much more force than the open position, but it limits our ability to work with two hands because one hand is usually occupied in supporting the head. In supported positions, we usually use leg floats only or no flotation devices. We can switch from a supported to an open position and back at any time during the session.

MRW in WATSU practice: Putting the map on the body

Concepts of manual myofascial release are widely used in clinical practice on the land (Stecco 2004; Schwind 2006; Richter & Hebgen 2007; Myers 2014). Practitioners from all over the world give very positive feedback about the results of practical applications of these techniques in many areas of manual and movement therapies. Aquatic therapy practitioners have started to use the concept, but in general, the MRW is not known in the hydrotherapy field yet. Since WATSU combines movement and manual techniques, MRW techniques seem to be a very useful tool to increase the effectiveness of the therapy. In MRW, the concept of connection of the body aids in understanding the behavior of a relaxed body that has been immersed in warm water and is being stretched, cradled and worked on with manual techniques. The holistic view of the body's distal relations aids in understanding the specific shape and patterns of the body and in applying appropriate manual and movement tools to unwind the patterns. *Distant stillness* is a WATSU technique in which the practitioner allows the body to have any movement coming from inside the body while applying minimal support and following any movement that occurs. It is pure movement exploration without knowing its source or where the movement will end up. Having knowledge about interrelationships, at least, will give us some picture of why the body moves in this way and ideas about what to do with the next techniques in order to address a specific issue. In combination, the myofascial connection map put on the body in each WATSU sequence will help us to achieve this.

WATSU stretching

WATSU was originally designed to stretch certain Shiatsu meridians, so stretching is an important component of the therapy. Obviously, besides meridians, we also stretch muscles, tendons, ligaments and whole chains of soft tissues (Decoster *et al.* 2005). Putting up the map of connections will give us more information about what we really affect during the application of the stretch. We need to remember that during stretching, we affect the whole myofascial unit, not only the muscle. Stretching resistance stems from two sources: fascia and muscle tension. In warm water, the tension of the muscle is significantly reduced and the main resistance to stretching comes from the fascia. In other words, in water we stretch more fascial components and on land we stretch muscle and fascia. Some WATSU techniques like simple offering, free spine, seaweed and distant stillness have a great diagnostic value and we can see where the restrictions are in the body. Adding the connection map will help us link these restrictions and plan a more effective strategy—where to put emphasis during stretching with a thigh press, twist over, sweep around or other techniques. Some of the WATSU stretches influence mainly one chain of connection, but most of the stretches influence multiple connections.

Adding manual techniques

In WATSU, there are not many manual techniques applied. We use Shiatsu point pressure, massage of areas holding tension, and mobilization of joints, soft tissues and nerves. MRW is a great addition here. Even if there is little time for manual work in a WATSU session and applying a massage can be considered as wasting the precious time of warm water immersion, adding a precise MRW technique to a critical spot can bring significant release. Knowing about connections, when we see areas with higher tension, we can expect they will affect neighboring tissues, spreading the tension to more distant parts. Applying the map of connections, we can anticipate where the tension will most probably go and we can be more effective with our intervention. For instance, if we have tension in the erector spinae group, we should address not only the muscles of the back, but also the neck muscles, hamstrings and calves.

Positioning ourselves in the water

The myofascial connection map explaining the transmission of forces is also very useful for the therapist when it comes to the ergonomics of the work, which has a direct and proportional influence on the quality and safety of the session. Any tension in the practitioner's body will travel along the main chain of connections and will end up in the client's body. The practitioner needs to constantly scan their own body in order to find and release any tension, as well as to look for positions that use minimal muscle engagement. Because there are bases, this scanning should begin with the feet and legs. The popular WATSU wide stance, which provides stability, is unfortunately a source of tension that originates in the foot and travels vertically through the *deep posterior compartment* and the adductor group. It continues via the *pelvis* to the *chest* and to the *arms* which hold the practitioner's body. To avoid this tension, the giver must adopt a more relaxed stance on their feet and abandon the wide stance habits learned from on-land activities, instead relying on core balance.

Support

This is critical for both your safety and the quality of the session. The way we hold someone's body in water is important because our support is the replacement of muscle activity, which holds the spine and bones on land, and here in water is significantly reduced due to the lack of gravity and relaxation.

The practitioner's role is to provide support using traction applied to specific points (for instance, *occiput*, *sacrum*) instead of applying pressure by squeezing the neck. This pressure involves our muscle activity and is associated with tension in the body, which we want to avoid. The pressure provides tension on the client's body and gives a feeling of discomfort or pain. This reduces trust in the practitioner or therapist and induces a general state of alertness in the client's body, as well as a higher overall level of tension—the polar opposite of the desired state of relaxation. The map of myofascial connections will help us to apply the correct points of support as well as the correct way of supporting the body, and achieve optimal conditions for relaxation.

Practitioner's movement

Besides the practitioner's posture and method of supporting the body, the way that the practitioner moves is also very important. Here, we need to look for the most simple and most energy-cost-effective way of moving, in order to avoid giving extra work and extra tension to our bodies (Sawicki, Lewis & Ferris 2009; Elphinston 2013). To achieve this, we need to apply the movement closest to the locomotion movement. If we need to walk 10km, we direct the whole of our body to the direction of the movement and we move in this direction. No side-to-side movements, no walking with the knee pointing to the side, no additional energy-consuming moves. Straight to the finish point. It is also similar in the water. If we need to do forward or back-and-forth movements, we need to point the whole of our body in the direction of the movement and use the most effective locomotor muscles. Any out-of-line placement of the leg will result in additional tension traveling along the connection chains. In the water, we must consider the water resistance forces that we are confronted with right in front of us. The more powerful and dynamic our movement, the more resistance we face from the water. On the other hand, we have an inertion force that helps us move, and we can use it for movements that are less energy consuming. As a result, we try to position and move our bodies in a way that reduces unnecessary tension while also utilizing the most effective muscle groups along the main myofascial connection chains.

Summary

Myofascial Release in Water is a concept that connects healing on land and in water, as well as allowing us to better understand the body, seen from a different perspective. It is an encouragement for land-based therapists to try another approach and widen their already broad horizon with new assessment and therapy tools. For water-based therapists, MRW gives the opportunity to learn specific manual techniques for land and water use, together with specific visual assessment skills, as well as the ability to see the body and its movement in a holistic aspect based on the biotensegral network of connective tissue.

Acknowledgment

I wish to express my gratitude to Harold Dull for creating WATSU, which has made profound changes in people's lives and gathered a network of individuals with different backgrounds and scopes of practice. The WATSU Water Family is a living connective tissue, which enriches the development and gives it its own momentum. I wish to thank all my teachers for their priceless knowledge and inspiration, and my students for their questions, giving me motivation to learn more and continue to share the fascial water work. Lastly, I wish to thank Mariusz Kurkowski for the inspiration to bring this work to the water.

References

Becker, B. & Cole, A. (2010). *Comprehensive Aquatic Therapy* (third edition). Pullman, WA: Washington State University Publishing.

Bordoni, B., Marelli, F., Morabito, B. & Castagna, R. (2018). A new concept of biotensegrity incorporating liquid tissues: Blood and lymph. *Journal of Evidence-Based Integrative Medicine*, 23: 2515690X18792838.

Bordoni, B. & Simonelli, M. (2018). The awareness of the fascial system. *Cureus*, 10(10): e3397.

Cameron, M. (2013). Hydrotherapy. In *Physical Agents in Rehabilitation. From Research to Practice* (fourth edition). St. Louis, MO: Elsevier.

Chaitow, L. (2014). *Fascial Dysfunction. Manual Therapy Approaches*. London: Handspring Publishing.

Decoster, L., Cleland, J., Altieri, C. & Russell, P. (2005). The effects of hamstring stretching on range of motion: A systematic literature review. *Journal of Orthopaedic & Sports Physical Therapy*, 35(6): 377–387.

Earls, J. & Myers, T. (2010). *Fascial Release for Structural Balance*. Chichester: Lotus Publishing.

Elphinston, J. (2013). *Stability, Sport and Performance Movement: Practical Biomechanics and Systematic Training for Movement Efficacy and Injury Prevention*. Chichester: Lotus Publishing and On Target Publications.

Fukashiro, S., Hay, D.C. & Nagano, A. (2006). Bio-mechanical behavior of muscle-tendon complex during dynamic human movements. *Journal of Applied Biomechanics*, 22(2): 131–147.

Gracovetsky, S. (2008). *The Spinal Engine*. Montreal, Quebec, Canada: Serge Gracovetsky.

Guimberteau, J.-C. & Amstrong, C. (2015). *Architecture of Human Living Fascia*. London: Handspring Publishing.

Magnusson, S., Langberg, H. & Kjaer, M. (2010). The pathogenesis of tendinopathy: Balancing the response to loading. *Nature Reviews Rheumatology*, 6(5): 262–268.

Myers, T. (2014). *Anatomy Trains: Myofascial Meridians for Manual and Movement Therapists*. Elsevier: Churchill Livingstone.

Richter, P. & Hebgen, E. (2007). *Triggerpunkte und Muskelfunktionsketten in der Osteopathie und Manuellen Therapie* (second edition). Hippokrates in MVS Medizinverlage Stuttgart: GmbH & Co. K.G.

Sawicki, G., Lewis, C. & Ferris, D. (2009). It pays to have a spring in your step. *Exercise and Sport Sciences Reviews*, 37(3): 130–138.

Scarr, G. (2014). *Biotensegrity: The Structural Basis of Life*. London: Handspring Publishing.

Schleip, R., Findley, T.W., Chaitow, L. & Huijing, P.A. (2012). *Fascia: The Tensional Network of the Human Body. The Science and Clinical Applications in Manual and Movement Therapy*. Edinburgh: Churchill Livingstone, Elsevier.

Schleip, R. & Muller, G. (2013). Training principles for fascial connective tissues: Scientific foundation and suggested practical applications. *Journal of Bodywork & Movement Therapies*, 17: 103–115.

Schultz, R.L. & Feitis, R. (1996). *The Endless Web: Fascial Anatomy and Physical Reality*. Berkeley, CA: North Atlantic Books.

Schwind, P. (2006). *Fascial and Membrane Technique. A Manual for Comprehensive Treatment of the Connective Tissue System*. Edinburgh: Churchill Livingstone, Elsevier.

Stecco, C. (2015). *Functional Atlas of the Human Fascial System*. Edinburgh: Churchill Livingstone, Elsevier.

Stecco, L. (2004). *Fascial Manipulation for Musculoskeletal Pain*. Padova: Piccin.

Vleeming, A., Mooney, V. & Stoeckart, R. (2007). *Movement, Stability and Lumbopelvic Pain. Integration of Research and Therapy*. Edinburgh: Elsevier.

Zagorski, T. (2014). Work on Fascia in Water: Benefits, Possibilities and Limitations of Application. In M. Bilska, R. Golonko & J. Soltan, *Movement Activities in Disabled Children and Youth* (pp.124–136). Biala Podlska: Akademia Wychowania Fizycznego Józefa Piłsudskiego w Warszawie. Wydział Wychowania Fizycznego i Sportu w Białej Podlaskiej.

Chapter 17

Moving into Clinical Frameworks Through the Heart of WATSU®

DR. JENNIFER OLEJOWNIK

Introduction

WATSU is a complex integrative therapy because it has many therapeutic dimensions. Integrative therapies are classified by the National Center for Complementary and Integrative Health (NCCIH) by the type of primary input, or how a therapy is administered or delivered. Using this framework, complementary health approaches fall under three main categories or a combination thereof including: nutritional, physical, and psychological (NCCIH 2022). WATSU is certainly a physical practice due to the way therapists glide and gently twist clients' bodies through water during a session. WATSU is also a psychological practice as clients are guided toward stillness, which provokes deep contemplative and meditative experiences. For these reasons, WATSU is considered both a physical and psychological category according to the NCCIH guidelines. Although the NCCIH has migrated away from using the five domains of integrative medicine—alternative medical systems, biologically based therapies, manipulative therapies, mind-body therapies, and energy medicine—the domains are a bit more appropriate for the practice of WATSU since they acknowledge the energetic and mind-body aspects of the therapy. Inspired by Zen Shiatsu, WATSU incorporates stretches that promote the flow of "chi" or life energy along the meridians. Simultaneously, the practice fosters stress reduction and personal growth due to the powerful stillness that invites receivers to pay attention to their interior landscape without interruption.

Beyond the NCCIH's categorization, it is also useful to examine the underlying tenets of WATSU to understand where it falls on a medical or healing paradigm continuum. A paradigm is a way of seeing the world and consists of the taken-for-granted theories, concepts, ideas, and methods belonging to a particular discipline. Paradigms are important to consider since they highlight the underlying philosophies, beliefs, and assumptions of a given discipline, and exploring paradigmatic constructs related to WATSU helps us understand where it fits in clinical and cultural contexts. Davis-Floyd and St. John (1998) identified three main paradigms through their research which explored why traditional medical providers were pivoting away from their philosophical and biomedical training to embrace instead a more holistic orientation. They conducted formal interviews with over 40 physicians to identify distinct healing paradigms as medical providers transitioned to becoming a holistic healer. Davis-Floyd and St. John's research identified three main paradigms that describe medical or healing practices in the United States: technocratic medicine, humanistic medicine, and holistic medicine (see Table 17.1). Providers in their study did not fall neatly under one paradigm and instead adopted tenets, concepts, and ideas across each of the three paradigms. The same holds true for WATSU as it resides somewhere between the humanistic and holistic aspects of the continuum.

Table 17.1: Tenets of technocratic, humanistic, and holistic medicine (Davis-Floyd & St. John 1998, reproduced with kind permission from Rutgers University Press)

Technocratic Medicine	Humanistic Medicine	Holistic Medicine
Mind-body separation	Mindy-body connection	Oneness of body-mind-spirit
The body as machine	The body as organism	The body as an energy system interlinked with other energy systems
The patient as object	The patient as a relational subject	Healing the whole person in whole-life context
Alienation of practitioner from patient	Connection and caring between practitioner and patient	Essential unity of practitioner and client
Diagnosis and treatment from outside in	Diagnosis and healing from the outside in and from the inside out	Diagnosis and healing from inside out
Hierarchical organization and standardization of care	Balance between the needs of the institution and the individual	Networking organizational structure that facilitates individualization of care
Authority and responsibility inherent in practitioner, not patient	Information, decision-making, and responsibility shared between patient and provider	Authority and responsibility inherent in each individual

cont.

Technocratic Medicine	Humanistic Medicine	Holistic Medicine
Supervaluation of science and technology	Science and technology counter-balanced with humanism	Science and technology placed at the service of the individual
Aggressive intervention with emphasis on short-term results	Focus on disease prevention	A long-term focus on creating and maintaining health and well-being
Death as defeat	Death as an acceptable outcome	Death as a step in the process
A profit-driven system	Compassion-driven care	Healing is the focus
Intolerance of other modalities	Open-mindedness towards other modalities	Embrace of other modalities

These paradigms are a useful framework to consider for many therapies, disciplines, and practices that fall under the umbrella of integrative health. The terms "alternative," "complementary," and "integrative" are constantly evolving and changing, and the NCCIH provides the most current and relevant terminology relevant to this discussion. According to the NCCIH, integrative health:

> brings conventional and complementary approaches together in a coordinated way. Integrative health also emphasizes multimodal interventions, which are two or more interventions such as conventional health care approaches and complementary health approaches in various combinations, with an emphasis on treating the whole person rather than, for example, one organ system. Integrative health aims for well-coordinated care among different providers and institutions by bringing conventional and complementary approaches together to care for the whole person. (NCCIH 2022)

A distinctive feature of integrative health is that it brings conventional and complementary care together in a coordinated and intentional way targeting the whole person.

Until the integrative revolution in the late 1990s, many integrative therapies including acupuncture, naturopathy, and WATSU were *not* included in conventional, western, or allopathic institutions because the paradigms were largely oppositional, antagonistic, or incongruent with mainstream medicine. Prior to the integrative movement spanning from the 1990s to 2000s, integrative and complementary therapies mostly existed and operated outside conventional medicine. Most still do today, for a variety of reasons. As a vestige of the Flexner Report, many institutions that prepared and trained non-biomedical providers were forced to close due to Flexner era mandates, which marked a separation from pluralistic medicine in our society. During this time, philanthropists only funded biomedical schools receiving excellent evaluations from the Flexner Report while heterodox medical schools were denied philanthropic support (Baer 2001, p.37). Heterodox or unconventional schools, therapies, and approaches possessed different philosophical lenses, viewpoints, concepts, and ideas that were outside the main paradigm of western medicine. Eventually, the medical establishment gained control over licensing boards in the late 1900s and stipulated that only graduates from institutions deemed acceptable by the American Council on Medical Education were granted licensure. These decisions sealed the fate of many heterodox institutions as many were forced to close. Those that remained still feel the lasting impact of the Flexner Report as many of these disciplines today do not have the robust funding, library, and research support found in traditional medical academic settings. Because many of the heterodox schools were outside mainstream or conventional medicine, they were largely viewed antagonistically by biomedical providers in practice and also in prestigious medical journals (Winnick 2005).

Eventually, this began to change with the integrative medicine movement in the late 1990s–early 2000s which was born as a result of the creation of the NCCIH (formerly the National Center for Complementary and Alternative Medicine), the increased participation of major academic centers belonging to the Academic Consortium for Integrative Medicine and Health, and the inclusion of holistic (sometimes referred to as alternative or complementary) therapies in conventional clinical models. These changes represented an experimental blending of the tenets across the spectrum of technocratic, humanistic, and holistic paradigms of medicine. As holistic providers entered biomedical or technocratic settings, they found themselves in an entirely different culture of medicine comprised of new occupational structures, expectations, patient-provider relationships, rates of reimbursement, collegiality, and status. Differences related to how the body was viewed and constructed also existed, which impacted the delivery of care, diagnostic procedures, and how outcomes were measured. As integrative therapies aligned with biomedicine during this phase, providers pivoted or adapted to the biomedical tenets which at times compromised or contradicted some of the values and tenets of holistic healing.

The technocractic, humanistic, and holistic tenets are still timely to consider because they represent a snapshot of our own culture's changing perspectives on medicine. The views expressed in this book support the notion that WATSU incorporates both humanistic and holistic elements when applying the paradigm typologies as a lens to appraise healing systems (Table 17.2). Based on the content of this book, Table 17.2 shows where WATSU falls on the paradigmatic continuum of healing systems. WATSU is mostly a holistic approach, but it occasionally overlaps with some of the humanistic tenets as outlined below. Although technocratic tenets most often pertain to biomedicine, some clinical aspects of the practice align with biomedical practices and procedures.

When WATSU does align with biomedicine it is mostly due to providers having additional credentials in fields in medicine as well as the setting in which it is delivered. As the field of WATSU continues to grow and professionalize, it is possible that it may adopt additional tenets on the technocratic end of the continuum while simultaneously adding new tenets to the holistic dimension.

Since Davis-Floyd and St. John's research was conducted in 1998, it is most certain that another paradigm shift is occurring since complementary and integrative therapies have become more mainstream for the last 20 years. It is realistic to consider the possibility that new tenets and paradigms have likely emerged through the heightened visibility and popularity of the integrative professions, but these tenets have yet to be formally studied or identified. The University of Arizona, one of the most renowned and pioneering institutions of integrative medicine, provides a list of the principles of integrative medicine, to use as a guide or framework for how to apply these principles in practice. This list provides a glimpse of the current tenets of integrative medicine. Most of these are in alignment with holistic tenets and convey a commitment to research and self-exploration, which are central to both the art and science of WATSU (see Table 17.2). This chapter highlights some of the emergent tenets as viewed through the lens of WATSU in practice as well as suggesting where WATSU might fall on the paradigmatic continuum of medicine.

Table 17.2: Tenets of WATSU

(Note: There was not enough information to place WATSU for the tenet pertaining to organizational structure so this category was omitted.)

Humanistic Medicine	Holistic Medicine	WATSU	Example
Mind-body connection	Oneness of body-mind-spirit	Oneness of body-mind-spirit	The mind is located throughout the body
The body as organism	The body as an energy system linked with other energy systems	The body as an energy system linked with other energy systems	Breath, interoception
Patient as a relational subject	Healing the whole person in whole-life context	Healing the whole person in whole-life context	Focus on other factors—emotional regulation, meeting patients where they are at
Connection and caring between the practitioner and patient	Essential unity of practitioner and client	Connection and caring between the practitioner and patient	Mirroring, witnessing, deep listening, empathy

Diagnosis and healing from outside in and from inside out	Diagnosis and healing from inside out	Diagnosis and healing from inside out	Recognition that interrelated factors contribute to disease; trust wisdom of clients' bodies
Information, decision-making, and responsibility shared between patient and provider	Authority and responsibility inherent in each individual	Authority and responsibility inherent in each individual and information, decision-making, and responsibility shared between patient and provider	Respond to client's lead; high degree of collaboration between provider and client
Science and technology counter-balanced with humanism	Science and technology placed at service of the individual	Science and technology placed at service of the individual	High touch, use of scales and intake procedures as appropriate
Focus on disease prevention	A long-term focus on creating and maintaining health and well-being	A long-term focus on creating and maintaining health and well-being	Recognition that health and wellness is a process that is cultivated through body awareness over time
Death as an acceptable outcome	Death is a step in the process	Death as an acceptable outcome	WATSU as component of palliative care
Compassion-driven care	Healing is the focus	Compassion-driven care Healing is the focus	Heart-centered care with support for journey towards wellness
Open-mindedness towards other modalities	Embrace of other modalities	Embrace of other modalities	Recognition that WATSU is part of the constellation of therapies

Defining principles of integrative medicine:

1. Patient and practitioner are partners in the healing process.
2. All factors that influence health, wellness, and disease are taken into consideration, including mind, spirit, and community, as well as the body.

3. Appropriate use of both conventional and alternative methods facilitates the body's innate healing response.
4. Effective interventions that are natural and less invasive should be used whenever possible.
5. Integrative medicine neither rejects conventional medicine nor accepts alternative therapies uncritically.
6. Good medicine is based in good science. It is inquiry-driven and open to new paradigms.
7. Alongside the concept of treatment, the broader concepts of health promotion and the prevention of illness are paramount.
8. Practitioners of integrative medicine should exemplify its principles and commit themselves to self-exploration and self-development.

Integrative framework

Integrative therapies and disciplines view the body holistically, and in the most simplistic terms this conveys an understanding that there is a connection between the mind, body, and spirit. Prior to the 1990s, this view was broadly understood and recognized through contemplative traditions, but emerging research and scholarship spanning a variety of topics such as psychoneuroimmunology, somatics, and polyvagal theory provide scientific credence to the notion that the brain is not merely located in the head, but rather is experienced throughout the body via the central nervous system. Holism is central to the heart of WATSU philosophy, techniques, and practices and stands in stark contrast to the reductionist and Cartesian assumptions of biomedicine which maintains that body and the mind are distinct entities. The NCCIH's definition of integrative medicine recognizes the value of treating the whole person as opposed to focusing on isolated organ systems. More precisely, the NCCIH (2022) defines whole-person health as "helping individuals, families, communities, and populations improve and restore their health in multiple interconnected domains—biological, behavioral, social, environmental—rather than just treating disease." Many ideas postulated in this book emphasize the notion that WATSU is a whole-person approach to care and as such, it can be viewed as an integrative framework or orientation.

Chapter 11 describes the way WATSU and the work of WaterDance can be viewed as a link between contemplative traditions and scientific perspectives. This chapter describes how breath in WATSU is a vital link to the individual self and universal soul, touching on the spiritual elements of the tenets of holistic medicine. Parasympathetic response and vagal tone are improved through the fluctuations in and rhythm of the breath. Focused attention on breathwork is a signature activity of many contemplative and somatic practices, and is a prominent feature of the eight-limbs of yoga, also known as *pranayama*. Because WATSU, and its other aquatic bodywork modalities like WaterDance, combines physical manipulations of the body in conjunction with breath control, it satisfies the NCCIH's definition of integrative health since it includes multimodal interventions. Chapter 11 acknowledges the acceptance and embrace of other systems of medicine by describing how the four elements—earth, water, air, and fire—apply to aquatic bodywork. The four elements are pan cultural because they are central to other medical systems such as Ayurvedic medicine, traditional Chinese medicine, and indigenous medicine. The four elements are timeless and identifying and incorporating them in practice means that providers strive to provide a balanced range of activities so that receivers are not over-prioritizing any one aspect of themselves. The four elements represent a powerful analogy for how to engage the whole person physically, emotionally, psychologically, and spiritually.

One of the differences that separates healing paradigms from one another is the way the body is viewed or constructed. For example, the machine metaphor is often associated with biomedicine as the body is viewed as a series of parts that can be repaired or replaced. Holistic or integrative therapies use generative, holographic, or natural metaphors to describe how the body is understood. In Chapter 13, the author provides additional justification for placing WATSU and its related aquatic bodywork modality Aquatic Integration within an integrative framework due to the way the body is viewed and constructed. Practitioners of aquatic bodywork view the body as a natural landscape, which implies that humans are a part of nature, and as such our bodies fluctuate through different seasons, cycling through conditions that lead us in and out of harmony and balance. The implication here is that a state of balance is not static or fixed, but is impermanent and changing. This view of the body encourages practitioners to see the uniqueness of each individual and to be alert to provide authentic responses tailored to the needs of each client. Chapter 2 further supports this orientation by reminding providers to "remember that each client is a unique individual who will respond according to a multitude of factors. Every session with each client will develop according to the needs of the client throughout the session." Seeing the uniqueness of each body unites theory and practice in an integrative worldview and also impacts how biology and behavior are interpreted as well. Chapter 13 provides a concrete example:

> As practitioners, we must remember that the psyche and body are not separate entities, and whatever has caused a shift in structure, muscle, bone, mood, behavior, belief has a direct effect on the whole organism. These shifts will show up in the physical form as holding patterns or habituated postures.

Here, WATSU practitioners are clearly instructed to adopt a whole-systems approach while working with clients. An integrative orientation includes a deliberate and intentional focus on somatic fluctuations. Another way to consider this is that some integrative therapies, such as WATSU, expand Engel's biopsychosocial model to include concepts that represent the wisdom of the body, such as embodiment and interoception. Very few systems of healing discuss the importance of one's kinesthetic sense, somatic awareness, or how the body is perceived from within. Often, somatic awareness is folded generically into categories that pertain to the physical dimension, which usually relates to exercise or diet, or to the emotional realm and managing one's feelings and interactions with others. Currently, there are nine dimensions of wellness, but these categories are merely another attempt to view the body through a reductionist lens as none of these categories points to the relationship we have to our interior experience (Melnyk & Neale 2018). Chapter 9 compares WATSU to life coaching and explains why incorporating somatic aspects to the wellness paradigms is important to expand the behavioral, psychological, and emotional aspects of healing:

> The whole body is concerned about leading to better self-awareness in the somatic coaching approach. Somatic coaching aims to deepen understanding of self and enable clients to explore faulty thinking and hidden emotion at a deeper level, which is a key to change in coaching, whereas deepening understanding of self and emotions is the key to healing in WATSU.

Furthermore, including aspects of the body not valued in conventional medicine, such as the relevance of fascia, fluids, and phenomenology as described in Chapter 15, expands the limitations of the eight dimensions of wellness or the biopsychosocial model.

Elevating wisdom of the body: Towards a somatic scope of practice

Related to an integrative framework or orientation is the way the practice of WATSU elevates the wisdom of the body. Reducing, discounting, muting, and ignoring messages from the body to privilege cognitive functioning is a complicated remnant of Cartesian dualism. Although this legacy has persisted for hundreds of years, WATSU clearly moves away from this orientation and provides a way to amplify, reorient, and reclaim a context for information that originates from the body. Acknowledging the wisdom of the body is achieved by both the provider and the client through several key strategies and techniques.

Meditation

Because Cartesian dualism has dominated healing paradigms for centuries, orienting clients to messages from the body requires a deliberate approach and container for this type of exploration. Although contemplative practices have existed in religious places in our society, the steady decline of the institution of religion has moved people away from embodied awareness. With this decline, contemplative practices, like yoga and meditation, have been on the rise. In 2017, the National Center for Health Statistics evaluated the use of complementary and integrative health practices in the United States and reported that yoga and meditation were the most commonly used approaches for adults and children (Clarke *et al.* 2018). Although these figures have grown since 2012, they represent a small portion of the population, which means that only a small percentage of the population is likely to be familiar with embodied practices and how to recognize and learn from messages communicated from the body.

During WATSU sessions, clients are given the opportunity to experience the body from within using a variety of techniques that are often learned through contemplative practices. The experience of being immersed in the stillness and silence of water creates a context for and an expectation of a meditative experience. Quieting the mind is important because it allows one to listen to and pay attention to somatic information. In Chapter 11, the author explains how quieting the mind occurs effortlessly through aquatic bodywork:

> I soon realized how quickly and effortlessly I entered a deep state of silent meditation when being moved harmoniously underwater. There was a feeling of expansion and opening, and the contact of the water with my skin was no longer perceptible. Water and body seemed to merge into an energetic unity. From deep meditations I already knew I could enter a space where suddenly everything became very quiet and peaceful.

During meditation, a person strives to acknowledge or observe the thoughts, sensations, feelings, ideas, and perceptions that emerge without getting attached or entangled with any one of them. Throughout the course of a meditative experience, people practice how to notice what sensations are alive and present in each moment while watching how these unfold and change. They pay attention to how they are feeling, and, most importantly, they allow and accept the different sensations that come across their body-mind to be there without attempting to change, fade, or fix them in any way. After prolonged periods of deliberate concentration immersed in water, clients may experience a sense of dissolution, or loss of the sense of self that often accompanies meditative experiences or flow states (Csikszentmihalyi 1990). Other times, as described in Chapter 5, clients may experience non-ordinary states of consciousness beyond those felt in everyday life. WATSU as a medium allows clients to naturally mute outside distractions so that the focus can reside solely on the body-mind and one's interior landscape. The meditative experience also applies to providers. Chapter 13 describes the importance of aquatic providers to accept, educate, and allow clients' bodies to respond to invitations to a heightened awareness of the inner experience of the self. WATSU and other aquatic therapies provide a meditative container for clients and practitioners alike to reclaim and orient to the wisdom that emanates from the body.

Interoception

Another prerequisite for recognizing the wisdom from the body is interoception, or the sense of reflecting on the self by journeying inward. The decline of the role of religion amounts to fewer dedicated and intentional places to experience the expressions of our interior landscape. The digital age has ushered in a variety of gadgets to compete for our attention and to distract us further from our interior sense. In several chapters throughout this book, authors discuss how WATSU helps to develop a client's sense of interoception as part of the meditative process. Interoception involves self-reflection directed inward to explore one's thoughts and feelings and the practice of WATSU invites clients to go a step further to cultivate, not only a relationship to body and emotional awareness, but a curiosity as well. The act of interocepting leads to an appreciation of the inner world which allows one to notice and observe sensations from the body. Chapter 9 discusses the importance of the ability to look inward to identify the root causes of emotions, to address impulsivity control, and to help mitigate careless decisions and judgments. Chapter 11 explains how combining WATSU with WaterDance leads to deeper states of interoception and brings to the surface memories of attachment and developmental formation.

Other chapters explain the importance of interoception, or "the representation of the internal world of an organism," which "includes the processes by which the organism senses, interprets, integrates, and regulates signals from within itself" as a component of health and healing (NCCIH n.d.). As an example, the author in Chapter 15 points out that interoceptive awareness, or sustained attention to internal bodily sensation, is essential for the regulation and experience of emotions. While contemplative traditions have historically recognized and valued the importance of interoceptive awareness, biomedicine has just started to explore through research at the NCCIH the processes of interoception through the central nervous system, helping to translate these ancient practices into a language scientists recognize and understand.

Emotional regulation

The paradigms of biomedicine and holism view the body in philosophically oppositional ways. The machine metaphor is often used to reflect reductionist views of biomedicine which sees the body as a series of parts that can be repaired or replaced. Holistic or integrative approaches rely on a more expansive and holographic view of the body which acknowledges that there are interconnected domains creating health. The NCCIH classifies integrative therapies into three main categories: nutritional, physical, or psychological, which may overlap for some therapies. Relevant to this discussion is the psychological category which includes spiritual practices, mindfulness, and psychotherapy. By combining the physical category with the psychological category, mind-body therapies, such as meditation, breathing exercises, yoga, Tai Chi, and others, are created. WATSU clearly falls into the psychological/physical or mind-body category because it combines physical manipulation of the body with purposeful awareness. Similar to the introspective aspects of meditation, the practice of WATSU invites receivers to journey inward to contemplate sensations, thoughts, and emotions that arise within. In general, contemplative practices teach adherents how to weather, watch, and witness internal fluctuations of the body-mind which manifests as the rumination of thoughts, emotional states, or persistent physical sensations (hunger, pain, temperature, etc.). Like meditation, WATSU provides an opportunity for receivers to refine emotional processing skills as discussed in Chapter 9. Here, the authors describe how emotional regulation is truly an interplay among afferent inputs across sensory systems (auditory, visual, gustatory, olfactory, tactile, vestibular, proprioceptive, and interoceptive). WATSU disrupts input across many of these systems and allows receivers to amplify inward attention, which results in increased mindfulness and self-awareness.

Non-verbal awareness

Providers of WATSU elevate the wisdom of the body through their interactions with receivers through non-verbal awareness, somatic psychology, and presence. Many bodywork providers develop and refine a certain set of skills that sets them apart from biomedical providers through the repeated act of holding space for clients. Although biomedical providers have done much over the last few decades to improve bedside manner and to strengthen provider-patient relationships, the ability to witness a client on their introspective journey requires a kind of self-reflection and appraisal that often accompanies contemplative practices (meditation, yoga, Tai Chi, journaling, etc.). To recognize the path in oneself creates the awareness and ability to hold space for others on their journey. WATSU providers cultivate a keen sense of non-verbal awareness while working with receivers, since the therapy is delivered to clients who are fully immersed in water. Without verbal communication, providers must look for other markers and cues that communicate how a client is progressing during a session. Biomedical professionals are aided by devices to monitor internal states of patients, yet WATSU providers must rely on interpreting the art of touch, breath, and movement. In Chapter 12, the author explains the art of mirroring through the intake process, posturing, gaze, breath, and motion. Kinetic mirroring requires that a provider is sensitive and attuned to a client's position in water, as influenced by size, shape, flexibility, and gravity, to attend to a client's comfort, limitations, and wishes. Non-verbal communication increases attunement, rapport, and connection between client and provider.

Chapter 15 highlights the principles that shape the development of trust between the client's inner knowledge of the body and the therapist. The principles that apply to administering craniosacral therapy outlined by John Upledger apply to other systems of bodywork too, especially manipulations of the body that impact fascia. Taken together, these principles serve as a foundation outlining the meditative stance a provider adopts when interacting with a client. Similar to the meditative process described above, a provider must also be open, prepared, and confident to receive whatever manifests during a session. To achieve this openness, a provider strives to let go of belief systems, expectations, or pre-conceived outcomes pertaining to what might or should occur for the client during a session. The provider aims to maintain a non-judgmental orientation toward themselves and also toward the client. The provider recognizes that their role is to serve as a facilitator and to create a container for the experience so that clients are able to take agency and responsibility for their own health and wellness. Clients' somatic responses guide how providers deliver and apply WATSU techniques, so there is an element of reciprocal exchange in this client-provider relationship. Providers must also cultivate an awareness and willingness to change or utilize different strategies based on the feedback they witness while observing clients' responses to treatment. This requires providers to reflect on their own body awareness to determine if techniques are meeting clients' needs. Chapter 2 provides an example:

> If the client's body responds in a way that suggests something you did affected the client in a counter-productive way, ask yourself, "Why?" Then test your informed reasoning. Perhaps try doing the same thing but with less tension in your own body and more sensitive awareness of the client. Or perhaps try a movement that's nearly the opposite of what was previously tried but didn't yield positive results. Look at the client with fresh eyes and an open mind to discover a better path.

Embedded in this quote is a reminder to invoke aspects of meditation while working with clients. The breath is a vehicle for providers to establish a somatic scope of practice, as seen in Chapter 6:

> Being aware of our breathing patterns and learning to connect with those of the patient is the first step in creating a meditative (mindful) state during a session and really one of the foundations of our palliative aquatic programming. Harold's teachings emphasized that "the deeper you drop into the emptiness of the breath, the more it will feel as if your client is drawing you out of the void as the breath comes back in and the water lifts you without effort" (Dull 2004, P.22). What Harold continued to further highlight in his text is that connecting the breath with movement was an invitation to the receiver (client) to free the body and mind from physical and mental stressors.

Lastly, in Chapter 14, we learn the value of touch as a way to help clients cultivate a sense of their interior sensory experience as well as the importance of providers offering non-judgmental experiences. Remaining neutral and grounded are necessary meditative elements for providers to adopt, so that clients are able to safely sink into their process. Here, the concept of holding the edge is relevant.

> Training of somatic therapy practitioners requires helping them learn to "hold the edge"—show compassion and empathy without intruding on the client's process. When a practitioner can successfully hold an edge with a client, it allows them to feel, experience and express their sensations and feelings. This expression can feel like a pushing against, a pulling away, a reaching out or a drawing inward. The ability of the practitioner to provide safety, support and freedom is a critical function that allows a client to do their work. (Chapter 14)

Somatic providers refrain from interpreting or evaluating a client's internal experience as it is outside most providers' scope of practice unless they have additional mental health training or credentials.

All of this is to say that one of the latent side effects of being a WATSU practitioner is that bodyworkers develop a somatic awareness not only for and about their clients, but also for themselves. Collectively, the ability to read non-verbal cues, witness clients' introspection and interoceptive experiences, and provide opportunities to enhance emotional regulation amount to what I identify as a somatic scope of practice. Chapters 3 and 4 introduce the concept of interoceptive embodiment and provide detail about the somatic benefits related to the practice of WATSU, lending additional support and credence to the concept of a somatic scope of practice.

Presence

The art of WATSU has much to do with the sense of presence providers bring to a session. While the production of medical knowledge has greatly enhanced the treatment of disease, it has also impersonalized the delivery of care. Interpersonal interactions in clinical settings are opportunities to gather rich information beyond what is entered into electronic medical records. Zulman *et al.* (2020) performed a systematic review to identify practices that foster physician presence and connection with patients in the clinical encounter. In this research, presence is defined as "a purposeful practice of awareness, focus, and attention with intent to understand and connect with patients." The authors sought to identify evidence-based interpersonal interventions and also observed physician-patient interactions in three diverse settings. While the research team thoughtfully included observations and interviews with nonmedical professionals, they did not include integrative providers. Results identified a set of five practices that could enhance physician presence and meaningful engagement with patients in clinical encounters. These recommendations include: 1) prepare with intention, 2) listen intently and completely, 3) agree on what matters most to the patient, 4) connect with the patient's story, and 5) explore emotional cues. Because integrative providers were excluded from this study, the researchers missed an opportunity to capture the value of somatic interactions that shape and impact patient encounters. As described in the previous section on meditation, a somatic scope of practice is related to the art of presence. As clients tune inward to observe their own somatic fluctuations, providers also tune inward and partake in some of the same behaviors, strategies, and rituals while guiding clients. Presence in WATSU includes the five recommendations identified by Zulman and colleagues and yet goes beyond the act of witnessing since providers are mindful of their own somatic resources. In Chapter 6, we learn that WATSU providers follow respiratory patterns as a way to understand clients' non-verbal states and this helps explain the connection between somatic regulation and presence:

> When practitioners are fully present, we pay close attention to the rise and fall of their patients' chests, observing in detail the degree of tension, facial expressions, respiratory effort and breathing patterns. In practice, the respiratory pattern is one of the keys to understanding the non-verbal child's state of being and connecting with the patient one-to-one, which is an essential element of presence.

Connecting with clients in the moment without an agenda is a guiding principle of WATSU and highlights another element of presence which is markedly different from interpersonal interventions often found in biomedicine.

Presence also conveys a profound sense of connection and caring between the provider and client. The origins of WATSU can be found in the extreme closeness between the provider and client prior to the addition of flotation devices. Holding space with equanimity is another element of presence. As described in Chapter 2, presence requires a steadfast and unwavering ability to recognize the newness and raw unfolding of each moment: "Frequently sessions evoke old sorrows, injuries and psychological wounds, sometimes very strongly with tears, laughter and movement. As practitioners, we are there to hold the space with calm, unconditional acceptance, without intervening, giving advice, 'mothering' or rescuing." By following a client's natural rhythms through breath and movement, embodied connection is established.

> When we feel them getting lighter on that arm as they breathe, the therapist's breath is drawn up. Then, we drop back into the emptiness at the bottom of the breath and do nothing. Being drawn up out of that emptiness again and again, up through our core in this *Water Breath Dance*, engages our whole body and establishes a connection that continues through our moves and stretches born in that rhythm. (Chapter 1)

Here, presence and connection contribute to a full-bodied experience that is linked with movement created in the moment.

Information, decision-making, and responsibility shared between patient and provider

In technocratic medical paradigms, decision-making and authority have traditionally been associated with the provider (i.e., a physician) making decisions on behalf of the patient. While the advent of the person-centered care movement has challenged some of the assumptions of this tenet by placing more decision-making in the hands of the patient, it seems that WATSU resides somewhere between the humanistic and holistic paradigms. WATSU emphasizes both a caring connection as well as a shared responsibility between patient and provider. As discussed above, some of this connection pertains to the way non-verbal information is conveyed and interpreted during a session and another part of it relates to acceptance and allowing clients to have voice and agency throughout the course of their experience.

Central to the idea of a shared responsibility is the ability of providers to meet clients where they are on their unique healing journey. As providers strive to practice meditation in the moment, they refrain from having a goal or expectations for the client during the session, and they allow somatic processes to unfold. The skill associated with acknowledging where patients are, as explained in Chapter 2, is learning how to manage or interact with the silent pauses that occur during a session. For example:

> We need to give our client the time and peaceful space to share more than this. This often means quietly waiting during times of silence without a need to fill the silence. Many clients will then choose to share more about their physical and emotional pain and challenges. (Chapter 2)

As providers become comfortable with allowing silent moments to occur during interactions with clients, they give clients the ability to choose freely what they wish to share. Although this quote refers to the intake process for special needs patients, the notion of holding the silence or the pause also happens during segments of the session that involve movement: "Sometimes we give the body an invitation for movement. We listen carefully, yet we are unattached to whether or not the client's body chooses to follow our invitation" (Chapter 2). In this instance, providers engage in deep listening and observation to pause and notice whether a client responds to a movement. Helping clients accept with grace the limitations of their neurobiology is yet another example of meeting clients where they are at with their growth and development:

> With implicit memories, it is important to encourage the client to recognize that it is their neurobiology that isn't supporting a life that pleases them, rather than something being wrong with them. Once a client can be lifted out of shame, a connection can begin. (Chapter 4)

In biomedical encounters, research has acknowledged that physicians interrupted the patients on average 18 seconds within the encounter, and this improved slightly when it was reported that doctors redirect their patient's opening statement after 23.1 seconds (Marvel *et al.* 1999). As a response, improving communication with patients has been an ongoing project, as evidenced by the creation of Presence: The Art & Science of Human Connection at Stanford as well as other initiatives focusing on medical humanism. The deep listening and empathetic witnessing that occurs during somatic therapies such as WATSU represents another model for patient engagement that may be an antidote to the 15-minute encounters clients experience with biomedical providers.

Allowing patients to make choices during a session emphasizes a commitment to shared decision-making strategies between the provider and the client. For example, Chapter 4 describes how giving choice to clients allows them to tap into their somatic awareness while forging relationship dynamics with the client:

> ...let the client choose where they wish to be in the pool. Find just the right place that makes them orient to safety and trust you as a practitioner. Circumambulate the client with a distance two arm lengths. You will note where the boundary of the client pulls you in and where the boundary pushes you away. This exploration is done at a snail's pace, with the practitioner keeping a close eye to changes in breathing, skin color and facial expressions.
>
> Do not move too close in, nor too far away. Having the client drop inside into their felt sense of the space around them can be an exciting first step to creating ease in the system. This is a great way to come into relationship with the client and also a way to palpate where the original breaches to the protective boundary occurred.

Chapter 9 describes how WATSU practitioners provide a safe container through emotional connection and physical support to allow clients to move towards greater awareness and emotional regulation. While practitioners give shape to the session through rapport-building activities including witnessing, touch, mirroring, and attunement, clients have the authority to interpret and make meaning of the experience for themselves:

> ...the client takes the lead invisibly, making the client feel/sense a high quality of emotional connection and physical support from the therapist's gentle and light touch. The emotional strain can be replaced with the most potent emotional forces for regulation and self-healing in these moments of connection. Feelings of gratitude, safety, trust, relaxation, self-awareness, and being understood are triggered in this connection. These positive emotions and their awareness empower the cognition that moves the clients into a higher meaning-making process. Validation and acceptance are also promoted in coaching and WATSU enhancing EI and leading the client into resourcefulness.

The experience of WATSU invites clients to be responsible for their own health and well-being.

Art of WATSU

The National Academies of Sciences convened a team of experts in 2018 to investigate the impact of single-subject learning on educational and career outcomes for undergraduate and graduate STEMM (science, technology, engineering, math, medicine) students (National Academies of Sciences 2018).

The American educational system, they argue, has become siloed by increased specialization and the team reasoned that adding humanistic and artistic learning experiences to STEMM programs might help develop valuably needed skills such as life-long learning, critical thinking, communication, and teamwork (p.ix). The focus on single-subject learning, another reductionist orientation, does not cultivate these skills among students, and instead an integrative approach is recommended to teach students how to make connections across disciplines. This document argues for greater support and inclusion of integrative approaches in education and provides a number of recommendations for stakeholders, institutions, and employers to consider to advance this agenda. There is a growing recognition that while we absolutely need outstanding clinicians in medicine, we equally need outstanding humanitarians in medicine, too. The Icahn School of Medicine has acknowledged this need through the creation of the FlexMed Program which recruits second-year humanities students for early entry into their medical program (Muller 2014). The School reserves half of its incoming seats for medical school for humanities majors to demonstrate its commitment to the value of integrative and interdisciplinary learning. If we are hoping to model holism in medicine, then it makes sense that holism and integration are also included in education to shape future medical providers.

The Association of American Medical Colleges (AAMC) is supporting this effort and published *The Fundamental Role of the Arts and Humanities in Medical Education* (Howley, Gaufberg, & King 2020) to "improve the education, practice, and well-being of physicians through deeper integrative experiences with the arts and humanities" (p.3). The report maps the field of incorporating arts and humanities into medical education and makes a number of recommendations (Table 17.3) for changing the culture of medicine for meaningful integration. Since the publication of the report, the AAMC has created resources and tools for integrating arts and humanities into medical education.

Table 17.3: AAMC recommendations

---

1. Assert that the practice of medicine is an art as well as a science, requiring a grounding in humanistic values, principles, and skills, including a deep understanding of the human condition.

---

2. Create more effective arts and humanities integrative models for competency-based teaching and learning in medicine.

---

3. Enhance the research and evaluation of courses and programs that integrate the arts and humanities into medical education and continuing professional development. Such research and evaluation should include measuring learner outcomes beyond satisfaction with the course or program and should follow sound scholarly practices.

---

4. Design approaches to enhancing trainee and physician well-being that integrate the arts and humanities into medicine.

5. Increase collaboration among scholars of higher education, medical professionals, arts organizations, creative arts therapists, artists, humanities scholars, learners, and patients.

6. Provide professional development offerings that enhance faculties' capacity to design curricula and facilitate the use of models that integrate the arts, humanities, and medicine in training.

7. Investigate effective integrative pedagogical practices and recognize an expansive view of scholarship in academic promotion and tenure processes.

The patient-centered care movement has been an attempt to place patient needs at the forefront of medical providers' minds for quality and safety assurance purposes. The National Academy of Medicine (formerly the Institute of Medicine) includes patient-centeredness as one of the six components needed to deliver quality care. Patient-centeredness is represented by six dimensions that must be "respectful to patients' values, preferences and expressed needs; coordinated and integrated; provide information, communication and education; ensure physical comfort; provide emotional support; and involve family and friends" (Tzelepis *et al.* 2015, p.831).

The patient-centered care movement is an attempt to fortify medical encounters with prescriptive humanism to ensure patients are in partnership with medical professionals. This is biomedicine's cognizant strategy to turn towards the humanistic or holistic paradigm to acknowledge the deep need for authentic connection between patient and provider. The patient-centered care movement arose out of the Planetree concept of care in the 1970s, was later popularized by the Institute of Medicine in 2001, and is now celebrated through the compassion in medicine and arts in medicine movement. While the intent of the compassion and patient-centered care movement has been a noble attempt to inject more humanistic and holistic tenets into biomedicine, what the patient-centered care movement in medicine is missing is an understanding of the role of the wisdom of the body.

Research on the various benefits of WATSU and the new forms of aquatic bodywork that grew from its innovation and are discussed elsewhere in this book confirms the physiological, physical, and somatic benefits of practice. WATSU is helpful for athletes, pregnant women, and special populations, as well as people with conditions such as PTSD and pain. Beyond the growing body of evidence showcasing the benefits of WATSU, there exists another branch of the practice, the artistic side of WATSU, that focuses on compassion-centric and heart-based care. Conventional medical care is consumed by diagnoses, aggressive interventions, and a profit-driven system that often competes with the compassionate and artful delivery of care. Previous chapters of this book provide an understanding of how WATSU is informed care that is delivered at the heart level. Since providers of WATSU often have other professional credentials and licenses, sessions may be informed by different scopes of practice. The implication is that some practitioners may have clinical skills and are able to understand medical terminology and diagnoses. What is distinctive about WATSU providers is that they are also good somatic listeners and have a repertoire of skills that enable them to witness clients while maintaining a quiet and grounding presence.

Dance is used as a metaphor in Chapter 11 to describe how the practice leads to self-exploration. WaterDance is understood as a dance, meditation, and spiritual practice: "...dance is an art, which always leaves imprints on the physical, emotional, and spiritual being that we are. Dance is therefore a *healing dialogue between the body and the soul*" (Chapter 11). WATSU, WaterDance, and other aquatic therapies are the mediums that allow a person to integrate many aspects of the self. Engaging in art often leads to an experience of flow, where one becomes immersed in a focused and enjoyable state where they often lose the familiar sense of self and are able to access different layers of consciousness (Csikszentmihalyi 1990). WATSU and WaterDance are indeed artful movement forms that guide, inform, and shape self-exploration. The metaphor of dance reminds us of the dynamic interplay between provider and client. Although the client is ultimately in charge of the session, the provider finds unison and attunement with the client through the breath, movement, and gesture.

The increasing role of technology in medicine creates more distance between the patient and provider in traditional healing encounters and disrupts the delivery of care. While machines, devices, and gadgets obtain useful information to peer inside the body, they are devoid of warmth and human connectivity. Abraham Verghese has written about the physical exam as a privilege and a sacred ritual and argues that the art of touch is a skill that goes beyond diagnostic capability (Costanzo & Verghese 2018). Touch is a gentle form of communication that provides support, reassurance, nurturance, and guidance. It allows providers to "read the body" in that it provides an opportunity to experience a felt sense of a person's context. Low-tech fields such as massage, rolfing, acupuncture and WATSU provide deeply intimate encounters through the art of touch.

Moving into clinical frameworks

This chapter highlights how the tenets of WATSU reside mostly along the humanistic-holistic side of the paradigmatic continuum. Practitioners of

WATSU who have additional credentials in the areas of physical therapy, occupational therapy, acupuncture, and other allied health areas will incorporate some aspects of biomedicine, thus representing a merging of paradigms, or at least an openness and tolerance of other modalities, frameworks, and orientations. Many signature elements of traditional healthcare, ranging from physiological data to case study reports, recommendations for working with clients who have challenging needs, and precautions and contraindications for aquatic bodywork, are showcased in Chapter 2. An emphasis on safety and preparedness for emergency is reminiscent of the Hippocratic notion of "do no harm" and connects with the National Academy of Medicine's charge to provide quality care. Use of a WATSU client screening questionnaire as part of safety considerations prior to a session is also discussed in Chapter 2, along with a reminder for providers to stay within their respective scopes of practice. The use of questionnaires has become a standard practice across many integrative disciplines, suggesting that many therapies have taken a biomedical turn and are more accepted as part of the fabric of the healthcare environment. Intake questionnaires are useful because they collect baseline information that can be compared over time. They also help providers gather more information about patients' medical conditions that may impact the delivery of care. Because WATSU is a quiet therapy with little or no dialogue, intake forms set expectations for what happens during a session and equip clients with tools and strategies to have a productive and meaningful session. Information obtained through intake forms provides the opportunity to collaborate with others. For instance, if a client indicates that they have experienced significant traumas in the past, a WATSU practitioner will likely refer the client to a mental health professional to ensure that the client has adequate support to process what may surface during a session. In this light, WATSU is understood as a part of a client's constellation of care for overall health and well-being.

WATSU in clinical practice

Because the five licensed integrative professions (acupuncture & Chinese medicine, chiropractic, naturopathic medicine, licensed massage therapy, and direct entry midwifery) had been operating mostly outside biomedicine prior to the early 2000s, a research gap developed between these professions and biomedicine. The creation of the National Center for Complementary and Integrative Health provided opportunities to address the gap by attempting to research the integrative fields, but this was mostly done through the lenses of biomedicine and reductionism. Historically, the integrative fields have been underfunded and have lacked the capacity and infrastructure to engage in research. Recently, however, the NCCIH has expanded its methodological approach to include whole-systems research which is in alignment with the values of integrative disciplines (NCCIH 2021). While more research exists than ever before about integrative therapies through the advancements of NCCIH, national research priorities have done little to capture or address the somatic or body-based aspects of integrative therapies.

Whole-systems research and mixed-method approaches are useful for studying somatic therapies. Chapter 14 provides an example of how researchers studied AMNION. Various scales were used (The Patient-Related Outcome Measure scale, Scale of Body Connection, The Experience of Close Relationship) along with semi-structured interviews to understand clients' experience of the AMNION session. This strategy utilized both qualitative and quantitative measures to document the experience of a somatic therapy. This chapter recognizes the need for measuring body awareness to understand how somatic therapies disrupt painful experiences as well as to investigate how trauma is metabolized in the body. These approaches suggest that future research on WATSU and other aquatic therapies should be methodologically diverse to capture the physical, physiological, somatic, and psychological aspects of these practices.

In clinical practice, WATSU may organically grow to be part of a constellation of care for those with a variety of conditions, but especially for those with trauma-based injuries. Because some WATSU providers have other professional credentials, there is some opportunity to broaden and extend the field to other biomedical and clinical settings. What is the ideal clinical setting for WATSU? Should it collaborate more deeply with biomedicine? With the explosive growth of integrative therapies in the United States, it is important to acknowledge that most of these therapies still reside outside biomedicine. True integration, where inter-professional collaboration between biomedicine and integrative medicine occurs, is actually quite rare. Because it has a strong emphasis on mind-body approaches, WATSU may have more in common with psychotherapy and social work than biomedicine. This might change, of course, as the NCCIH continues to explore the mechanics of interoception, which could elevate the value of somatic and mind-body approaches, including WATSU. Moreover, the clinical key and further advancement of the work lie in our continual exploration for best practices that seamlessly integrate existing allied health professions with the somatic scope and benefits of WATSU in daily practice.

Future directions for WATSU as a discipline and profession

As WATSU and other aquatic body-based therapies continue to blossom in the United States and around the globe, there are a number of ways the field might evolve. For example, with the rise of the arts in medicine movement, there could be opportunities for WATSU and aquatic providers to teach others about how to cultivate a somatic approach with clients. Movement is yet another narrative where clients' stories are revealed. WATSU providers are mindful of a patient's story, and future research may involve investigating how new narratives are created or change over time. It could be helpful to include some arts-based tools to gather phenomenological experiences that unfold during sessions (Mehling *et al.* 2011). Perhaps this could be accomplished in partnership with an art therapist to provide a container to process and interpret the meaning and significance of WATSU sessions.

With the growing national conversation on trauma-informed and trauma-sensitive approaches, there will likely be a greater need for somatic-based therapies. Using arts-based assessment in tandem with new scales that investigate the somatic experience will illuminate rich details of the practice while honoring the philosophical underpinnings of these therapies. There are a number of emerging somatic-based scales that could be relevant, including the Multidimensional Assessment of Interoceptive Awareness (MAIA) created by the NCCIH, or any of a number of scales devised by Stephen Porges and his team, including the Body Brain Center Sensory Scale of the Body Perception Questionnaire (BPQ).

References

Baer, H.A. (2001). *Biomedicine and Alternative Healing Systems in America: Issues of Class, Race, Ethnicity, & Gender.* Madison, WI: The University of Wisconsin Press.

Clarke, T.C., Barnes, P.M., Black, L.I., Stussman, B.J., & Nahin, R.L. (2018). Use of yoga, meditation, and chiropractors among U.S. adults aged 18 and over. *NCHS Data Brief.* Hyattsville, MD: National Center for Health Statistics.

Costanzo, C. & Verghese, A. (2018). The physical examination as ritual: Social sciences and embodiment in the context of the physical examination. *Medical Clinics,* 102(3): 425–431.

Csikszentmihalyi, M. (1990). *Flow: The Psychology of Optimal Experience.* New York, NY: Harper & Row.

Davis-Floyd, R. & St. John, G. (1998). *From Doctor to Healer: The Transformative Journey.* New Brunswick, NJ: Rutgers University Press.

Dull, H. (2008). *Watsu: Freeing the Body in the Water.* Middletown, CA: Watsu Publishing.

Howley, L., Gaufberg, G., & King, B. (2020). *The Fundamental Role of the Arts and Humanities in Medical Education (FRAHME): A National Strategic Initiative to Further Advance Curricular Integration of the Humanities and Arts into U.S. Medical Schools and Teaching Hospitals.* Association of American Medical Colleges.

Marvel, M.K. *et al.* (1999). Soliciting the patient's agenda. *JAMA,* 281(3): 283.

Mehling, W.E. *et al.* (2011). Body awareness: A phenomenological inquiry into the common ground of mind-body therapies. *Philosophy, Ethics, and Humanities in Medicine,* 6(1): 6.

Melnyk, B.M. & Neale, S. (2018). 9 dimensions of wellness. *American Nurse Today,* 13(1): 10–11.

Muller, D. (2014). FlexMed: A nontraditional admissions program at Icahn School of Medicine at Mount Sinai. *AMA Journal of Ethics,* 16(8): 614–617.

National Academies of Sciences (2018). *The Integration of the Humanities and Arts with Sciences, Engineering, and Medicine in Higher Education: Branches from the Same Tree*. Washington, DC: National Academies of Sciences.

NCCIH (n.d.). *National Center for Complementary and Integrative Health Strategic Plan 2021–2025*. Available at www.nccih.nih.gov/about/nccih-strategic-plan-2021-2025/top-scientific-priorities/interoception-research.

NCCIH (2021). *Methodological Approaches for Whole Person Research Workshop*. Available at www.nccih.nih.gov/news/events/methodological-approaches-for-whole-person-research.

NCCIH (2022). *Complementary, Alternative, or Integrative Health: What's In a Name?* Available at www.nccih.nih.gov/health/complementary-alternative-or-integrative-health-whats-in-a-name.

Tzelepis, F. *et al.* (2015). Measuring the quality of patient-centered care: Why patient-reported measures are critical to reliable assessment. *Patient Preference and Adherence*, 9: 831–835.

Winnick, T. (2005). From quackery to "complementary" medicine: The American medical profession confronts alternative therapies. *Social Problems*, 52(1): 38–61.

Zulman, D.M. *et al.* (2020). Practices to foster physician presence and connection with patients in the clinical encounter. *JAMA*, 323(1): 70.

Epilogue

WATSU grows within its unique creation, breath, movement, sequence and free flow. Demonstrating even the simplest moves of WATSU can evoke a deeper understanding of self and other that ignites our basic human need for connection, embodiment and oneness with equanimity and grace. Many of WATSU's unique benefits come from having the whole body held this way, a containment that makes it safe to go deep within. The more the holder engages their whole body, their whole being, their whole heart, the deeper those benefits. This engagement took me by surprise when I felt a *heart wrap* with whomever I floated at my heart, a wrapping from my heart out under and around their chest, a oneness, even with those I would not have imagined any oneness.

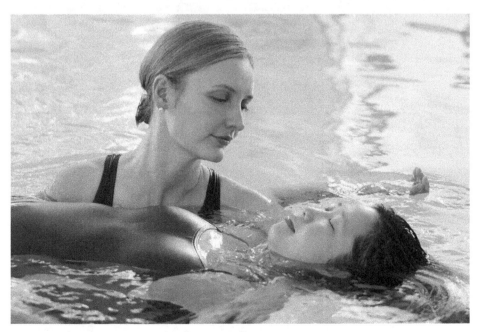

Figure E.1: Follow movement

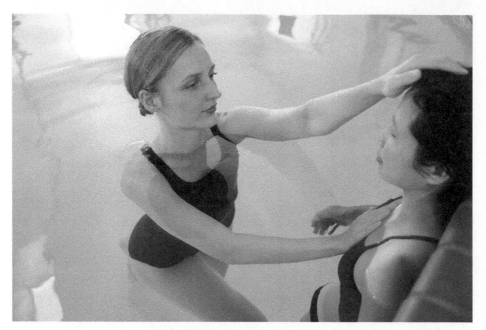

Figure E.2: Third eye and heart

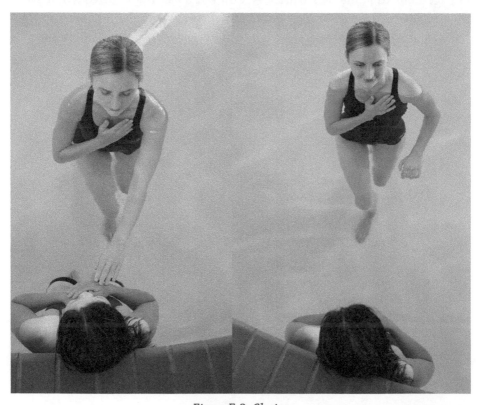

Figure E.3: Closing

We could build a WATSU machine or a robot that holds someone in the water and program it to execute all the moves of WATSU, but it is hard to imagine it engaged in a heart wrap. It would be equally hard to imagine it moving in a free flow, being drawn to those places that again and again we are told are those places where we are most needed. In the latest theories of emergence, every level of the universe engages in its creation. From my own experience, I like to think of our engagement in WATSU as a form of love.

Harold Dull

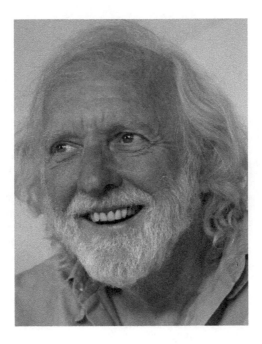

In Memoriam
Harold Dull
1935–2019

Index